Entomological Health and Safety for Ecologists and Environmental Professionals

Outdoor work for environmental professionals in ecological, engineering, or resource management settings frequently brings workers into contact with arthropods. Some are dangerous, many are disruptive, and most are overlooked in traditional safety planning. *Entomological Health and Safety for Ecologists and Environmental Professionals* offers a structured, field-focused guide to the medical and operational risks posed by insects, arachnids, and their allies. Combining insights from biology, health and safety, and practical field experience, it equips readers with the knowledge to anticipate, assess, and mitigate arthropod-related risks across a wide range of environments and occupations.

From mosquito-borne pathogens to venomous spiders, from allergic reactions to massive insect emergences that disrupt logistics, this guide goes beyond identification to evaluate risk through a clear exposure and severity framework. It is designed for field biologists, utility crews, safety officers, project managers, and anyone who plans or participates in outdoor work, especially where biological hazards are underappreciated but unavoidable.

Key Features:

- Practical exposure × severity risk model applicable to diverse arthropod encounters
- Structured entries for over 100 arthropod hazards, including arachnids, crustaceans, myriapods, and insects
- Operational insights into allergic responses, panic-inducing swarms, vector transmission, and field logistics
- Regionally variable risk considerations with support for SOPs (Standard Operating Procedures), JHAs (Job Hazard Analyses), and HASPs (Health and Safety Plans)
- Field-ready summaries, visual ID aids, and training support tools

Ideal for professionals in environmental consulting, land management, public works, and scientific fieldwork, this book empowers teams to plan confidently, reduce avoidable risk, and improve morale by understanding the entomological landscape of their job sites. Whether you're building a risk register or briefing a crew before deployment, this guide offers clarity, caution, and competence – without alarmism.

Entomological Health and Safety for Ecologists and Environmental Professionals

Grant D. De Jong

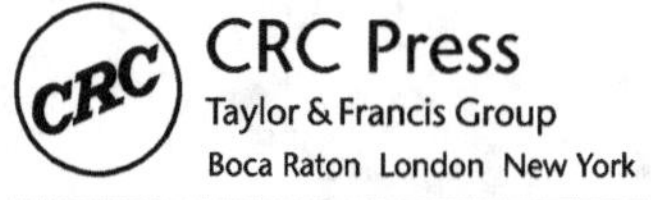

CRC Press
Taylor & Francis Group
Boca Raton London New York

CRC Press is an imprint of the
Taylor & Francis Group, an **Informa** business

First edition published 2027
by CRC Press
2385 NW Executive Center Drive, Suite 320, Boca Raton FL 33431

and by CRC Press
4 Park Square, Milton Park, Abingdon, Oxon, OX14 4RN

CRC Press is an imprint of Taylor & Francis Group, LLC

ISBN: 978-1-041-25227-6 (hbk)
ISBN: 978-1-041-25226-9 (pbk)
ISBN: 978-1-003-74570-9 (ebk)

DOI: 10.1201/9781003745709

Typeset in Times
By codeMantra

Contents

PART 2   The Arthropods

Preface

This guide was born from the field as I explored the places where environmental professionals spend much of their working lives and saw firsthand how the smallest organisms can have outsized impacts on safety, morale, and operations. After college graduation, I worked as an invertebrate ecologist for Chadwick Ecological Consultants, Inc., a small aquatic ecology firm, and GEI Consultants, Inc., a mid-size engineering firm, for a combined 22 years in streams and rivers all over the United States and in a couple of other countries.

My employer had a robust health and safety team, from the Corporate Health and Safety Officer to regional officers, down to each employee who recognized that safety was also an individual responsibility. Health and Safety Standard Operating Procedures (SOPs) were available for everything from ladder use to confined spaces to excavation and trenching; however, biological hazards (with the exception of bloodborne pathogens) were essentially ignored – just a mere statement that poisonous plants and venomous animals may exist. I realized that, despite the frequency of entomological encounters, we had nothing to address those hazards. So, I led a team in organizing and assembling a Health and Safety SOP for electro-fishing and ecological surveys, allowing at least some focus on entomology.

But Health and Safety SOPs are written only to be broad enough to address a general hazard, and they do work well at that level. Project Health and Safety Plans (HASPs) fill in the details for specific projects, but that is where information is not readily available; resources addressing entomological hazards are limited to technical medical entomology or parasitology textbooks or scattered primary literature. So, corporate mitigation advice against arthropods did not involve any education; it was just merely, "use bug spray."

This book was written to address that gap: to bring together biology, public health, and operational insight in one practical, field-ready resource for writing HASPs as well as Job Hazard Analyses (JHAs) and SOPs. It is not a field guide or diagnostic manual; it is not meant to tell medical professionals or legal experts how to do their jobs. It is, however, a tool for risk awareness and planning, designed to help professionals prepare for the realities of working outdoors, whether that be during a vegetation survey in fire ant country, a mosquito-heavy wetland delineation, or routine, but infrequent, engineering inspections near spider-prone structures.

While I love my dear arthropods, including the ones that bite me, I've aimed to present these organisms as real components of field safety. They are to be respected, not feared; understood, but not either over- or underestimated. The risks they pose vary by region, season, and circumstance, and this guide reflects that variability with structured entries, exposure × severity scales, and contextual notes.

My hope is that this guide will equip its users – ecologists, project managers, safety officers, forest rangers, linemen, summer camp directors, dam engineers, and others – with practical knowledge that enhances their safety protocols without breeding unnecessary alarm. Arthropods are part of the job (and for some, they *are* the job). Let's meet them with clarity, caution, and competence.

Let me also thank those who have helped me with this project, some unknowingly. Drs. Boris Kondratieff (Colorado State University, now deceased), W. Wyatt Hoback and Leon G. Higley (University of Nebraska), and Jerome Goddard and Florencia Meyer (Mississippi State University) were my mentors in academic entomology. Messrs. Jim Chadwick, Steve Canton, and Don Conklin, my supervisors at Chadwick Ecological Consultants, Inc. and GEI Consultants, Inc., provided so many opportunities to do field work through my employment there. Dr. Robin DeHate, Corporate Health and Safety Officer for GEI Consultants, Inc. (now retired), was instrumental in helping me navigate the world of corporate health and safety. From Pensacola Christian College, Dr. Troy Shoemaker (President) authorized this project, while Drs. Shane Smith and Aresia Watson (Chairs of the Department of Natural Sciences) provided health and safety opportunities and encouragement, respectively. For the book itself, Dr. Jerome Goddard suggested that I take my copious notes on the topic and turn them into a book, referring me to Alice Oven, Senior Editor for Life Science and Veterinary Medicine at Taylor & Francis/CRC Press, who is an example of professionalism in publishing and who helped me through so much of the publishing process. Anonymous proposal reviewers not only said the book idea was worthwhile but also made many comments that were incorporated and made it so much better. Taylor & Francis employees also aided immeasurably in typesetting, proofreading, graphic design, and production. My wife, Nikki, and daughters, Abby and Katie, are likewise thanked for their support in the preparation of this work.

DISCLAIMERS

The health and safety information provided in this guide is for general educational purposes only. It is not intended to diagnose, treat, or prevent any medical condition and should not be construed as medical advice. Individuals should consult a licensed medical professional regarding personal health concerns, insect bite or sting management, and the use of medical treatments or preventive measures.

The organizational policies, strategies, and recommendations described in this guide are also intended for general educational purposes only. They are not intended to constitute or substitute for legal advice. Organizations and individuals are responsible for evaluating their own circumstances and should consult qualified legal counsel when considering the incorporation of these practices into workplace policies or procedures. Employers must also ensure compliance with applicable federal, state, and local laws, including but not limited to the Americans with Disabilities Act (ADA) and the Health Insurance Portability and Accountability Act (HIPAA) in the United States and the Personal Information Protection and Electronic Documents Act (PIPEDA) in Canada.

Mention of specific brand names or trademarked products in this document does not imply endorsement by the author or affiliated organizations. Product names are included solely for clarity or illustrative purposes. Users should evaluate all products independently before use.

It is also understood by the author that the taxonomic organization of arthropods in this guide is generalized and may not adhere precisely to some understandings of arthropod taxonomy because higher-level arthropod taxonomy remains in flux. Relegation of organisms to a certain taxonomic class or order (e.g., designating crustaceans as a "class" instead of a subphylum or including Collembola as an insect order) is not intended to indicate formal taxonomic change, but to relate lay workers to arthropods in a traditionally recognized taxonomy.

About the Author

Grant D. De Jong, Ph.D., B.C.E., is an entomologist, ecologist, and educator with more than three decades of experience in field biology and environmental consulting. A Board Certified Entomologist and author of over three dozen peer-reviewed publications and two books, he has led ecological investigations in forests, streams, wetlands, deserts, and coastal systems across the United States and internationally.

Before entering academia, Dr. De Jong spent 22 years in environmental consulting, where he managed ecological field projects in urban and mining-impacted watersheds, led the development of health and safety protocols for ecological fieldwork and electrofishing operations, and provided technical taxonomic oversight for a biological laboratory. He now serves as Assistant Teaching Professor of Biology at Pensacola Christian College, where he teaches ecology, entomology, parasitology, and research methods and mentors undergraduate researchers.

Drawing on extensive field experience, Dr. De Jong brings a dual perspective of practical insight and scholarly rigor to Entomological Health & Safety, offering scientifically grounded guidance for professionals who work where arthropods and environmental risk intersect.

Part 1

Introduction to Arthropods and Their Role in Risk

Professionals who work outdoors routinely encounter arthropods, sometimes intentionally, sometimes not, but often in ways that affect the safety, morale, and operations. Chapter 1 introduces the concept of entomological health and safety hazards that are frequently overlooked or reduced to vague warnings in project health and safety protocols. Identifying who should be interested in this material, the guide's goal is to support risk awareness, preparation, and mitigation without sensationalizing these organisms.

To lay the foundation for hazard recognition, Chapter 2 introduces the major arthropod groups of health and safety relevance. It provides basic taxonomy and distinguishing features for arachnids, crustaceans, myriapods, and insects, as well as an "Entomology 101" overview to orient users who may not have a formal biology background. The chapter emphasizes that while these organisms may play ecological roles as parasites, vectors, or simply as incidental fauna, their impact depends on specific environmental and occupational contexts. This framing helps users understand why certain taxa are included in the guide and prepares them to interpret later entries with biological nuance.

Chapter 3 builds on this foundation by introducing a practical framework for risk evaluation. The concept of risk is broken into two components: exposure and severity. Exposure considers how likely one is to encounter a given arthropod based on habitat, behavior, and seasonal patterns. Severity reflects potential outcomes, from mild irritation to serious medical or operational consequences. Using these two dimensions together, readers are encouraged to assess relative risks using a simple

DOI: 10.1201/9781003745709-1

matrix. This helps prioritize planning efforts and avoid over- or under-reacting to particular hazards.

Together, the first three chapters set the tone for the remainder of the guide. They provide conceptual scaffolding, define the scope, and explain the logic behind the structured entries that follow in Part 2. Rather than overwhelming users with exhaustive identification keys or technical entomology, the early chapters aim to equip readers with enough background to understand the relevance of each hazard, evaluate it in context, and integrate appropriate precautions into field protocols. In doing so, the guide fosters not just safety compliance but also ecological literacy and informed judgment.

1 Introduction

The *Entomological Health and Safety* guide is intended to serve as a practical, field-oriented resource for recognizing, anticipating, and managing the hazards posed by insects, arachnids, and other arthropods in North America. Its primary purpose is to inform risk assessment, safety planning, and operational decision-making for those who work in outdoor, ecological, or remote environments. By systematically cataloging entomological threats and organizing them by type of exposure, severity of outcome, and ecological context, this guide equips professionals to make informed choices about fieldwork, equipment, training, and emergency preparedness.

This guide is designed with field personnel, project managers, and health and safety professionals in mind, especially those working in ecological consulting, environmental engineering, natural resource management, and related fields. It provides a structured framework to assess potential entomological hazards before work begins, during daily operations, or when responding to incidents. Whether planning a vegetation survey in tick-heavy woodlands, conducting wetland delineation in mosquito-prone marshes, or installing monitoring equipment in areas with stinging insects, users will find detailed information on what risks to expect and how to prepare for them.

However, it is important to emphasize what this guide is not.

It is not a taxonomic field guide or insect identification manual. While common names and general descriptions are provided to aid recognition, this book does not replace entomological keys, dichotomous guides, or visual identification tools such as Johnson and Triplehorn (2004), Ubick et al. (2005), or Darsie and Ward (2005). Users looking to positively identify unknown arthropods should consult reputable field guides, scientific keys, extension services, or professional entomologists. The organisms covered here are described primarily in terms of their health and safety relevance, not their full ecological or morphological characteristics.

This guide cannot in any way be comprehensive. Attention is given to about a hundred of the most common entomological health and safety hazards, since space simply does not allow full treatment of every potential hazard. Frankly, any arthropod could feasibly cause harm, just as the "friendliest" pet dog could bite under the right circumstances. For example, there are several beetles that bore into construction timber or chew on electrical wire insulation and could feasibly cause equipment failures, and some of our largest beetles could fly along a busy roadway, hit a motorcyclist, and cause a motor vehicle accident, but these instances are incredibly rare.

Likewise, this guide only broadly addresses non-entomological health and safety concerns that might arise during ecological or environmental work. For example, environmental exposure to heat or cold or lack of water is a major concern for ecologists and environmental professionals but has little to do with entomology. On the other hand, some workers may function within enclosed spaces or on ladders (not addressed in this guide), with their attendant entomological hazards – which

DOI: 10.1201/9781003745709-2

might include wasps nesting within structures or in trees (addressed in this guide). Likewise, the guide is limited to arthropods; other organisms with which contact may occur, such as dogs, cats, cattle, horses, wildlife, jellyfish, corals, cone shells, etc., are not addressed in this guide even though they may be incidental in the areas where entomological hazards do occur.

While this guide references typical medical outcomes and common treatment approaches, such as using antihistamines for minor stings or seeking antibiotics for specific bacterial infections, it is not to be considered a substitute for professional medical advice. The inclusion of medical terminology or first aid references is intended solely to provide context for health and safety planning. This guide should not be purported to offer medical diagnosis or treatment recommendations, and it should never be used as a replacement for consultation with licensed healthcare providers. Medical entomology and parasitology textbooks exist to address those more specific issues, as well as detailing life history, anatomy, and physiology of arthropod vectors, pathogens, and human hosts (e.g., Service 2012; Moraru and Goddard 2019). Users experiencing symptoms must refer cases to appropriate medical personnel without delay.

The guide also does not attempt to provide legal, regulatory, or insurance guidance related to occupational health standards except to point out the following. The United States Occupational Safety and Health Administration (OSHA) does not specifically address entomological hazards in 29 CFR. Threats from arthropods may fall within the "General Duty Clause" (Section 5(a)(1)), in which employers are required to protect employees from known hazards. Entomologically, this would include tick-borne diseases in field workers, mosquito exposure, fire ant infestations, wasp nests at worksites, and similar scenarios. In fact, interpretation letters from OSHA have acknowledged tick exposure in forestry, yellowjacket hazards at construction sites, and mosquito-borne disease risk during outbreaks, always within the purview of the General Duty Clause. Furthermore, OSHA includes non-regulatory guidance on its website, which includes webpages on mosquitoes and Zika virus, ticks and Lyme disease, and stinging insects.

Other entomological aspects that could arise and which to some degree would be covered by OSHA regulations include the requirement for employers to provide appropriate personal protective equipment (PPE) for workers (29 CFR 1910.132). This could include, for example, permethrin-treated clothing, insect repellants, head nets, or bee suits. Additionally, Hazard Communication Standards (29 CFR 1910.1200) would kick in when chemicals, such as insect repellants or fumigants and other insecticides, are employed. The Hazardous Waste Operations and Emergency Response (HAZWOPER, 29 CFR 1910.120) standard requires hazard assessments, training, PPE availability, site control, and monitoring at appropriate worksites.

So, while this guide may support the development of safety plans or job hazard analyses, it also follows protocol in that it leaves up to industry how to interpret regulatory frameworks such as OSHA standards or state-specific guidelines. Users are responsible for ensuring that any mitigation strategies developed from this guide comply with relevant laws and organizational policies.

While this guide provides detailed information on arthropods of medical and occupational concern, it is important to emphasize that its purpose is to promote informed, balanced, and practical caution – not undue fear. Many of the organisms described herein are capable of inflicting painful bites or stings, triggering allergic reactions, or transmitting life-threatening pathogens. Some individual people may even be hyper-sensitive to bites, stings, or contact allergens, in which case, they may find themselves at more risk than the average worker. However, in most field settings, such outcomes are uncommon and typically occur only under specific or exceptional circumstances.

The vast majority of tick, mosquito, and other arthropod bites encountered by environmental professionals result in minor irritation or no symptoms at all. Serious medical consequences, such as central nervous system (CNS) invasion, coma, or death, are astonishingly rare when compared to the number of entomological agents in nature, and they often depend on factors such as existence of a reservoir, geographic region, seasonality, length of exposure, and host susceptibility. A single tick or mosquito bite does not equate to a high likelihood of infection or life-threatening illness.

That said, during periods of heightened risk or outbreak, such as surges in tick-borne disease incidence or local arboviral transmission, increased vigilance and adherence to preventive protocols are warranted. This guide aims to support such informed decision-making by providing credible, field-relevant information rooted in biological understanding and public health principles.

By equipping workers and safety officers with accurate knowledge and reasonable expectations, this guide seeks to foster a culture of risk awareness without alarmism, one in which entomological hazards are recognized, respected, and managed effectively within the broader context of field health and safety.

Furthermore, this guide focuses on arthropods that are already recognized as pre-senting some degree of health or safety risk in occupational or environmental set-tings. While it is true that nearly any arthropod could feasibly become a hazard under the right circumstances, this guide does not attempt to catalog every theoretical risk. Instead, it prioritizes species and groups that have a documented history of causing bites, stings, noxious exudates, allergic reactions, disease transmission, infestations, psychological trauma, or other adverse effects relevant to ecological fieldwork and environmental operations.

In short, the guide is a risk communication tool (National Research Council 1989), a planning resource, and a supplement to safety protocols; it is not a diagnostic manual, medical handbook, or field ID reference. It exists to fill a crucial, but often overlooked, gap in environmental and occupational safety: the real-world effects that arthropods can have on personnel, gear, logistics, and morale. By focusing on these practical concerns, and by being allowed to remain within its defined scope, the guide aims to be a trusted, responsible, and actionable companion for professionals working in the field. Note, however, that the information in this guide is for educa-tional purposes only. It should not be taken as medical or legal advice. Individuals should consult qualified medical professionals for health concerns and licensed legal counsel for workplace policy decisions.

SCOPE AND AUDIENCE

This *Entomological Health and Safety* guide is designed as a practical reference for ecological and environmental professionals who work in environments where interactions with insects, arachnids, and other arthropods are unavoidable. Its primary audience includes ecologists, environmental scientists, and field technicians conducting biological surveys, habitat assessments, site remediation, endangered species monitoring, and related fieldwork in terrestrial, freshwater, and even wadable marine and estuary habitats. For these individuals, knowing what arthropods may be encountered and what hazards they pose can make the difference between a routine outing and a medical incident or logistical disruption. Admittedly, some individuals in these occupations probably took classes in ecology or entomology and are well aware of the animals discussed herein. Some ecologists and entomologists may actually love ticks, mosquitoes, wasps, fire ants, and flies more than they like their fellow humans!

However, familiarity may not necessarily translate into caution and awareness. Sometimes it ventures into unnecessarily risky, cavalier behavior. See Box 1.1. Plus, other environmental professionals may have focused on engineering or botany or vertebrates and did not necessarily take entomology courses in which they would have been introduced to these animals. Therefore, this guide is designed to help users (both those who are experienced and knowledgeable and those who are inexperienced and naïve) anticipate entomological risks, prepare appropriately, and make informed decisions in the field.

BOX 1.1

So much of this book is born out of personal experience – cavalier behavior despite knowledge. Some examples are provided:

- In college, a buddy and I were collecting insects on Horsetooth Mountain just outside Fort Collins, Colorado, for an entomology class when we encountered a *Scolopendra* centipede under a rock. We clumsily tried to catch it, and it jabbed me under my thumbnail with its venomous front legs. See "Centipedes" section in Chapter 5
- For a college club outreach, we conducted cockroach races, and I always came home feeling itchy. A skin prick test years later informed me that I am, indeed, allergic to cockroaches. See "Cockroaches" section in Chapter 7
- My Ph.D. dissertation involved elucidation of the relative roles of fire ants and blow flies in carrion decomposition in Mississippi and Florida. Probably needless to say, but I got stung nearly a hundred times over a six-week time period. See "Fire Ants" section in Chapter 4. And the flies that had just fed on dead, decaying pig carcasses were landing on me. See "Filth Flies" section in Chapter 8
- Conducting a fish community survey in several streams just north of the Black Hills in South Dakota, I and others in our crew were bitten frequently on our fingers by *Ambrysus mormon* bugs hiding in vegetation. See "Aquatic True Bugs" section in Chapter 5

- While dredging for benthic invertebrates in a shallow reservoir in the Dominican Republic at the end of a very long day, we switched on the lights on our boat, only to be swarmed by a bazillion non-biting midges. By the time we could don handkerchiefs to mask our faces, I had inhaled at least a dozen of the gnats. I sneezed three of them out four days later! See "Non-Biting Gnats" section in Chapter 9
- When collecting samples from an automatic water quality sampler along a stream in Idaho, we disturbed several nests of *Polistes* paper wasps just inside the door. I got stung; everyone else made it away safely. See "Stinging Flying Wasps" section in Chapter 4
- At an elevation of 4,191 m near the top of Mount Blue Sky, Colorado, while conducting a carrion succession study, I was swarmed by thousands of hungry *Aedes* mosquitoes. I clapped my hands in the air to see how many I could kill at once – seven – just like Mickey Mouse in *Brave Little Tailor* (1938)! See "Mosquitoes" section in Chapter 6
- In Uganda, I was fascinated by a *Macrotermes* termite mound that was being excavated, especially knowing that the adults were frequently used as food by the Ugandan nationals. The armored soldiers have formidable mandibles. And they bite. And they draw blood. Our North American species do not get large enough to bite, but they cause serious structural damage. See "Termites" section in Chapter 9
- I was trapping insects at a blacklight and sheet just south of Mobile, Alabama, for about two hours after nightfall, happily collecting cool beetles and moths. In the morning, I counted over 400 no-see-um bites on my hands and arms. See "Biting Midges/No-See-Ums" section in Chapter 5
- Despite so much time in the field, the only ticks I've ever had clamp down on me were two *Ixodes* in the Hell Hole Bay Wilderness in the Francis Marion National Forest just outside Charleston, South Carolina. See "Ticks" section in Chapter 6. On the other hand, I've gotten chiggers in 12 different states. See "Chiggers" section in Chapter 5.Thankfully, I haven't experienced any arthropod-borne diseases. But see a list of potential diseases in Chapters 6 and 8

Beyond the field team, the guide is intended for use by project managers who are responsible for planning and deploying field crews. These professionals are often not entomologists or ecologists themselves, but they are tasked with developing site safety plans, allocating resources, and ensuring team readiness. This guide gives them an accessible, scientifically grounded reference for understanding entomological risks associated with different regions and site types, helping them plan logistics, choose appropriate PPE, and communicate realistic expectations to staff and subcontractors.

Health and safety professionals, including those working at the corporate, regional, or local levels, will also find this guide valuable when writing or reviewing health and safety plans (HASPs), job hazard analyses (JHAs), and standard operating procedures (SOPs), and conducting safety briefings. Entomological hazards are often overlooked or under-characterized in standard safety documents. This guide fills that gap by systematically categorizing exposure levels, severity ratings, and types of impact, whether medical, logistical, or psychological. These ratings allow safety professionals to quantify entomological risk in a standardized way, promoting consistency across job sites and work crews.

Regulatory and government personnel, such as state and federal biologists, park rangers, public land managers, and natural resource officers, are another important user group. These professionals often interact with the public and may need to communicate arthropod-related risks clearly to visitors, contractors, or community stakeholders. In many cases, they are responsible for responding to complaints, assessing exposure risks, and writing guidance documents for field operations. The guide gives them a ready-made framework for understanding which arthropods are most relevant to their jurisdiction and how best to respond to them.

The military, particularly units that conduct training, environmental assessment, or infrastructure work in remote or ecologically sensitive areas, may also benefit from the guide. As my Ph.D. advisor told me, "Bugs have killed more soldiers than bombs or bullets." Military planners and medical officers can use the guide to identify regional threats, evaluate health risks to personnel, and support the development of preventive medicine protocols. Given the potential for vector-borne diseases and environmental stressors during training and upon deployment, the military has long been aware of entomological hazards to warfighter protection (e.g., Bowles and Swaby 2006); however, this guide provides an additional resource to support the same types of operational planning.

Other potential users include forestry personnel, wildfire response teams, utility inspectors, construction crews, and infrastructure engineers working in natural or semi-natural areas. Groundskeepers in urban and suburban locations may encounter arthropods in landscaping. These professionals may encounter entomological hazards as a secondary concern during their primary work. For instance, linemen restoring power after a hurricane where mosquito presence is increased, or wildfire crews working in tick- or wasp-infested areas, would benefit from the situational awareness this guide provides. Understanding the range of possible arthropod-related impacts, from venomous bites to mechanical nuisances, can improve crew safety and operational efficiency.

Ecologists, environmental engineers, or natural resource professionals may find themselves using as shelter or inspecting various buildings or structures across different landscapes. They can run the gamut from barns and sheds to pump houses and irrigation control stations, field cabins, fire lookout towers, remote outhouses and pit toilets, stream or river gaging station boxes, water quality monitoring huts, dam spillway control rooms, weather station enclosures, remote generator shacks, field storage containers or trailers, utility substations, transformer boxes, communication towers, relay stations, and more. Any low-use or intermittently occupied building in remote, rural, forested, or even aquatic landscapes can serve as a refuge for nuisance or hazardous arthropods. Because these structures are often small and unsealed, and contain heat or light sources, they are especially attractive to overwintering insects, spiders, or nesting pests.

Camp staff at youth camps, summer retreats, and outdoor recreation facilities, particularly those located in wooded, rural, or semi-natural environments, can benefit from this guide by gaining insight into the identification, prevention, and management of entomological risks that might otherwise go unnoticed or unreported. Unlike traditional workplaces, these settings involve not only staff, but also children and adolescents who may be more vulnerable to arthropod-related hazards due to their behavior, lack of awareness, or increased time spent outdoors during high-risk periods (e.g., dawn and dusk). Even when cabins are clean, air-conditioned, and well maintained, children and camp staff may still encounter hazards during daily and evening outdoor activities. Activities such as hiking, fishing, swimming, sitting around campfires, or playing games in grassy or wooded areas can increase contact with biting insects, stinging arthropods, or hidden vectors like ticks and chiggers. Here, practical instruction is provided for directors, counselors, groundskeepers, and medical personnel on how to protect both staff and campers through proper clothing, repellant use, habitat awareness, and emergency response protocols. It also helps in distinguishing harmless but fear-inducing arthropods from those that may require medical attention, supporting both education and reassurance in potentially anxious situations. In this way, the guide not only contributes to individual safety but also supports risk management policies for camp administration, helping ensure regulatory compliance, incident prevention, and peace of mind for families.

Educators and trainers may also use the guide as a supplementary resource in university field courses, safety certification programs, or workplace training modules. The inclusion of medically important arthropods, vector-borne disease summaries, and standardized exposure/severity ratings makes it suitable for use in preparing students and employees for fieldwork. It may also be used to raise awareness of entomological safety in industries where such knowledge has traditionally been passed on informally or inconsistently.

Emergency medical providers, particularly those in rural or resource-limited settings, may find the guide useful in recognizing less common but medically significant arthropod-related injuries and conditions. Paramedics, field medics, and rural health officers often encounter insect stings, bites, or infestations without specialized entomological training. The guide's symptom summaries, exposure mechanisms, and illustrative descriptions can assist in rapid triage or referral.

In short, this guide is not limited to any one profession or industry. While its core is built around the needs of field ecologists and environmental professionals, particularly in consulting, engineering, and regulatory contexts, it serves a much broader role in supporting health, safety, and operational awareness wherever humans and arthropods intersect (Goddard 2012; Duval et al. 2023). Whether used in a corporate safety office, a ranger station, or a mobile command center, it provides a grounded, field-tested resource for anticipating, understanding, and managing entomological risks.

REFERENCES

Bowles DE, Swaby JA. 2006. *Field Guide to Venomous and Medically Important Invertebrates Affecting Military Operations: Identification, Biology, Symptoms, Treatment.* U.S. Air Force Institute for Operational Health, Brooks City-Base, TX.

Darsie Jr RF, Ward RA. 2005. *Identification and Geographical Distribution of the Mosquitoes of North America, North of Mexico.* University Press of Florida, Gainesville, FL.

Duval P, Antonelli P, Aschan-Leygonie C, Moro CV. 2023. Impact of human activities on disease-spreading mosquitoes in urban areas. *J. Urban Health* 100: 591–611.

Goddard J. 2012. *Public Health Entomology.* CRC Press, Boca Raton, FL.

Johnson NF, Triplehorn CA. 2004. *Borror and DeLong's Introduction to the Study of Insects,* 7th Edition. Cengage Learning, Independence, KY.

Moraru GM, Goddard J II. 2019. *The Goddard Guide to Arthropods of Medical Importance.* CRC Press, Boca Raton, FL.

National Research Council. 1989. *Improving Risk Communication.* National Academies Press, Washington, DC.

Service M. 2012. *Medical Entomology for Students,* 5th Edition. Cambridge University Press, Cambridge, UK.

Ubick D, Paquin P, Cushing CE, Roth V. 2005. *Spiders of North America: An Identification Manual.* American Arachnological Society, Keene, NH.

2 Arthropod Overview

OVERVIEW OF THE MAJOR ENTOMOLOGICAL GROUPS

This book addresses a wide range of medically and operationally significant arthropods, with particular attention to those groups that pose direct health risks or disrupt field activities. Presentation of entomological groups is primarily done at one of two methods: taxonomic or ecological. Both presentations are important because environmental workers often recognize entomological groups by a common name – spiders, bugs, flies, wasps, etc. – but from a health and safety perspective, ecological groupings better define how each group can potentially cause harm. Further, taxonomy and ecology do not always line up one-for-one; for example, workers in the southern United States generally tend to associate all ant mounds with fire ants (which sting), but there are many ant species that do not sting and are harmless, and there are some species that, instead of direct medical harm, cause operational hazards – and some that do both.

Taxonomy is the science of how organisms are classified by name. Each organism fits within a hierarchy of classification levels, much like a corporate organizational chart (although the function is not administrative). The broadest, or highest, levels (like the C-suite officers) are the domain and kingdom, and the narrowest, or lowest, level is the species. Between these levels are multiple middle levels such as the phylum, class, order, family, and genus. Names are in Latin, so they often have weird spellings.

All entomological organisms are in the domain Eukaryota, which indicates that the internal parts of their cells have membranes; this separates them from things like bacteria, in which the intracellular parts are not membrane-bound. All entomological organisms are also in the kingdom Animalia (which means that they are animals) and the phylum Arthropoda (which means that they have exoskeletons and jointed legs).

It is at this next level that entomological organisms of health and safety interest differentiate. These organisms fall into five major taxonomic classes: Arachnida, Crustacea, Chilopoda, Diplopoda, and Insecta. The "Entomology 101" section that follows will go through each of these classes and discuss their distinguishing characteristics, behaviors, and typical mechanisms of harm.

A couple of quick notes about taxonomy that will hopefully help non-biologists use this guide more effectively. Although most people use common names like "tick" or "mosquito," biologists tend to use scientific names because they are more precise. Biologists also use particular conventions when using the scientific names of organisms. Species names have two words (a genus name and a specific epithet), and they are italicized, like *Ixodes scapularis*, a deer tick. If the genus name has already been mentioned recently and the word is not at the beginning of a sentence, the genus might be abbreviated, like *I. scapularis*. If only the genus name is given but refers to multiple species, the abbreviation "spp." may be used instead of the species names.

DOI: 10.1201/9781003745709-3

From an ecological standpoint within the health and safety perspective, entomological organisms tend to be parasites, pathogens, vectors, or agents. The "Ecological Roles" section that follows "Entomology 101" discusses characteristics and the mechanism of harm for each of these classifications.

ENTOMOLOGY 101

As mentioned above, the arthropods are divided into Arachnida, Crustacea, Chilopoda, Diplopoda, and Insecta. Arachnids include spiders, scorpions, ticks, mites, whip scorpions, and solifuges (sun/wind/camel spiders). Arachnids typically have two body regions (cephalothorax and abdomen) and eight legs. Some arachnid groups, like ticks and mites, are small and easily overlooked but may transmit pathogens. Others, such as spiders or scorpions, are not vectors for pathogens but may deliver medically significant bites or stings, though most species are relatively harmless. Learning to broadly distinguish arachnids from other arthropods is vital, since their risks and management strategies may differ.

While crustaceans are not traditionally central to most entomological work, they are arthropods and are occasionally encountered during environmental and ecological field operations. The crustacean group is broad and diverse, but the kinds most commonly encountered by ecologists and environmental professionals are isopods (often referred to as pill bugs, sow bugs, or roly-polies) and certain decapods such as crabs and crayfish. Isopods are small, segmented animals typically found under logs, rocks, or leaf litter in moist environments. They feed primarily on detritus and pose no health risk, though large aggregations can emit a pungent, unpleasant odor if disturbed. Crabs and crayfish are aquatic decapods often encountered in freshwater streams, ponds, or wetlands. Although generally not aggressive, they can be audacious if threatened and are equipped with large front claws, called chelae, capable of delivering a surprisingly firm pinch.

Chilopoda and Diplopoda are often lumped together in a group called the Myriapoda, which means "many-legged organisms." Chilopoda are centipedes, fast-moving predators with one pair of legs per body segment; they can "bite" using modified front legs, delivering venom that causes localized pain. Diplopoda are millipedes, slow-moving animals with two pairs of legs per segment and which generally just eat leaf litter and other detritus; while millipedes do not bite, they can secrete irritating chemicals that may blister skin. Both groups are common in leaf litter and soil environments, and while rarely dangerous, they are worth recognizing.

Insects are the largest group of arthropods, with incredible diversity. They are recognizable by their three body regions (head, thorax, abdomen), six legs, and usually one or two pairs of wings. Insects include familiar groups such as flies, beetles, butterflies, moths, ants, bees, and wasps. Some insects are major vectors of disease (e.g., mosquitoes, fleas), others are nuisance biters (e.g., horse flies, black flies), while the vast majority are entirely harmless. Insects are grouped by order (e.g., Diptera = flies, Coleoptera = beetles, Lepidoptera = butterflies and moths).

For professional entomologists, these distinctions are second nature. For other environmental professionals, however, the ability to tell "spider" from "insect," or "beetle" from "bug," is not always obvious – in many cases, they are all "bugs."

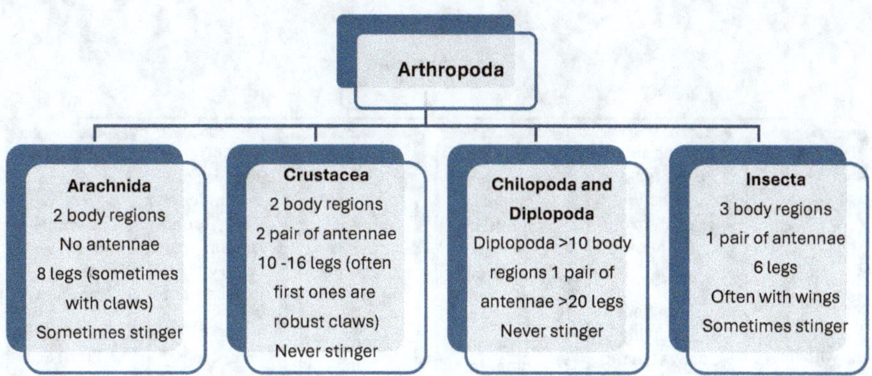

FIGURE 2.1   Class-level organization of the Arthropoda, with characteristics of each group.

However, misidentification usually leads to unnecessary fear but sometimes can underestimate a true risk. A basic grasp of arthropod diversity empowers managers to guide workers confidently, provide accurate instruction, and avoid costly overreactions. Figure 2.1 is a high-level "field orientation" to arthropod groups, laying the groundwork for the more detailed hazard discussions that follow.

ARACHNIDS

The arachnids are a diverse group of arthropods distinguished by their eight legs, two main body regions (cephalothorax and abdomen), and an absence of wings or antennae. While often overshadowed by insects in both abundance and public attention, arachnids play outsized roles in ecological systems and human health. Their diversity is striking, ranging from microscopic mites to formidable scorpions. For ecological and environmental professionals working in North America, the most important arachnid groups include ticks, mites, spiders, scorpions, whip scorpions (vinegaroons), and sun/wind/camel spiders (solifuges).

   Collectively, arachnids represent a spectrum of hazards that range from nuisance exposures to envenomation to life-threatening diseases. Their biology and ecology overlap with the daily tasks of ecological and environmental professionals: conducting field surveys, handling soil or vegetation, managing wildlife, and working in remote areas. An understanding of their diversity, behavior, and risks provides the foundation for effective prevention and mitigation strategies (Figure 2.2).

Ticks

Ticks are blood-feeding ectoparasites belonging to the subclass Acari, which also includes mites (discussed separately). Unlike insects, ticks have eight legs, a flattened oval body, and lack wings and antennae. They go through several life stages, and each active stage requires a blood meal to develop to the next. Ticks attach firmly to their hosts using specialized mouthparts, including a barbed hypostome, and can remain embedded for several days as they feed. Most are found in grassy, brushy, or wooded habitats, where they seek hosts through a behavior known as questing.

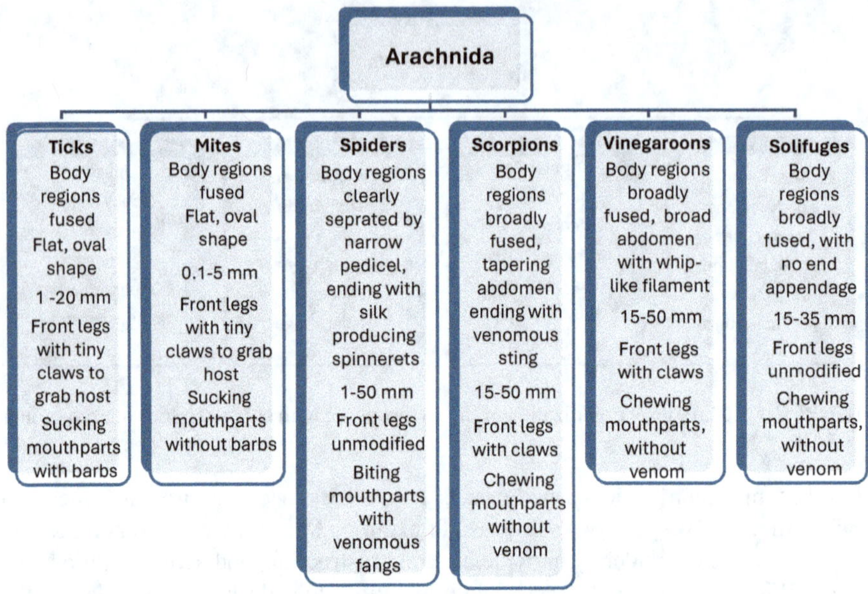

FIGURE 2.2   Order-level organization of the Arachnida, with characteristics of each group.

Ticks are medically significant because they are vectors of numerous pathogens, including bacteria, viruses, and protozoa. Among the most notorious is Lyme disease, caused by the bacterium *Borrelia burgdorferi*, and transmitted primarily by *I. scapularis* in the eastern United States and *Ixodes pacificus* in the west. If left untreated, Lyme disease can cause serious neurological and joint complications. Other serious bacterial infections transmitted by ticks include Rocky Mountain spotted fever (*Rickettsia rickettsii*), ehrlichiosis, anaplasmosis, and tularemia, all of which can be severe or even fatal without prompt medical treatment.

Ticks are also responsible for transmitting several viral diseases, some of which have emerged or expanded in recent years. These include Powassan virus, a rare but potentially deadly encephalitic virus carried by *Ixodes* species; Heartland virus and Bourbon virus, recently discovered in the central United States; and Colorado tick fever, a viral illness of the Rocky Mountain region. Due to the growing range of multiple tick species and increasing human-tick interactions, the public health threat from tick-borne viruses continues to evolve.

In addition to pathogen-mediated diseases, ticks can also cause significant illness through non-infectious mechanisms. Alpha-gal syndrome is a red meat allergy that results from a sugar molecule introduced by the bite of the lone star tick (*Amblyomma americanum*). It can lead to delayed, and sometimes severe, allergic reactions after consuming mammalian meat. Another non-pathogen condition is tick paralysis, caused by a neurotoxin present in the saliva of certain female ticks (especially *Dermacentor variabilis* and *Dermacentor andersoni*). This rare but potentially life-threatening syndrome can lead to progressive paralysis, which typically resolves upon tick removal.

Recognizing the wide range of diseases and syndromes associated with ticks, it is critical for environmental professionals, field biologists, and outdoor workers to implement preventive strategies, such as protective clothing, repellents, and habitat awareness. Refer to Box 2.1 on "How to Perform a Tick Check" for post-exposure best practices, and Box 2.2, the "Tick Removal" guide, for safe extraction in case of attachment. Awareness and early intervention are key, as many tick-borne illnesses can be effectively treated if diagnosed in time.

As climate change, land use patterns, and wildlife movements continue to influence tick ecology, tick-borne diseases are expected to rise in both geographic range and incidence. Understanding the biology, behavior, and risks associated with ticks is therefore an essential component of entomological health and safety in North America.

BOX 2.1   HOW TO PERFORM A TICK CHECK

Conducting a thorough tick check is a critical step in reducing the risk of tick-borne illness and avoiding complications such as tick paralysis. Tick checks should be done as soon as possible after returning from tick-prone environments, such as forests, brushy fields, or areas with tall grass. Ideally, the check should occur within 2 hours of exposure, as prompt removal reduces the chance of disease transmission.

Begin by examining clothing before entering a vehicle or indoor space. Ticks often cling to fabric before finding a path to the skin. Shake out clothing vigorously, and, if possible, place exposed garments in a hot dryer for at least 10 minutes to kill any unseen ticks. When possible, shower soon after exposure to help wash off unattached ticks and facilitate a full-body check.

Next, conduct a systematic visual and tactile examination of your entire body. Use a full-length mirror and a handheld mirror to inspect all surfaces, or enlist a partner for hard-to-see areas. Check in and around the following key locations where ticks are most likely to attach:

- Hairline and scalp (especially behind ears and at the nape of the neck)
- Underarms and behind knees
- Around the waistline and belt area
- Inside the belly button
- In groin and buttocks region
- Between toes and under fingernails

Run your fingers gently over your skin to detect any small bumps or attached ticks. Some ticks, especially in the nymphal stage, can be as small as a poppy seed, so take your time and examine closely under good lighting. Use a fine-tooth comb to check through hair.

BOX 2.2   HOW TO REMOVE A TICK PROPERLY

If a tick is found attached to the skin, it should be removed as soon as possible. Use a pair of fine-tipped tweezers or a specialized tick removal tool. Grasp the tick as close to the skin's surface as possible, ideally at the point where the mouthparts enter the skin. Pull away from the skin perpendicularly with steady, even pressure. Do not twist, jerk, or squeeze the tick's body, as this can cause the mouthparts to break off or squeeze fluids back into you.

If part of the mouth remains embedded in the skin after removal, do not dig with needles or knives. Instead, clean the area with soap and water and let the body expel the remnants naturally. If several days go by and the mouthparts remain, consult a health care provider. After removal, disinfect the bite site with antiseptic, and wash hands thoroughly.

Do not use folklore remedies such as applying petroleum jelly, nail polish, alcohol, or heat (e.g., matches or hot pins) to try to "suffocate" or "burn out" the tick. These methods are ineffective and can cause the tick to regurgitate, increasing the risk of disease transmission. Likewise, squeezing the tick's abdomen can inject pathogens directly into the wound. These methods can also kill the tick and make it even more difficult to remove the embedded mouthparts.

If possible, save the tick in a sealable plastic bag or container with the date and location of the bite. This can assist with species identification and medical diagnosis if symptoms develop. Monitor the bite site and general health over the next few weeks. Seek medical attention if you develop fever, rash, fatigue, or signs of paralysis.

Mites

Mites are small, often microscopic arthropods in the subclass Acari, closely related to ticks. While the vast majority of mite species are free-living and ecologically beneficial as decomposers, predators, or plant feeders, a small number have medical or veterinary significance. These medically relevant mites can act as ectoparasites, allergens, or vectors of pathogens. Due to their small size and cryptic habits, mite infestations often go unnoticed until clinical signs appear, such as skin irritation, dermatitis, or respiratory symptoms.

One of the most well-known mite-related conditions is scabies, caused by *Sarcoptes scabiei var. hominis*. This mite burrows into the skin, leading to intense itching and a rash, and spreads primarily through direct, prolonged skin-to-skin contact. Outbreaks can occur in communal living or health care settings. Another medically significant group of mites is the chiggers, which do not burrow but inject digestive enzymes into the skin, causing intensely itchy, inflamed lesions. Particularly frustrating is the fact that the chigger actually leaves the body of its host before the itching starts! In some parts of the world, chiggers transmit scrub typhus, but in North America, their impact is largely limited to dermatitis and secondary infection from scratching.

Mites have also been implicated as vectors or reservoirs of pathogens in rare but notable cases. Rodent mites, such as *Ornithonyssus bacoti*, may feed opportunistically on humans, especially in buildings with rodent infestations. These mites can cause bites and localized skin reactions and have been occasionally associated with the mechanical transmission of diseases like murine typhus. Additionally, tropical rat mites and bird mites may bite humans when their primary hosts are removed or nests are disturbed.

Though often overlooked due to their size, mites should be recognized as potential occupational hazards in certain environments – especially during work in attics, abandoned buildings, rodent-infested structures, or wildlife handling scenarios. Awareness of mite-associated health risks, coupled with appropriate hygiene, pest control, and personal protective equipment (PPE), can help prevent infestations and minimize discomfort or disease transmission in field and indoor settings alike.

Spiders

Spiders (order Araneae) are a diverse and ecologically important group of arachnids found throughout North America. Over 3,500 species have been described from this region, occupying nearly every terrestrial habitat from deserts and forests to grasslands and urban environments. Despite their ubiquity and often fearsome reputation, the vast majority of spiders are harmless to humans and play beneficial roles in controlling insect populations.

Of the thousands of species of spiders that exist, only a small handful (fewer than a dozen!) are considered of medical significance in North America. The most notable include the widow spiders (*Latrodectus* spp.), known for their neurotoxic venom; the brown recluse spider (*Loxosceles reclusa*), which may cause necrotic skin lesions; and, to a much lesser extent, species such as sac spiders (*Cheiracanthium* spp.), which are sometimes implicated in minor envenomations. Hobo spiders (*Eratigena agrestis*) have historically been reported to be dangerous, but current empirical evidence suggests that they are at most a very minor cause of necrotic envenomation. Tarantulas, though large and intimidating, are not medically dangerous, and their bites rarely result in more than local pain and swelling.

Tracking the true epidemiological incidence of spider bites is difficult. Unlike vector-borne diseases or poisonings, spider bites are not systematically reported or confirmed, and a large percentage of attributed cases are misdiagnosed or lack verification of the actual spider involved. Many skin lesions caused by infections, insect bites, or environmental irritants are mistakenly blamed on brown recluse or other spiders, and this is frustratingly common in areas where the suspected species does not even occur. As a result, epidemiological data on spider envenomation are limited and likely inflated in public perception.

For most environmental professionals and field personnel, the risk of serious spider envenomation is extremely low. However, understanding which species are of concern, where they are found, and how to recognize potential exposure is still valuable for risk assessment, especially in areas where venomous spiders are endemic or when working in spaces such as crawlspaces, storage sheds, woodpiles, or remote shelters where human-spider encounters are more likely.

Other Arachnids

Scorpions, vinegaroons, and solifugids are non-spider arachnids belonging to distinct taxonomic orders within the class Arachnida. These organisms are most commonly encountered in the southern and southwestern United States, particularly in arid or semi-arid environments. While less diverse than spiders, these groups are nonetheless important for occupational safety in outdoor and remote settings, especially where fieldwork takes place under rocks, logs, debris, or in infrequently accessed structures. Across North America, there are approximately 90–100 species of scorpions, a few species of vinegaroons, and about a dozen species of solifugids, many of which are localized and rarely encountered.

Of these, scorpions are the only group with documented medically significant envenomation. Most North American scorpion stings result in localized pain, swelling, and mild systemic symptoms, similar to a bee or wasp sting. However, in the southwestern United States, particularly Arizona and New Mexico, the Arizona bark scorpion (*Centruroides sculpturatus*) poses a greater risk.

Vinegaroons and solifugids are non-venomous and pose little direct medical threat to humans. Vinegaroons, also called whip scorpions, can spray a defensive mist of acetic acid when threatened, producing a mild burning sensation or irritation if it contacts eyes or mucous membranes. Solifugids, sometimes sensationalized as "camel spiders," may bite defensively with their large chelicerae, but their bites are rare and typically no more serious than a superficial wound. Both groups are generally shy, nocturnal, and unlikely to interact with humans unless disturbed in their daytime retreats.

While bites and stings from these arachnids are infrequent and often exaggerated in folklore, awareness of their presence is valuable for risk management, especially in desert, scrubland, or dry forest environments. Field personnel working at night, moving rocks or logs, or accessing understructure areas in these habitats should be trained to recognize these arachnids and take basic precautions. As with spiders, incidence data are not systematically collected, and most exposures go unreported or are treated symptomatically without species-level identification. Nonetheless, these groups deserve mention in entomological safety planning due to their regional significance and potential for painful, if rarely serious, encounters.

CRUSTACEANS

Crustaceans are a group that includes familiar animals such as crabs, crayfish, shrimp, and lobsters. Although most crustaceans do not pose significant risk to humans and are not commonly considered in the same health and safety categories as arachnids, myriapods, or insects, some species encountered in freshwater, estuarine, or littoral zones where ecologists and environmental professionals may work can cause injury through pinching or crushing mechanisms. Their inclusion in this guide is warranted due to their occasional but notable presence in fieldwork settings, particularly when ecological professionals are sampling aquatic habitats, handling debris near water, or working in environments with submerged infrastructure.

Crayfish and many freshwater or estuarine crabs are equipped with robust claws (chelae) capable of delivering a painful pinch. While not venomous, these injuries can break the skin, cause bruising, or, in rare cases, become secondarily infected, particularly if the water source is contaminated. Crayfish and crabs are often faster than expected and may instinctively clamp down and hold fast when threatened. While most individuals will quickly release if placed back in water, others may hold tightly, especially if handled improperly or in high-stress situations. Field workers lifting submerged logs, reaching into crevices, or clearing intake grates should be aware that crustaceans may be hiding underneath or inside these features.

Certain amphipod species, especially those in the family Talitridae, have been reported to "nibble" at exposed human skin in estuarine or freshwater environments. These bites are typically not medically serious but can cause minor skin irritation, redness, or itching, small abrasions that could become secondarily infected if exposed to contaminated water, and a psychological nuisance, especially when occurring in dense swarms. These types of bites are typically reported by waders, beachcombers, or field workers sampling shallow waters, estuaries, or detritus-rich zones.

Amphipods can also reach explosive population densities in certain aquatic systems, particularly around decomposing organic material, wastewater outflows, or nutrient-rich sediment. Their large numbers can clog field sampling equipment, overwhelm laboratory tanks or aquatic mesocosms used in ecological research, and cause minor slip hazards if swarming near boat ramps, docks, or shorelines.

Crustaceans are not vectors of disease through biting or stinging, and they are not blood feeders. However, some species could feasibly act as mechanical carriers of pathogens or parasites, especially in water bodies affected by agricultural runoff or sewage contamination. These risks are low in North America, but they are of greater concern in tropical waterways.

Myriapods

Myriapod means "many-legged" and includes the centipedes and millipedes, elongate, multi-segmented invertebrates that are commonly encountered in soil, leaf litter, under logs, and within decaying organic matter. Although often overlooked in discussions of arthropod-related health and safety, these organisms can pose minor but potentially noteworthy risks to field personnel, especially in warm, humid, or forested environments. Centipedes are predators equipped with venomous forcipules (modified front legs) that can puncture skin and inject venom, resulting in localized pain, swelling, and, in rare cases, systemic effects. Millipedes, while non-venomous and incapable of biting, can secrete irritating defensive chemicals, including benzoquinones and hydrochloric acid derivatives, which may cause skin staining, blistering, or eye irritation.

In North America, there are over 1,000 described species of centipedes and millipedes, with most posing minimal threat to humans. However, larger centipede species, particularly those in the genus *Scolopendra*, can deliver painful bites if handled or trapped against the skin. Millipede secretions are usually more of a chemical nuisance than a serious hazard, but they can create operational issues when these animals congregate in large numbers in damp field gear, boots, or under structures. While bites and chemical exposures are not tracked systematically and rarely result in medical intervention, they remain relevant for occupational health planning in

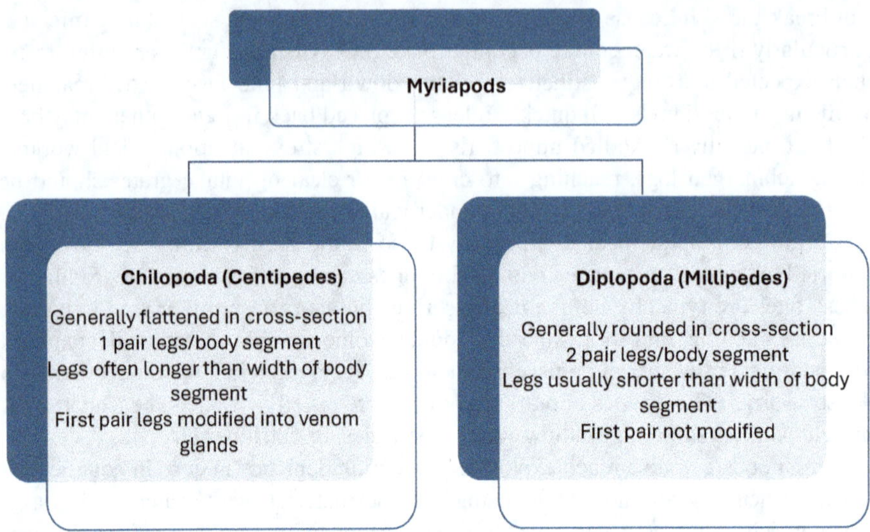

FIGURE 2.3 Class-level organization of the myriapods, with characteristics of each group.

regions where myriapods are abundant. Field workers should be advised to avoid handling them unnecessarily and take precautions when working in areas with moist organic ground cover or debris where these organisms may be concealed (Figure 2.3).

INSECTS

The insects are the most diverse and numerous group of arthropods, characterized by six legs, segmented bodies with three main regions (head, thorax, abdomen), and typically one or two pairs of wings. Unlike arachnids, insects possess antennae and undergo a range of developmental strategies, which influence their behavior, ecology, and potential to interact with humans. From wingless springtails to charismatic butterflies, insects inhabit every terrestrial and freshwater habitat encountered by ecological and environmental professionals.

Insects present a wide range of potential health and safety concerns, from minor nuisances like fly bites or ladybug-induced dermatitis to more serious exposures involving stings, allergic reactions, or vector-borne diseases. Their ubiquity in natural and built environments means that encounters are often unavoidable, particularly in field-based work involving water, soil, vegetation, or wildlife. Furthermore, the diversity of insect form and function demands an understanding of their biology and seasonal activity patterns to properly assess risks. Whether investigating aquatic ecosystems, managing forested landscapes, or conducting long-term biological monitoring, professionals in the field benefit from recognizing which insect groups may pose hazards and how best to avoid or mitigate those risks.

To help organize this broad taxon, I am grouping them according to their growth patterns: (1) ametabolous, in which the newly hatched young look just like the adults, but smaller, (2) hemimetabolous, in which the young look somewhat like the adults

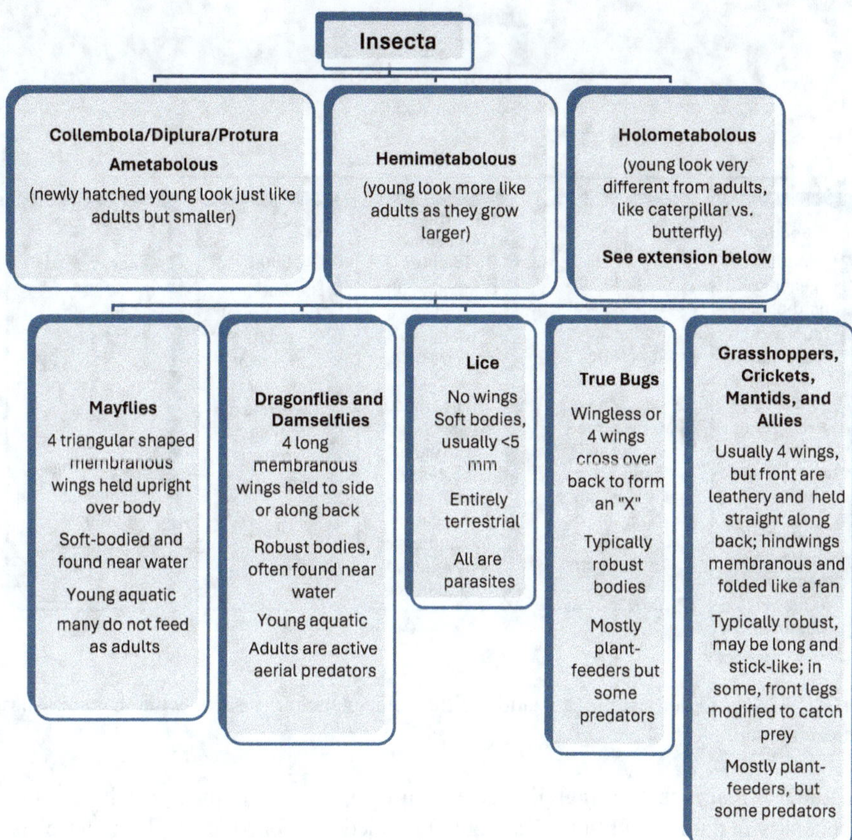

FIGURE 2.4 Order-level organization of the insects, including the ametabolous insects and hemimetabolous insects, with characteristics of each group.

and resemble them more and more as they age, and (3) holometabolous insects, in which the young look nothing like the adult and go through a metamorphosis to turn into the adult. Then, each of the growth pattern groups is further divided into the various groups covered in this guide (Figures 2.4 and 2.5).

Collembola, Diplura, Protura

These three groups that primarily dwell in soil and leaf litter have traditionally been considered to be insects; however, they have recently been split out of the insects to form their own small group. They are primarily differentiated from the true insects in that they have mouthparts that are enclosed within folds of their head capsule. In contrast, insects have exposed mouthparts. These organisms are generally tiny (often less than 5 mm) and are rarely noticed unless present in large numbers, but they play important roles in soil ecology through decomposition and nutrient cycling.

Of the three groups, only the Collembola could reasonably be considered to be of occupational concern. While they do not bite or sting or pose any other direct

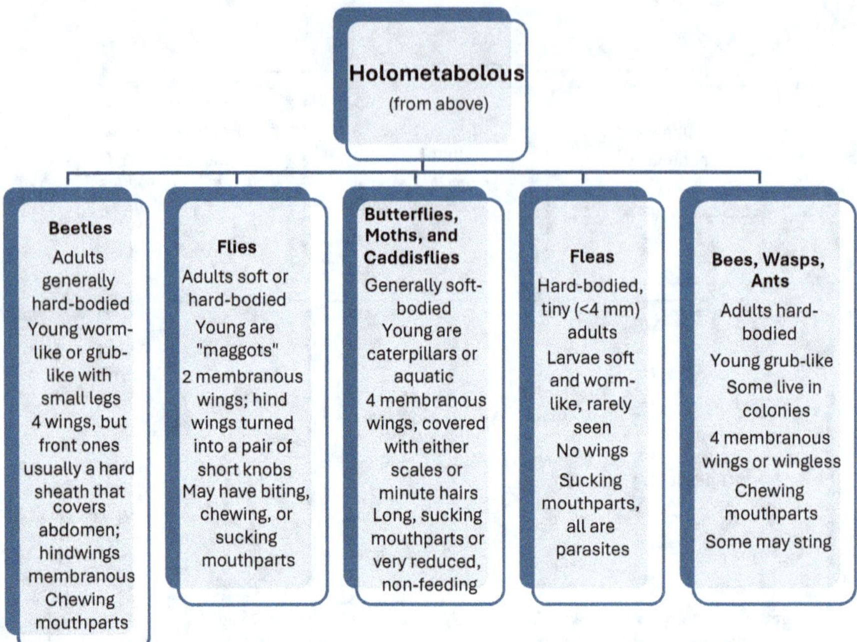

FIGURE 2.5   Order-level organization of the holometabolous insects, with characteristics of each group.

medical threat, some springtail species can occur in exceptionally high densities, especially in damp conditions, leading to nuisance-level encounters. There have also been anecdotal reports linking springtails to skin irritation or psychological stress, though such associations remain poorly substantiated. Field personnel working in moist, shaded environments such as wetlands, riparian zones, or forest floors may encounter springtails in high numbers on equipment, skin, or clothing, warranting their occasional inclusion in entomological health and safety considerations.

Mayflies

Mayflies are delicate, soft-bodied insects. The immature stages of mayflies live in streams, rivers, ponds, and lakes, and the adults leave the water to fly around. Mayflies can occasionally pose logistical or nuisance hazards, especially during mass emergences of the adults near large bodies of water. Adult mayflies are short-lived, often surviving only a day or two, and do not bite, sting, or carry diseases.

In regions near rivers, lakes, or reservoirs, large, synchronized hatches of mayflies can result in extreme swarming events, covering vehicles, roadways, lights, and structures in dense, slippery layers. These swarms can reduce visibility, create hazardous driving conditions, clog air intakes or filters, and even cause temporary shutdowns of bridges or industrial equipment. While harmless to human health (except for persons who are allergic to them), the sheer biomass of mayfly emergences has made them a notable concern for environmental and transportation safety managers working near aquatic systems during peak emergence seasons.

Dragonflies and Damselflies

Dragonflies and damselflies are both in the order Odonata. Most people are familiar with dragonflies, large aerial predators that feed on smaller flying insects. Damselflies are similar to dragonflies, but generally smaller and daintier. Although some people have a fear of dragonflies, the Odonata pose medical concern only to the extent that some larger species can bite if mishandled.

Lice

Lice (order Phthiraptera) are obligate ectoparasites of birds and mammals, including humans. Unlike many other arthropods of medical importance, lice are wingless, dorsoventrally flattened insects that spend their entire life cycle on a host. Lice are extremely species-specific, and those that infest humans are adapted exclusively to that host. There are three types of lice that infest humans: the head louse (*Pediculus humanus capitis*), the body louse (*P. humanus corporis*), and the pubic louse (*Pthirus pubis*).

Head lice are most commonly associated with children and communal living environments, and while they can be transmitted through shared headgear or close contact, they are more of a nuisance than a health threat. In contrast, body lice live in clothing and bedding, moving to the skin to feed. They are associated with poor hygiene and crowded conditions and are the only human louse known to transmit pathogens, including epidemic typhus (*Rickettsia prowazekii*), trench fever (*Bartonella quintana*), and relapsing fever (*Borrelia recurrentis*). Although rare in modern field conditions, body lice infestations have been reported in disaster zones, among unsheltered populations, and in overcrowded facilities, making them a potential concern during post-disaster assessments and building inspections.

Pubic lice (*P. pubis*) are a sexually transmitted ectoparasite with no relevance to occupational or environmental exposure. As such, infestations with this species fall under personal health rather than field safety protocols and are not considered within the scope of this guide.

While most lice are host-specific, a few species associated with animals can opportunistically bite humans. These zoonotic lice do not typically establish long-term infestations on people but may cause discomfort, localized irritation, or confusion during pest investigations. One such example is *Haematopinus suis*, the hog louse, which has been known to bite humans working in close contact with infested swine. Likewise, poultry workers may encounter *Menacanthus stramineus*, the chicken body louse, or *Lipeurus caponis*, the wing louse, particularly in poorly maintained coops or during direct animal handling. In rural or agricultural field settings, especially where wildlife and livestock interface, lice may be encountered on deer, cattle, goats, or other mammals, although cross-species transmission remains extremely uncommon. Animal lice are not typically vectors of human disease; however, they may introduce secondary skin infections through scratching or be mistaken for other ectoparasites such as mites or fleas.

In general, lice are unlikely to pose a significant risk to ecologists or environmental professionals conducting routine fieldwork. However, personnel working in overcrowded, unsanitary, or infested indoor environments, such as during structural evaluations or wildlife removal in abandoned homes, should be aware of lice transmission risks. Wearing disposable coveralls, minimizing contact with fabric surfaces, and maintaining good hygiene can reduce potential exposure. Suspected infestations should be reported to a supervisor and evaluated by medical professionals for appropriate treatment.

True Bugs

The order Hemiptera, commonly referred to as the "true bugs," includes a diverse array of species with varied ecological roles. While most true bugs are plant feeders, several families include species of medical or public health significance, particularly those that bite humans or live in close association with human dwellings and activities. Hemiptera are characterized by piercing-sucking mouthparts and hemelytra – forewings with a thickened base and membranous tip. Their ability to exploit a wide range of environments means that both aquatic and terrestrial hemipterans may be encountered during environmental or ecological fieldwork.

Several aquatic hemipterans are known to bite defensively when handled or inadvertently disturbed. While not medically dangerous, their bites can be sharply painful, and some species, like the giant water bugs, are large enough to cause brief localized swelling. These insects may be encountered in freshwater systems during invertebrate sampling and should be handled with care.

Among the terrestrial hemipterans, kissing bugs (*Triatoma* spp., family Reduviidae) are of particular concern due to their role in transmitting Chagas disease, caused by the protozoan *Trypanosoma cruzi*. These nocturnal blood feeders defecate during or after feeding, and transmission occurs when feces are rubbed into the bite site, eyes, or mucous membranes. While Chagas disease is more common in Latin America, several *Triatoma* species occur in the southern United States, and autochthonous cases have been documented. Other blood-feeding hemipterans, such as bed bugs (*Cimex lectularius*) and swallow bugs (*Oeciacus vicarius*), do not transmit disease but can cause significant irritation, secondary skin infections, and psychological stress in infested environments.

Though the majority of hemipterans encountered in the field are harmless, awareness of medically significant species is important, especially when working in tick- or bat-infested buildings, handling wildlife, or performing aquatic biomonitoring. Preventive measures such as using gloves during sampling, minimizing skin exposure during insect-rich seasons, and recognizing signs of infestation in field housing or equipment can help reduce unwanted interactions with these true bugs.

Orthopteroids (Cockroaches, Earwigs, Grasshoppers, Katydids, Crickets, Stick Insects, Praying Mantids)

The orthopteroid insects are a diverse assemblage of orders characterized by chewing mouthparts, leathery forewings, and incomplete metamorphosis. While many orthopteroids, such as grasshoppers and crickets, are primarily ecological indicators or agricultural pests, a few groups contain species of entomological health significance, particularly due to mechanical transmission of pathogens, nuisance swarming, or non-venomous (but painful) bites. These insects are generally ground-dwelling or associated with vegetation and often interact with humans through field work, agriculture, or habitation in rustic shelters.

Medically or occupationally relevant orthopteroid orders include the Blattodea (cockroaches), Dermaptera (earwigs), and, to a lesser extent, Orthoptera (grasshoppers and katydids). Cockroaches, especially *Periplaneta americana* and *Blattella germanica*, are significant in urban and field environments for their role in mechanical transmission of bacteria and parasites, as well as their ability to trigger asthma and allergic responses via airborne feces, cast skins, and saliva. Earwigs, while often feared due to their pincers, are harmless in terms of venom but may deliver pinching bites and serve as minor mechanical vectors (Jeong et al. 2021). Large katydids and lubber grasshoppers occasionally bite defensively when handled and can become locally abundant, interfering with equipment or operations, particularly in warm and vegetated habitats.

Although cockroaches do not transmit systemic disease in the same manner as ticks or mosquitoes, their high mobility, resilience, and association with unsanitary conditions make them relevant in occupational health planning, particularly in field housing, latrine areas, food storage, and during nighttime activities when many species are active. For environmental professionals, understanding their role as mechanical vectors, allergen sources, and nuisance pests is critical to effective risk assessment and mitigation.

Beetles

Beetles (order Coleoptera) represent the most diverse group of insects on Earth, with over 350,000 described species worldwide and thousands in North America alone. They occupy nearly every terrestrial and aquatic habitat and serve a wide range of ecological roles – from pollinators and decomposers to predators and pests. While the overwhelming majority of beetles are harmless or even beneficial to humans, a handful have characteristics that warrant attention in health and safety planning due to their capacity to bite, secrete irritants, or cause allergic reactions. Field professionals may encounter these beetles during soil excavation, vegetation surveys, in stored materials, or when working in abandoned structures or near decomposing organic matter.

Some beetles have chemical defenses that can cause direct harm or discomfort. Bombardier beetles (e.g., *Brachinus* spp.) are notable for their ability to eject a boiling, noxious chemical spray from their abdomen, producing a popping sound and a painful burn upon contact with skin or eyes. Similarly, blister beetles (family Meloidae) excrete cantharidin, a potent blistering agent that can cause severe skin irritation. Cantharidin exposure is most often a concern when beetles are crushed against the skin or contaminate food, forage, or bedding materials.

Other beetles present risks through biting or allergic response. Some of the ground beetles, such as fiery searchers (*Calosoma scrutator*) or other Carabidae, may secrete irritating substances if handled carelessly. *Dermestid* beetles (family Dermestidae), often encountered in carcass work, food storage facilities, or neglected indoor spaces, are not dangerous themselves, but their larval hairs and shed skins can cause allergic reactions and dermatitis in sensitized individuals. The multicolored Asian lady beetle can also bite, emit foul-smelling defensive compounds, and trigger allergic responses, particularly during mass aggregations indoors in fall and winter.

Additionally, mealworms (larvae of *Tenebrio molitor* and other tenebrionid beetles) and other stored product beetles may be found in food storage or composting systems. While not dangerous, their presence can indicate sanitation issues, and prolonged handling may result in skin irritation or allergen exposure. Overall, while beetle-related risks are generally minor, field personnel should be aware of specific genera or environments where noxious, stinging, or allergenic beetles may be encountered, and take care when handling beetles manually or working in infested structures.

Butterflies, Moths, and Caddisflies

The orders Lepidoptera (butterflies and moths) and Trichoptera (caddisflies) are best known for their ecological importance and aesthetic appeal rather than for posing direct threats to human health. Both groups undergo complete metamorphosis and are commonly encountered in terrestrial and aquatic environments, respectively. While most adult Lepidoptera are harmless nectar feeders, and most caddisflies do not feed at all in the adult stage, certain larval and adult forms can cause irritation, allergic responses, or rare envenomation in specific occupational settings.

In the Lepidoptera, health risks primarily stem from contact with the larvae (caterpillars) of certain moth species that bear urticating hairs or venomous spines, such as the puss caterpillar (*Megalopyge opercularis*), saddleback caterpillar (*Acharia stimulea*), or io moth (*Automeris io*). These hairs can penetrate the skin and cause localized pain, swelling, rash, or, in some individuals, systemic reactions. Caterpillars may be found on foliage, low vegetation, or even accidentally encountered during sampling. In some species, detached hairs or scales may also become airborne and cause respiratory or ocular irritation. While adult moths and butterflies are generally harmless, some can produce irritating scales or powders that cause mild reactions upon close contact.

Caddisflies, on the other hand, are a common component of aquatic biomonitoring work and are regularly collected in benthic samples. Adult caddisflies are often abundant near water bodies and may swarm lights at night, but they do not bite or sting. The swarming species are of most concern, since they can become a nuisance by their sheer numbers or can cause logistical or equipment failures.

True Flies

The order Diptera (the true flies) is one of the most ecologically and medically significant groups of insects. Characterized by a single pair of functional wings and a pair of halteres (modified hindwings used for balance), flies occupy a vast range of ecological niches and are found in nearly every terrestrial and aquatic environment. Many species play beneficial roles as pollinators, scavengers, or predators, while others are known for their association with filth, decay, or disease. In the context of health and safety, certain dipteran families are important not only for their annoyance factor but also for their capacity to bite, cause allergic reactions, infest wounds, or transmit pathogens to humans and animals.

Nearly everyone knows what a mosquito is! Mosquitoes (family Culicidae) are among the most medically significant arthropods in the world due to their role as vectors of disease. They are slender, long-legged flies with elongated mouthparts adapted for piercing skin and sucking blood. Only female mosquitoes feed on blood, which they require to produce eggs. Males feed exclusively on nectar. Mosquitoes breed in standing water – from ponds and marshes to temporary puddles, ditches, and artificial containers – and are most active during dawn, dusk, or nighttime, depending on the species.

In North America, several genera of mosquitoes pose public and occupational health risks, most notably *Culex*, *Aedes*, and *Anopheles*. These mosquitoes are capable of transmitting viruses like West Nile virus, St. Louis encephalitis, eastern equine encephalitis (EEE), and La Crosse virus; protozoans such as *Plasmodium* spp., the cause of malaria; and parasitic worms, such as *Dirofilaria immitis*, the dog heartworm. *Aedes aegypti* and *Aedes albopictus* – introduced species now established in much of the southern and eastern United States – are vectors of diseases such as dengue, zika, and chikungunya in tropical regions and may pose a risk during outbreaks or travel. However, it is important to note that most mosquito bites in North America result in only local irritation and do not lead to disease.

Field personnel working near water bodies, wetlands, or shaded vegetation during mosquito season should take standard precautions, including the use of Environmental Protection Agency (EPA)-registered repellents (e.g., DEET, picaridin), long-sleeved clothing, and, where needed, head nets or permethrin-treated gear. While the risk of severe mosquito-borne disease varies by region and season, proactive prevention remains the most effective strategy for minimizing exposure and maintaining health during field operations.

True flies other than mosquitoes can also be implicated in health and safety scenarios. Key families covered here include Tabanidae (horse and deer flies), Simuliidae (black flies), Ceratopogonidae (biting midges), Asilidae (robber flies), Muscidae (house flies and stable flies), Calliphoridae and Sarcophagidae (blow flies and flesh flies), Oestridae (bot flies), and others. These flies may be encountered in a range of field settings, including forests, grasslands, wetlands, urban waste areas, and animal enclosures. Depending on the species, they may bite, feed on secretions or open wounds, lay eggs on exposed tissue or clothing, or serve as mechanical vectors of bacteria and parasites.

While not all flies pose a direct threat to health, several are responsible for significant occupational hazards. For example, black flies and biting midges can cause painful bites and allergic reactions, while stable flies can disrupt fieldwork with persistent blood-feeding behavior. Blow flies and flesh flies may contaminate food or instruments, and, in rare cases, cause myiasis – the infestation of live tissue with fly larvae.

Additionally, some flies are a nuisance because of sheer numbers and their tendency to congregate near humans or other landmarks. Even without biting, they can cause psychological stress or, under extreme circumstances, equipment failure and hazardous environmental conditions.

A few families include large flies that may be encountered during fieldwork in forests, wetlands, or near streams and rivers. Among these, large robber flies (Asilidae) are normally predatory on other insects and are generally beneficial, but some larger species (up to 50 mm/2 in) may bite defensively if captured or handled. These flies are fast-flying and often rest on sunlit vegetation or bare ground while hunting. Snipe flies (Rhagionidae) and watersnipe flies (Athericidae) include species whose females may occasionally bite humans, particularly in damp, shaded, or riparian environments.

Bites are typically brief and mildly painful, comparable to those of a deer fly, but these flies are generally not aggressive and do not transmit disease. Because their bites are almost always in response to rough handling, I did not include an entry for them here, Workers should simply avoid handling large flies barehanded, and bites, if they occur, should be cleaned and monitored for signs of secondary infection.

Understanding the biology and seasonality of these flies is essential for minimizing exposure. Appropriate preventive strategies, such as protective clothing, repellents, and environmental sanitation, can substantially reduce the risk of discomfort, infection, or work disruption associated with dipteran encounters in the field.

Fleas

Fleas (order Siphonaptera) are small, laterally compressed, wingless insects that are specialized blood-feeding ectoparasites of mammals and birds. Their strong hind legs allow them to jump considerable distances relative to their body size, making them highly mobile between hosts or from environment to host. Fleas are frequently encountered in association with rodents, small mammals, and domestic animals, and, while many species are host-specific, some will opportunistically bite humans when their preferred hosts are unavailable.

In North America, the most medically significant flea is the oriental rat flea (*Xenopsylla cheopis*), the primary vector of plague (*Yersinia pestis*), which persists at low levels in wild rodent populations in the western United States, particularly in parts of New Mexico, Colorado, Arizona, and California. Fleas may also transmit murine typhus (*Rickettsia typhi*), especially in areas where rodents and opossums (*Didelphis virginiana*) coexist near human settlements. Other flea-borne concerns include cat scratch disease (via *Bartonella henselae*) and the dog and cat tapeworm (*Dipylidium caninum*), with fleas playing a role in transmission between cats while humans become infected secondarily. Although currently rare in North America, flea-borne pathogens can cause serious or life-threatening illness, particularly if not recognized and treated early.

Fleas may be encountered occupationally when working in rodent burrows, abandoned buildings, wildlife dens, or when handling mammals during trapping, necropsy, or habitat assessments. Bites, which may not even have pathogens present and so are merely a nuisance, often present as clusters of itchy, inflamed papules, typically on the ankles or lower legs. To minimize exposure, field personnel should wear long pants tucked into socks, use insect repellents labeled for fleas, and avoid disturbing rodent habitats unnecessarily. Following fieldwork, clothing should be laundered promptly, and any signs of flea infestation or unusual febrile illness should be reported for medical evaluation.

Ants, Wasps, and Bees

The order Hymenoptera includes a diverse array of insects, many of which have direct implications for human health and occupational safety. Medically significant hymenopterans fall primarily into three groups: ants (Formicidae), bees (Apidae and related families), and wasps (Vespidae, Mutillidae, and others). These insects are unified by traits such as membranous wings, chewing or modified mouthparts, and a venomous sting apparatus in females, derived as a modified ovipositor.

Among the ants, we distinguish fire ants (*Solenopsis invicta, Solenopsis richteri,* and hybrids), which are aggressive and venomous, capable of inflicting multiple stings in rapid succession. Their stings often result in pustules and localized inflammation and may trigger allergic reactions in sensitive individuals. Other stinging ants, such as harvester ants (*Pogonomyrmex*) and various native woodland or desert species, also pose a risk, though they are less aggressive and more limited in distribution. Non-stinging ants, while medically harmless, are still relevant due to their sheer abundance and potential to disrupt fieldwork through equipment interference, food contamination, or psychological stress.

Wasps, particularly members of the Vespidae family (e.g., yellowjackets and paper wasps), are among the most common causes of stings in North America. These insects are highly defensive of their nests and can deliver multiple stings, making them a notable risk for field workers conducting vegetation surveys, clearing brush, or working in semi-urban environments. Velvet ants (actually wingless female wasps in the family Mutillidae) also deserve mention; though rarely encountered, they are capable of delivering an extremely painful sting and are nicknamed "cow killers" in the southern United States.

Bees constitute another key group of hymenopteran health concerns. While honey bees (*Apis mellifera*) are typically non-aggressive, accidental contact or defensive behavior can lead to painful stings and, in allergic individuals, systemic reactions or anaphylaxis. Africanized honey bees, present in the southern United States, pose a more serious threat due to their heightened aggression and tendency to swarm in large numbers. Other bees – such as bumble bees, carpenter bees, and sweat bees – are generally docile but may sting when provoked or disturbed at a nest site. Unlike honey bees, which die after stinging, most other bees can sting multiple times.

From an epidemiological standpoint, Hymenoptera stings account for the majority of venom-related medical emergencies in the United States. According to the U.S. Centers for Disease Control and Prevention (CDC) data, an average of 72 deaths per year in the United States are attributed to hornet, wasp, and bee stings combined, with 788 fatalities recorded from 2011 to 2021. An estimated 5%–10% of the population may experience systemic allergic reactions upon being stung, and thousands of emergency department (ED) visits occur each year due to hymenopteran stings. Most cases involve localized pain and swelling, but anaphylaxis remains a critical risk in susceptible individuals, underscoring the need for medical preparedness in field operations.

Given the combination of frequency of contact, potential severity of envenomation, and geographic ubiquity, Hymenoptera represent an important entomological health consideration for ecologists, field technicians, utility workers, and other outdoor professionals. Awareness, prevention, and early response protocols are essential components of any health and safety plan where these insects are present.

ECOLOGICAL ROLES

In the ecological context of entomological health and safety, understanding the distinctions and relationships between *parasites, pathogens, vectors,* and *entomological agents* is critical for evaluating risk, planning field operations, and mitigating harm. These categories overlap in complex ways but serve distinct roles in the transmission and manifestation of disease and other hazards caused by insects and other arthropods.

PARASITES

Parasites are organisms that live on or within a host and derive nutrients at the host's expense, often causing harm in the process. Usually, a parasite sucks its host's blood to provide itself with protein for its own egg maturation. In an entomological context, this category includes both ectoparasites such as lice, fleas, and ticks that attach externally to the body, and endoparasites like bot flies or warble flies, whose larvae develop inside host tissues. Thus, even though we often think of "parasites" as being internal, it should be recognized that some are external. Parasitic relationships can cause a range of outcomes from mild irritation to severe pathology depending on host susceptibility, parasite load, and duration of exposure. Insects and other arthropods may themselves be parasites, or they may transmit parasitic organisms such as filarial nematodes or protozoans.

PATHOGENS

Pathogens are microorganisms, typically bacteria, viruses, fungi, or protozoa, that cause disease. These disease-causing agents often require an arthropod vector to reach a human host. For example, the bacterium *B. burgdorferi* causes Lyme disease but cannot spread without the tick vector *I. scapularis*. Some pathogens, like *R. rickettsii* (Rocky Mountain spotted fever), rely heavily on specific vector relationships for persistence in nature. Importantly, the pathogen itself is the cause of the disease, not the arthropod, though without the arthropod the disease may not reach the human population at all.

VECTORS

Vectors are delivery systems – arthropods capable of acquiring and transmitting parasites or pathogens to a susceptible host. In the entomological health context, a vector may be biological (supporting replication of the pathogen, such as mosquitoes in malaria transmission) or mechanical (simply transporting the agent from one surface or organism to another, such as house flies spreading bacteria from feces to food). These mechanisms of transmission are discussed more thoroughly in the following section. Understanding the role of vectors is crucial not just for medical treatment but also for designing public health interventions, predicting outbreak potential, and deploying appropriate gear or repellents in the field.

ENTOMOLOGICAL AGENTS

Beyond these medically significant roles, the term "entomological agent" is used in this guide to encompass any arthropod that presents a risk or hazard, even if it does not transmit a known pathogen, parasite, or venom. This broader category includes insects and arachnids that might inflict non-venomous bites (such as black flies or biting midges), provoke allergic reactions (e.g., urticating hairs on caterpillars or cockroach allergens), or cause psychological stress (such as delusory parasitosis, entomophobia, or recurring irritation from persistent biting flies).

Entomological agents may also create logistical or operational hazards. Swarms of mayflies or lovebugs, for example, can obscure windshields or clog machinery, creating safety risks during transportation. Ground-nesting wasps near campsites or field stations may disrupt operations even without stinging, due to the need to avoid provoking them. In such cases, the presence of the arthropod itself, regardless of venom, pathogen, or bite, is enough to impact health and safety planning.

Some entomological agents also interfere with equipment function and field gear. Ants nesting in electrical equipment, beetles boring into wood supplies, or tiny insects infiltrating sensitive optical instruments can compromise field research or industrial operations. Entomological agents can thus have an outsized impact in environments where equipment reliability is critical even without any direct biological harm to humans.

Environmental and ecological considerations must also be factored in. Insect outbreaks driven by weather, climate, or land use changes can turn low-risk species into sudden threats. For instance, non-biting midges may become overwhelming in riparian areas during breeding booms, affecting water quality and causing mass nuisance. Even species that do not interact physically with humans may alter field conditions enough to influence safety, morale, and productivity.

In sum, parasites, pathogens, vectors, and entomological agents represent a spectrum of health and safety concerns. While traditional public health focuses primarily on disease-causing organisms and their transmission, the broader framework presented here allows for the inclusion of indirect effects – mechanical, psychological, logistical, or allergic. This approach ensures that the full impact of arthropods on human well-being and operational safety is assessed and documented across a variety of field and industrial settings.

MECHANISMS OF ENTOMOLOGICAL HAZARDS

When people think of dangerous arthropods, their minds often go first to stings and bites. While these are indeed important sources of hazard, the reality is more nuanced (Kar et al. 2022). Entomological hazards encompass a wide range of interactions between humans and arthropods. Some cause pain or allergic reactions, others spread pathogens, and some are little more than startling distractions that still have real safety implications. For ecological and environmental professionals, recognizing these distinctions is the foundation of effective health and safety planning.

Stings, delivered primarily by bees, wasps, ants, and scorpions, inject venom that can cause localized pain, swelling, or severe allergic reactions. Non-pathogenic bites, by contrast, come from arthropods with strong mandibles or piercing mouthparts but they do not transmit disease. These bites are painful and may cause irritation, yet they remain essentially mechanical injuries.

Potentially pathogenic bites from mosquitoes, ticks, and other vectors provide a direct route for microorganisms into the body, making them the most significant health concern in terms of disease. Others act as contact irritants or allergens, like urticating caterpillars, dermestid larvae, or cockroaches, provoking rashes or respiratory issues. Still others are potentially pathogenic contact agents such as house flies and dung beetles that can mechanically transfer bacteria, protozoa, or helminth eggs onto food or surfaces. While the mechanisms differ, the common thread is that each of these hazards stems from close contact between humans and arthropods.

Finally, not all hazards stem from venom, disease, or irritation. Some arthropods are harmless even though they seem to induce panic: dragonflies, large ichneumonid wasps, crane flies, or moths may frighten workers without posing any direct health risk, yet fear can lead to distraction or accidents. Similarly, swarming arthropods can become transportation, equipment, or operational hazards, clogging air intakes, shorting electrical systems, or rendering roadways impassable. In these cases, the insects themselves are not the problem so much as the secondary consequences of their numbers and behavior.

Taken together, these categories, discussed more fully below, show that entomological hazards are diverse and multifaceted. In fact, some entomological hazards may legitimately fall into two or more categories (e.g., tarantulas, mayflies, and Mormon crickets can cause transportation or operational hazards during mass events, but both tarantulas and Mormon crickets can also bite – mildly – while some people are highly allergic to mayflies). Here they are classified by the most likely hazardous conditions, and a few are listed twice when hazards are very divergent.

By classifying entomological health and safety hazards into stings, non-pathogenic bites, pathogenic bites, contact irritants and allergens, pathogenic contact agents, harmless panic inducers, and logistical hazards, ecologists and environmental professionals can more clearly understand the risks they face and adopt strategies tailored to each.

In addition to many scholarly journal articles and medical entomology/parasitology books, listed below, numerous web pages of the CDC were consulted. Many of these sites are regularly updated, so more recent visits to these sites may yield additional data that may reinforce or could feasibly conflict with data presented herein.

CDC sites included the following pages within the CDC website by filling in the listed word(s) in the blank in www.cdc.gov/____________: alpha-gal-syndrome, anaplasmosis, babesiosis, bartonella, bed-bugs, bourbon-virus, cache-valley, chagas, colorado-tick-fever, dengue, Dipylidium, dirofilariasis, eastern-equine-encephalitis, ehrlichiosis, fleas, heartland-virus, jamestown-canyon, la-crosse-encephalitis, leishmaniasis, lice, lyme, malaria, myiasis, niosh/asthma, niosh/outdoor-workers/ about/insects-and-scorpions, niosh/outdoor-workers/about/venomous-spiders, plague, Powassan, rocky-mountain-spotted-fever, scabies, sle, thelaziasis, ticks, tularemia, typhus, vector-borne-diseases, wee, west-nile-virus, zika.

STINGS

Arthropods that sting, particularly bees, wasps, and ants, use a modified ovipositor, or egg-laying structure, connected to venom glands. Scorpions simply have a dedicated structure at the end of the abdomen for stinging. When an arthropod stings, the stinger punctures the skin and injects venom. Venom contains a variety of compounds such as enzymes, peptides, and biogenic amines that cause pain, swelling, and sometimes systemic immune reactions; however, venoms vary in their mode of action and pain intensity and vary by species (Schmidt 2016). Bee venom includes melittin, a peptide that disrupts cell membranes and activates pain receptors; wasp venom often includes acetylcholine and serotonin, which quickly stimulate nerve endings; and both include chemicals like phospholipase A2, kinins, and mastoparans that exacerbate cell damage and induce inflammation, swelling, and redness.

Venom also includes chemicals that trigger histamine release, which in turn may trigger allergies. Due to individual variation in allergic reactions to stings, some individuals may experience some minor swelling, whereas others may go into anaphylactic shock (Kausar 2018). In honeybees, the stinger is barbed and often left behind with the venom gland attached, continuing to pump venom until removed; since it famously tears a significant portion out of the abdomen of the bee, it will almost always die. Wasps, hornets, and many ants can sting repeatedly because their stingers are smooth.

Scorpions and some wasps use their stings offensively to subdue prey items such as caterpillars, crickets, grasshoppers, or other animals smaller than themselves. Stings on humans are strictly defensive behaviors rather than predatory attacks. Social insects such as honeybees, yellowjackets, hornets, and fire ants sting to defend their colony, nest, or food sources. Individual encounters (e.g., a wasp tangled in clothing or a bee accidentally stepped on) can also trigger defensive stings.

Workers can minimize sting risk through both preventive behavior and environmental awareness. Avoid wearing bright floral colors or perfumes that mimic flowers. Stay calm around bees and wasps; sudden movements increase the chance of stings. Watch for signs of nests in soil, trees, or structures; avoid disturbing them. Wear protective clothing (long sleeves, gloves, boots) in known sting-prone areas. Keep food and drink covered when outdoors, since sweet scents often attract stinging insects.

During health and safety training, it should be emphasized that stings are usually preventable and that knowledge reduces fear. Training should:

- **Normalize calm responses**: Teach employees that most stinging insects do not attack unless provoked
- **Promote situational awareness**: Encourage routine scanning of work areas for nests and instruct employees to report the potential hazard rather than trying to handle it recklessly
- **Model best practices**: Supervisors should demonstrate calm behavior around bees or wasps, showing workers that retreat and avoidance are preferable to swatting or panic
- **Plan for medical contingencies**: Remind employees that while most stings are mild, workers with known allergies must carry their prescribed epinephrine auto-injector and know how to use it. Employers should ensure first-aid resources are available and coworkers are trained in assisting with severe reactions

Non-Pathogenic Bites

Not all arthropod bites carry the risk of disease transmission. Many invertebrates are capable of biting simply because of their anatomy (powerful mandibles, piercing mouthparts, or grasping appendages), yet they are not vectors of pathogens and pose no systemic risk beyond localized trauma. Examples include large insects with crushing mandibles (large beetles, mantids, grasshoppers) or true bugs with piercing mouthparts (giant water bugs and other aquatic bugs); bed bugs (*C. lectularius*), which feed on blood but are not established vectors of disease; head lice (*P. humanus capitis*), which cause itching but do not spread pathogens. Included in this group are the crabs and crayfish, which can pinch very painfully with the chelae on their expanded front legs.

In fact, ticks and mosquitoes, which can be vectors of diseases, may also simply bite and not spread a pathogen if they themselves were never exposed to a pathogen. If so, then their bite is non-pathogenic.

Insects and other arthropods may bite as a form of defense when handled, crushed, or startled. Their mandibles or piercing mouthparts can break the skin and cause pain, minor bleeding, or irritation. Some species that are normally predatory on other small animals may inject saliva that affects nervous or muscle tissue and results in greater pain than simply being bitten. Blood-feeding species such as bed bugs or head lice cause irritation because of saliva proteins that trigger immune responses, not because they transmit infections.

One minor area of concern besides the physical trauma of a bite is the risk of tetanus. Tetanus is caused by *Clostridium tetani*, an anaerobic bacterium commonly found in soil, dust, and animal feces. The risk is primarily associated with deep puncture wounds, wounds contaminated with soil or organic matter, and crushing injuries where oxygen-poor environments allow bacterial spores to thrive. Most insect bites, pinches, and superficial arthropod injuries (e.g., a crayfish pinch or beetle bite) are not ideal environments for *C. tetani*, unless they break the skin and occur in dirty environments. Tetanus vaccination is often a normal part of the schedule of childhood vaccines and is frequently required in workplaces, so management of this risk may simply be a matter of making sure employees' tetanus vaccinations are up to date.

It should be recognized that most of the time, bites are defensive. Large insects bite to protect themselves when handled. Insects caught in clothing or handled during sampling may bite reflexively. And some insects like bed bugs and head lice feed on blood but have no known pathogen transmission cycle in North America.

Like avoidance of stings, use preventive behavior and environmental awareness. Brush off large insects gently and wear protective clothing in habitats where these kinds of organisms live. Health and safety managers should normalize these encounters and provide clear, calm guidance, differentiating nuisance from danger (emphasize that while such bites can hurt, they are not medically dangerous), training workers in safe handling (encouraging use of tools rather than bare hands for insect collection or removal), and providing reassurance (for example, "That beetle can pinch, but it cannot make you sick"). Primarily, health and safety around these kinds of arthropods is about prevention of escalation. Workers who are less fearful of bites and stings are less likely to panic and injure themselves or others.

POTENTIALLY PATHOGENIC BITES

Arthropod vectors exploit the blood of vertebrate hosts to obtain proteins for their own egg maturation. However, unlike nuisance bites that cause only temporary irritation, potentially pathogenic bites occur when an arthropod transmits microorganisms during feeding. This can give pathogens a direct route into the bloodstream or skin tissues.

Ticks, mosquitoes, sand flies, fleas, kissing bugs, and some lice can act as vectors: they ingest a pathogen from one host, the pathogen survives or multiplies inside or on the arthropod, and it is then transmitted to another host during a subsequent blood meal. This process allows diseases such as Lyme disease, anaplasmosis, West Nile virus, and plague to persist in natural cycles among animal populations and spill over into human populations. Furthermore, the saliva of these arthropods contains compounds that can suppress clotting, dull pain, and modulate the immune response.

The arthropod is not just a passive syringe; it is part of a dynamic ecological cycle in which pathogens, vectors, and vertebrate hosts interact. Pathogen transmission is therefore the result of a complex biological relationship.

Mechanisms of Pathogen Transmission

Pathogens, whether viral, bacterial, protozoan, or helminthic, rely on various transmission routes to move between hosts and establish infection. Integral to the transmission of any disease, however, is the presence of an existing reservoir.

Some vector-borne diseases, such as malaria, depend entirely on human hosts and their mosquito vectors for transmission. In these cases, the pathogen completes its life cycle between humans and a specific type of mosquito, like *Anopheles* mosquitoes for *Plasmodium* parasites. This means that if malaria is eliminated from the human population in a given area, even the continued presence of vector-competent mosquitoes poses no risk of transmission. There simply is no parasite to spread. As such, public health interventions that reduce human cases to zero, combined with vector control, can break the cycle of transmission entirely.

In contrast, diseases like Lyme disease involve complex zoonotic cycles in which animals serve as reservoirs for the pathogen. The bacterium *B. burgdorferi*, which causes Lyme disease, normally circulates in populations of small mammals and deer. Ticks, such as *I. scapularis*, become infected when they feed on these reservoir hosts, and can then transmit the infection to humans. Crucially, even if no human in a region is currently infected, the presence of infected animal hosts and competent tick vectors means that Lyme disease can reemerge at any time. This makes eradication much more difficult, as control efforts must account not only for the vectors, but also for the persistent reservoir of infection in the environment.

When arthropods serve as vectors in these processes, their role can be categorized broadly as either biological or mechanical transmission. Understanding the distinction between these two modes is crucial for assessing the risks arthropods pose to human health and for implementing effective control strategies.

Biological transmission occurs when a pathogen undergoes development or reproduction within an arthropod vector before being transmitted to a vertebrate host. This interaction is often highly specific, with the pathogen exploiting the biology of the vector to complete part of its life cycle. Examples include *Plasmodium* parasites developing inside *Anopheles* mosquitoes to cause malaria, or *B. burgdorferi* multiplying within *Ixodes* ticks before causing Lyme disease. These relationships are typically obligate for the pathogen; without the vector, transmission cannot occur.

Biological transmission often involves a delay, called the extrinsic incubation period, during which the pathogen matures to an infectious form inside the vector.

In contrast, mechanical transmission does not involve any biological interaction between pathogen and vector. Instead, the arthropod acts as a passive carrier, transporting pathogens on its body surfaces, mouthparts, or feces. These are presented in the section on potentially pathogenic non-biting contact.

In mechanical transmission, the pathogen remains externally located and does not multiply within the vector. Mechanical transmission can occur rapidly, often immediately after the vector contacts contaminated material. A classic example is the house fly (*Musca domestica*) landing on feces or decaying matter, then contaminating food surfaces or utensils with pathogenic bacteria like *Shigella*, *Salmonella*, or *Escherichia coli* carried on its feet, body hairs, or regurgitated fluids.

One of the most significant public health concerns related to mechanical transmission involves gastrointestinal pathogens that are normally transmitted via the fecal-oral route, such as *Shigella* spp., *Salmonella* spp., *E. coli* (especially enterotoxigenic and enterohemorrhagic strains), *Campylobacter jejuni*, and protozoans like *Giardia* and *Cryptosporidium* (Graczyk et al. 2005). Synanthropic arthropods (those that thrive in close association with humans) such as house flies, blow flies, and cockroaches have long been implicated in the spread of these agents. These insects frequently breed in fecal matter, garbage, and decaying organic waste, where they come into contact with high concentrations of pathogens. They then move to kitchens, food preparation areas, and dining surfaces, depositing infectious agents on human food or directly onto hands or utensils.

Although these arthropods do not serve as biological vectors for gastrointestinal pathogens, their role in mechanical transmission can significantly amplify the spread of disease, particularly in environments with poor sanitation, high population density, or inadequate food safety practices. For example, during outbreaks of cholera or dysentery, increased fly populations have been shown to correlate with higher infection rates. Similarly, cockroach infestations in hospitals and urban housing have been linked to the spread of multidrug-resistant bacteria. In such settings, even low-severity pathogens can pose serious risks to vulnerable populations, including children, the elderly, and immunocompromised individuals.

Potentiality

The word "potentially" is used intentionally because not every bite will or even can result in transmission of a pathogen. In order for the cycle to continue, a whole host of circumstances must occur:

The tick or mosquito or other arthropod needs to have previously fed on an infected host (which means that geographically and temporally the host and pathogen must both be present)

and

acquired the pathogen from that host,

and

the pathogen needs to be situated in the arthropod in a way that allows
transmission (by reproduction or maintenance within the host to a
transmissible life stage and moving to the mouthparts or salivary glands),

and

the bite has to occur on a person susceptible to the pathogen,

and

the bite has to be prolonged enough to allow transmission.

If any of those circumstances do not occur, transmission is curtailed.

Hard ticks are significant because they feed slowly (sometimes for days!), giving pathogens time to transfer from tick to host. Soft ticks, in contrast, feed quickly and can transmit pathogens quickly. Likewise, mosquitoes feed quickly but are highly mobile and abundant, making them efficient transmitters of viruses. Fleas and other biting insects may also regurgitate or defecate while feeding, leaving pathogens on the skin that can be rubbed into the wound.

For ecologists and environmental professionals, training workers to manage the risks of potentially pathogenic bites is essential. While some of these pathogens may cause minor, temporary symptoms, it is a fact that some can cause lifelong, debilitating effects or even death, particularly if untreated. If it is likely that potentially pathogenic bites may occur, managers need to address these potential risks, taking into account the relative risk that each disease has.

Refer to the relative risk diagrams for each arthropod and pathogen listed in Part 2 to get an idea of how likely any given pathogen is to occur. Note that the entries for pathogens are shortened and do not include information on how to minimize exposure and what to do if infected; these are covered adequately for the vector arthropod.

To help employees manage these risks, employers can do the following:

- **Educate on Vectors and Disease Risks**: Provide employees with clear, regionally relevant information about which arthropods transmit pathogens in their work areas
- **Train in Personal Protection Practices**: Reinforce the consistent use of insect repellents, protective clothing, and post-work hygiene (e.g., daily tick checks)
- **Normalize Prompt Reporting**: Encourage employees to report bites and stings, especially from ticks or unusual insect exposures, so that potential medical evaluation can occur early, as soon as symptoms are experienced
- **Incorporate Vector Awareness into Site Planning**: For example, limit work at peak mosquito activity times, or establish procedures for checking clothing and gear for ticks
- **Develop Emergency Readiness**: Ensure field teams know how to recognize the early symptoms of vector-borne illness and when to seek medical help

Managers should frame training in a calm, factual, and empowering manner. Emphasize that while pathogenic bites are possible, relative risk is often minimal, and most exposures can be prevented with simple precautions. Encourage employees to treat arthropod awareness as part of professional fieldwork – just as important as proper footwear or hydration. Avoid using fear as a motivator; instead, stress confidence through knowledge and routine practice.

By presenting pathogenic bites as a manageable occupational hazard, health and safety managers help reduce both the real medical risks and the unnecessary anxiety that can arise from working in arthropod-rich environments.

PHYSICAL IRRITANTS AND ALLERGENS

Some arthropods can injure skin not through biting or stinging, but by direct contact with specialized hairs or spines. Millipedes have noxious exudates that they use as a defensive mechanism but can stain or even irritate skin. Carpet beetle larvae are covered in hairs that readily break off and can embed in skin, causing irritation, rashes, and sometimes pustules. These hairs can also become airborne, irritating the respiratory tract if infestations occur indoors.

A perhaps surprising group associated with physical irritants are the caterpillars of some moths. Slug caterpillars and the puss caterpillar are equipped with venomous spines or urticating hairs that deliver painful stings on contact, often resulting in welts or localized dermatitis. Other urticating caterpillars (e.g., buck moth larvae, saddleback caterpillars) have setae can break off into the skin, causing rashes, welts, or more severe dermatologic reactions.

Most of the several million species of insects produce potential allergens that can exacerbate asthma, rhinitis, or skin reactions (Kausar 2018). Depending on the individual, allergic reactions to these potential allergens may range from minimal, with perhaps a runny nose and teary eyes, to severe and life-threatening anaphylaxis. For cockroaches, their shed skins, saliva, and feces contain potent allergens that have been implicated as a major factor in allergies in urban areas. (The author of this book has, in fact, tested positive to cockroach allergens!) These are well-documented contributors to asthma, especially in urban environments. House dust mites are microscopic mites whose fecal pellets are among the most common indoor allergens. Many storage pests (e.g., flour beetles, grain moths) can produce dust and fragments that trigger allergic reactions in workers handling infested materials.

Logistically, these hazards may cause problems secondarily as they contaminate workspaces and even dead insects or their remains are irritants and allergens, reducing productivity by causing persistent itching, rashes, or respiratory discomfort. Furthermore, their presence may lead to misdiagnosis or confusion with more serious conditions (e.g., mistaken for infectious rashes).

Managers and workers can usually anticipate when workspaces that may potentially contain entomological physical irritants or allergens are present. Dry, dusty workspaces may require the use of PPE in the form of gloves, long sleeves, dust masks, or even respirators. Environmental hygiene may include vacuuming with high-efficiency particulate air (HEPA) filters, regular laundering of contaminated fabrics, and removal of infested foodstuffs or specimens. Known infestations by cockroaches, dermestid beetles, or other allergen producers may require implementation of pest management protocols.

Potentially Pathogenic Non-Biting Contact

As mentioned before, some entomological health and safety issues are due to mechanical transfer of pathogens. Instead of injecting pathogens during feeding, these insects pick up microorganisms externally on their body surfaces, legs, or mouthparts (or internally in their digestive tracts) and then transfer them onto food, surfaces, or directly onto people. This mode of transmission is especially important for gastrointestinal diseases, where the pathway is fecal material → arthropod → food or surface → human ingestion.

House flies (*M. domestica*) and similar species are the most notorious examples. They feed and breed in manure, garbage, carrion, and other unsanitary substrates, acquiring bacteria, protozoans, and even intestinal worm eggs. Flies transfer these pathogens mechanically when they walk across food or utensils with contaminated legs, regurgitate digestive fluids during feeding, and defecate on surfaces they land upon. This makes them important contributors to diarrheal disease transmission in both urban and rural environments.

Other flies that can transfer pathogens include blow flies and flesh flies. Normally associated with carrion, they can also transfer pathogens from decaying material to food surfaces. Likewise, even dung beetles, while ecologically beneficial in manure breakdown, have been occasionally found to harbor and transport parasites or bacteria, though the risk is much lower compared to flies. Though these insects are not efficient vectors compared to house flies, and especially in comparison to mosquitoes or ticks, their ubiquity and close association with human environments make them important contributors to contamination risks.

Usually, workers are already repulsed by the presence of flies around their workspaces, so these kinds of hazards are often minimized under most circumstances. However, outbreaks of gastrointestinal illness may stem from unnoticed fly activity around food, waste, or work areas or when there "just doesn't seem to be time" for proper sanitation. This makes preventive sanitation, food safety, and vector exclusion critical in occupational settings.

It therefore becomes incumbent on workers, for their own safety, to promptly dispose of garbage, fecal material, and organic waste to reduce fly breeding sites, while keeping food sealed, and avoiding preparation of meals in fly-infested areas. Organizations can use engineering controls such as air curtains, window screens, and self-closing doors in field stations or kitchens and by employing sticky traps, UV light traps, or bait stations that can reduce fly presence in enclosed areas.

Harmless Panic Inducers

One of the purposes in addressing entomological health and safety is not only to explain how to mitigate *real* hazards but also to address *perceived* threats. When arthropods occur in tremendous mass emergence or migrations, the sheer number of individuals can cause distraction, stress, or panic among employees. While all arthropods could feasibly bite or irritate under unusual conditions, some of these groups are essentially harmless to humans and do not warrant alarm. Instruction in this area helps employees distinguish between genuine hazards and benign encounters, building confidence and reducing unnecessary disruptions in the field.

For some examples, mayflies (order Ephemeroptera) can create large swarms that can be a nuisance near water, but mayflies also lack biting mouthparts (some lack mouthparts altogether!) and pose no health risk, except to people allergic to them. Similarly, caddisflies (order Trichoptera) are attracted to lights and are common and can sometimes swarm near rivers; they resemble small moths but do not bite or sting. Dragonflies and damselflies (order Odonata) are large, fast-flying insects that often zoom close to people. Despite their intimidating appearance, they neither bite nor sting humans. In fact, they are beneficial predators of mosquitoes and gnats.

Some large, slender ichneumonid wasps (e.g., the genus *Megarhyssa*) have dramatic ovipositors exceeding 50 mm (2 in.) in length and look dangerous, but they are exclusively parasitoids of wood-boring insects and pose no threat to humans. Their ovipositors are not stingers. Miller moths (family Noctuidae) have erratic flight patterns and suddenly appear indoors (especially in the fall) which make them unsettling to some people, yet they cannot bite, sting, or transmit disease. Often mistaken for "giant mosquitoes," crane flies (Family Tipulidae) do not bite at all and are completely harmless.

Harvestmen, sometimes called "daddy-long-legs" (order Opiliones), are often confused with spiders because of their long, gangly legs – and there is even a persistent urban myth that they could bite people except their fangs aren't long enough; however, these arachnids actually lack venom glands and are harmless to humans.

As health and safety managers consider entomological risks to their workers, they should coach employees on calm, practical responses when encountering these arthropods. Key points include the following:

- **Reassure, Don't Ridicule**: Acknowledge fear as natural, then provide clear facts ("That insect certainly does look like a wasp, but it doesn't sting people")
- **Promote Situational Awareness**: Teach staff to identify harmless groups at a glance, reducing uncertainty and panic
- **Model Calm Behavior**: Supervisors should demonstrate measured responses, gently brushing away a moth or pointing out dragonflies as beneficial mosquito-eaters
- **Encourage Entomological Tolerance in the Workplace**: While removing nuisance insects is appropriate, unnecessary killing or panic should be discouraged in favor of education

Even non-hazardous arthropods can distract workers, escalate stress, or cause accidents if panic sets in at the wrong moment. By providing employees with accurate knowledge and simple response strategies, organizations empower their teams to work safely and confidently. Clear instruction reduces overreaction, builds professionalism, and ensures that attention remains focused on genuine occupational hazards rather than imagined ones.

A special case in which panic can occur is in delusory parasitosis, also known as Ekbom syndrome, which is a psychological condition in which individuals have a fixed false belief that their immediate environment, and sometimes their body, is infested with parasites or crawling with small arthropods. Despite the absence of physical evidence, the conviction persists, often accompanied by intense itching at crawling or biting sensations known as formication. Those affected may have self-inflicted skin lesions from scratching or picking. Although extreme conditions are rare, very mild forms are seen when someone talks about "bugs" and the audience unconsciously feels "itchy."

Delusory parasitosis most often affects middle-aged or older adults, with a higher prevalence reported among those with a background of social isolation or chronic medical illness. However, it can occasionally arise among professionals working in pest control, public health, or environmental services in which they have had prolonged exposure to infested environments or repetitive handling of pest-related materials. This heightened awareness, when combined with fatigue, stress, or anxiety, can sometimes lead to misinterpretation of normal skin sensations (dryness, static, mild dermatitis) as signs of infestation.

If a worker should show symptoms suggestive of delusory parasitosis, managers should respond with professional empathy and discretion. Dismissive or confrontational approaches often deepen mistrust. Instead, managers can acknowledge the individual's symptoms (e.g., "I understand you're experiencing these sensations") while emphasizing evidence-based investigation. After ruling out real infestations through inspection and laboratory confirmation, individuals should be encouraged (not forced) to seek medical evaluation, ideally beginning with a general physician or dermatologist. These professionals can screen for secondary causes and, when appropriate, refer the person for psychiatric assessment. Maintaining confidentiality, avoiding ridicule, and providing factual reassurance can prevent escalation while upholding workplace dignity and safety.

TRANSPORTATION, EQUIPMENT, AND OPERATIONAL HAZARDS

Large swarms or mass movements of arthropods can create conditions hazardous to transportation. Mayflies, caddisflies, Mormon crickets, and tarantulas are all documented as causing slick, impassable, or obstructed roadways in North America. When crushed in large numbers, these animals produce a slippery film that reduces tire traction and increases the risk of motor vehicle accidents. In addition, dense swarms of mayflies, caddisflies, and love bugs can block headlights, obscure windshields, and overwhelm vehicle wipers, severely impairing driver visibility.

Ants and other swarming insects may also invade vehicles stopped for prolonged periods, damaging wiring or interfering with electrical systems. Airborne insects drawn to lights at night (e.g., moths, mayflies, aquatic insect hatches) can cluster so densely around lamps or headlights that they block illumination or attract predators (such as bats) that further distract drivers.

Beyond roads and vehicles, arthropod swarms can interfere with permanent installations and field gear. Mayflies, midges, and other aquatic insect emergences are notorious for clogging ventilation systems, air intakes, and radiators on vehicles and machinery. Clogged filters or intakes can cause overheating, reduced airflow, or engine failure. Electrical systems may also be compromised as insects drawn to lights can accumulate around fixtures, leading to short circuits or fires if moisture or organic material builds up. Wasps may build nests and reclusive spiders may build webs in permanent buildings that are not frequently used, leading to potential hazards from stings and bites, as well.

In field equipment, insects may infiltrate sensitive instruments such as weather stations, pumps, water samplers, or electrical boxes. Insects can infiltrate communication gear, reducing function of cameras and transponders. Ants are especially problematic, as they nest inside warm, enclosed spaces and chew through insulation or wiring. This can result in equipment downtime, data loss, or costly repairs.

Arthropod swarming events may also affect worker logistics more broadly. Swarms around floodlights or headlamps can obscure work areas and distract crews. Increased need to clean and maintain ventilation or lighting systems drains time and resources. Mass insect emergences near camps can contaminate food preparation areas, requiring enhanced hygiene measures.

Mitigation of these risks through planning and education can involve anticipating and monitoring seasonal and regional swarm events (e.g., mayfly hatches, Mormon cricket migrations) and scheduling field work accordingly, training employees to recognize conditions where swarms are likely and to adjust travel speed, lighting, or routes to maintain safety. Vehicles should be well-maintained with good tire tread and lighting, as well as regular cleaning of windshields, lights, and air-intake manifolds during high-risk periods. Power facilities can be designed strategically to reduce attraction to swarming insects (for example, using yellow-spectrum lights where possible) or to provide redundancies in case of temporary outages.

Exposure × severity graphs are not produced for organisms of Transportation, Equipment, and Operations hazards, since they are entirely incidental. When swarming or causing problems, there will likely be thousands of individuals; otherwise, they will be rare and of minimal consequence.

By recognizing that swarming arthropods are more than a health nuisance – they can involve real transportation and equipment hazards – everyone involved in health and safety (which is everyone!) can prevent accidents, protect valuable gear, and maintain safe, efficient field operations.

ENTOMOLOGICAL GROUPS AND HAZARDS

See Tables 2.1–2.4.

TABLE 2.1
The Orders of Arachnids, with the Mechanisms of Health and Safety Importance

Order	Common Names	Stings	Non-Pathogenic Bites[a]	Potentially Pathogenic Bites	Physical Irritants/ Allergens	Potentially Pathogenic Contact	Transportation/ Operations Risk
Acari: Ixodidae	Ticks		✓*	✓*	✓*		
Acari: Mesostigmata, Prostigmata, Astigmata	Mites		✓*	✓*			
Araneae	Spiders		✓*		✓*		✓*
Scorpiones	Scorpions	✓*					
Solifugae	Sun/camel spiders		✓*				
Thelyphonida	Vinegaroons/whip scorpions				✓*		
Pseudoscorpiones	False scorpions						
Opiliones	Harvestmen/daddy longlegs						
Palpigradi, Ricinulei, Schizomida	Micro whip scorpions, hooded tick-spiders, short-tailed whip scorpions						

A check mark indicates that at least some of the organisms in the order may be of health and safety importance; an asterisk means that the group is addressed in at least one entry in Part 2. Lack of a checkmark indicates that the mechanism is absent (e.g., stings) or extremely unlikely (albeit still possible, like non-pathogenic bites).

[a] Includes pinches.

TABLE 2.2

The Orders of Crustaceans, with the Mechanisms of Health and Safety Importance

Order	Common Names	Stings	Non-Pathogenic Bites[a]	Potentially Pathogenic Bites	Physical Irritants/ Allergens	Potentially Pathogenic Contact	Transportation/ Operations Risk
Decapoda	Crayfish, freshwater crabs, shrimp, lobsters		✓*				
Isopoda	Pill bugs, sowbugs				✓		
Amphipoda	Scuds, beach fleas		✓*		✓		✓
Cirripedia	Barnacles (sessile)						✓

A check mark indicates that at least some of the organisms in the order may be of health and safety importance; an asterisk means that the group is addressed in at least one entry in Part 2. Lack of a checkmark indicates that the mechanism is absent (e.g., stings) or extremely unlikely (albeit still possible, like non-pathogenic bites). Remipedia, Cephalocarida, Mystacocarida, Branchiura, Ostracoda, Copepoda, and others are excluded because they occur in deep waters or are of very little potential health and safety risk in North America.

[a] Includes pinches.

TABLE 2.3

The Classes of the Myriapods, with the Mechanisms of Health and Safety Importance

Class	Common Names	Stings	Non-Pathogenic Bites[a]	Potentially Pathogenic Bites	Physical Irritants/ Allergens	Potentially Pathogenic Contact	Transportation/ Operations Risk
Chilopoda	Centipedes		✓*				
Diplopoda	Millipedes				✓*		

A check mark indicates that at least some of the organisms in the order may be of health and safety importance; an asterisk means that the group is addressed in at least one entry in Part 2. Lack of a checkmark indicates that the mechanism is absent (e.g., stings) or extremely unlikely (albeit still possible, like non-pathogenic bites).

[a] Includes pinches.

TABLE 2.4

The Orders of Insects, with the Mechanisms of Health and Safety Importance

Order	Common Names	Stings	Non-Pathogenic Bites[a]	Potentially Pathogenic Bites	Physical Irritants and Allergens	Potentially Pathogenic Contact	Transportation/ Logistics/ Operations
Collembola	Springtails						✓*
Diplura	No common name						
Protura	No common name						
Archaeognatha	Jumping bristletails						
Zygentoma	Silverfish, firebrats						
Ephemeroptera	Mayflies				✓		✓*
Odonata	Dragonflies, damselflies		✓				
Plecoptera	Stoneflies						
Blattodea	Cockroaches				✓*		✓
Mantodea	Mantises		✓*				
Orthoptera	Grasshoppers, crickets, katydids		✓*				✓*
Phasmatodea	Stick and leaf insects				✓*		
Psocodea	Lice, including ectoparasitic lice		✓*	✓*			
Zoraptera	Angel insects						
Dermaptera	Earwigs						
Isoptera	Termites						✓*
Hemiptera	True bugs (bed bugs, assassin bugs)		✓*	✓*			

(Continued)

TABLE 2.4 (*Continued*)

The Orders of Insects, with the Mechanisms of Health and Safety Importance

Order	Common Names	Stings	Non-Pathogenic Bites[a]	Potentially Pathogenic Bites	Physical Irritants and Allergens	Potentially Pathogenic Contact	Transportation/ Logistics/ Operations
Thysanoptera	Thrips						
Neuroptera	Lacewings, antlions						
Megaloptera	Alderflies, dobsonflies						
Raphidioptera	Snakeflies						
Coleoptera	Beetles		✓*		✓*	✓*	
Trichoptera	Caddisflies				✓*		✓
Lepidoptera	Butterflies, moths				✓*		✓
Diptera	Flies, mosquitoes, midges		✓*	✓*	✓	✓*	✓*
Siphonaptera	Fleas			✓*			
Hymenoptera	Bees, wasps, ants	✓*					✓*

A check mark indicates that at least some of the organisms in the order may be of health and safety importance; an asterisk means that the group is addressed in at least one entry in Part 2. Lack of a checkmark indicates that the mechanism is absent (e.g., stings) or extremely unlikely (albeit still possible, like non-pathogenic bites). Mantophasmatodea are excluded because they do not occur in North America.

[a] Includes pinches.

COLLECTION OF THE PURPORTED OFFENDING ENTOMOLOGICAL SPECIMEN

Proper identification of arthropods involved in suspected bites, stings, infestations, or disease transmission is critical for accurate diagnosis, appropriate treatment, and informed public health responses. In many cases, the presence or absence of a specific arthropod species can strongly influence the medical implications of a case. Misidentifying the culprit, or assuming an arthropod is responsible when it is not, can lead to ineffective treatment, unnecessary anxiety, or overlooked alternative causes.

In cases of venomous bites or stings, accurate identification can be pivotal. For example, differentiating between a brown recluse (*L. reclusa*) and a harmless cellar spider (*Pholcus phalangioides*) while working in a close-quarters crawlspace is essential. Brown recluse venom can cause necrotic skin lesions and requires monitoring for systemic symptoms, while the cellar spider is completely harmless. Misdiagnosis based on fear or misidentification may lead to unnecessary debridement, antibiotics, or even surgery. Similarly, identifying a stinging insect as a southern yellowjacket (*Vespula squamosa*) versus a honey bee (*A. mellifera*) matters, since treatment protocols for retained stingers and allergy management may differ.

In contrast, there are situations where identifying the arthropod is of limited value. For example, if a person develops a nonspecific rash and finds a tiny mite or gnat indoors, a physician may not benefit much from seeing the specimen unless it's a medically relevant species (like *S. scabiei* or Trombiculidae larvae). Many small insects found in homes, like booklice or fungus gnats, are incidental and unrelated to the symptoms. Likewise, scab or bite-like lesions blamed on insects may instead result from dermatitis, infections, or self-inflected injuries due to delusory parasitosis. In these cases, ruling out arthropods can be just as important as confirming their presence.

When an arthropod is suspected of playing a role in symptoms or disease, collecting a specimen can be very helpful – but only if done safely and appropriately. The best specimens are collected without risk to the person, such as capturing the arthropod in a jar or vial after it is found crawling or flying. Specimens should not be crushed or dried out, as intact bodies (especially mouthparts or wings) are important for identification. Sticky traps and alcohol-preserved vials can also aid collection.

However, it is not always wise to attempt collection. Trying to capture aggressive wasps, venomous spiders, or ticks embedded in sensitive skin areas can lead to further injury or exposure. In such cases, seeking medical attention is the priority, and describing the arthropod's appearance, behavior, and location may suffice. If biting or stinging occurred, photographing the arthropod (e.g., with a smartphone) may be valuable even if it cannot be collected. If a patient is able to remove and preserve a tick properly, as described in Box 2.2 on "How to Remove a Tick Properly," and then placing it in alcohol, identification can assist in evaluating risk for diseases like Lyme disease or ehrlichiosis. But hunting for elusive arthropods, especially at night or in tight spaces, can escalate stress without yielding useful specimens.

In conclusion, proper arthropod identification plays a vital role in guiding medical decisions, ruling in or out possible diagnoses, and reducing unnecessary treatments or concerns. Health professionals, pest control experts, and entomologists can collaborate to evaluate specimens when needed, but the decision to collect should always be balanced against safety and practicality. Knowing when identification is critical and when it is irrelevant helps individuals respond rationally and effectively to arthropod encounters.

REFERENCES

Graczyk TK, Knight R, Tamang L. 2005. Mechanical transmission of human protozoan parasites by insects. *Clin. Microbiol. Rev.* 18: 128–132.

Jeong H, Shin JE, Kim C-H. 2021. Earwig crawling in the ear: Myth or truth. *Cureus* 13: e14827.

Kar S, Yadav N, Bonde P, Verma V. 2022. Cutaneous diseases caused by arthropods and other noxious animals. Pp. 251–265 in: Smoller B, Bagherani N (eds.) *Atlas of Dermatology, Dermatopathology and Venereology*. Springer, New York City, NY.

Kausar MA. 2018. A review on respiratory allergy caused by insects. *Bioinformation* 14: 540–553.

Schmidt JO. 2016. *The Sting of the Wild*. Johns Hopkins University Press, Baltimore, MD.

3 Exposure and Risk

INTERPRETING ARTHROPOD-ASSOCIATED RISK

Understanding the risks posed by arthropods in fieldwork and occupational settings is essential for professionals working in environmental, agricultural, and outdoor contexts. This guidebook provides a consistent framework for evaluating those risks by combining scientific information with practical experience. Central to this framework are the exposure and severity scales provided for each arthropod group. These scales are not meant to alarm but to inform, offering a structured way to think about the likelihood of encountering a particular organism and the consequences that could follow.

The Exposure Scale reflects how often a person is likely to come into contact with a specific arthropod in the field. This includes considerations such as seasonal activity, behavior, and typical habitats. For example, a biting fly found only in remote swamps and active only for a few weeks each year would score low on exposure, while mosquitoes or ticks that thrive in suburban or rural areas and are active for most of the warm season would rate much higher. Sources for this information come from biological information on each arthropod group, along with incidence rates reflected in materials from the U.S. Centers for Disease Control and Prevention (CDC). Readers should consider how their own activities, such as vegetation type, region, time of day, and duration of exposure, might increase or decrease their actual likelihood of contact. Geographic distribution is not taken into consideration for the Exposure Scale; if the proposed work activity occurs outside of an organism's geographic distribution, the risk would be considered negligible.

The Severity Scale, in contrast, addresses the potential medical or occupational impact of an encounter. Not all arthropods that bite or sting pose a serious threat; many cause only minor irritation. However, others can inflict painful injuries, trigger allergic reactions, or serve as vectors for pathogens. As with the Exposure Scale, sources for this information come both from biological information on each group and the CDC. A higher severity rating suggests the possibility of serious consequences, though actual outcomes depend on many factors including individual health status, access to medical care, and the specific circumstances of exposure. Readers should understand that severity does not imply inevitability; it just indicates potential severity under certain conditions.

When assessing their own risk, readers are encouraged to consider both exposure and severity together, rather than in isolation (National Research Council 1989). For example, an arthropod with low exposure but high severity (such as a brown recluse spider or certain parasitic flies) may be worth taking precautions against in rare situations. Conversely, a widespread nuisance species with low severity (like black flies or biting midges) may pose more annoyance than real danger. Risk arises where high exposure and high severity intersect; but even in these cases, informed precautions can substantially reduce the likelihood of harm.

DOI: 10.1201/9781003745709-4

Beyond the numerical scales, each entry in this guide includes narrative details that help contextualize the risk. These include information about the arthropod's geographic distribution, behavior, preferred habitat, seasonality, modes of contact with humans, known health effects, and any medically or ecologically significant pathogens they may transmit. Readers should not rely solely on the numbers; instead, they should read the entire entry to understand the biological and ecological context in which these organisms interact with people. Again, if the organism does not even occur in the vicinity of the proposed work, the risk is already negligible.

While this guide provides detailed information on arthropods of medical and occupational concern, readers should view this guide not as a list of dangers but as a tool to promote informed, balanced, and practical risk management and preparedness. In most field settings, serious outcomes are uncommon and typically occur only under specific or exceptional circumstances.

As was stated earlier, the vast majority of tick, mosquito, and other arthropod bites encountered by environmental professionals result in minor irritation or no symptoms at all. Serious medical consequences are relatively rare and depend highly on factors such as geographic region, seasonality, length of exposure, and host susceptibility. A single tick or mosquito bite does not equate to a high likelihood of infection or life-threatening illness.

That said, during known disease outbreaks, especially when distribution of the vector is widespread and geographic distribution seems to be increasing, greater vigilance and adherence to preventive protocols are warranted. This guide aims to support such informed decision-making by providing credible, field-relevant information rooted in biological understanding and public health principles. By equipping workers and safety officers with accurate knowledge and reasonable expectations, this guide seeks to foster a culture of risk awareness without alarmism, one in which entomological hazards are recognized, respected, and managed effectively within the broader context of field health and safety.

For most environmental professionals, the goal is not to eliminate all contact with arthropods; not only is this an impossible task, but often the focus of each project may specifically be to collect and study these organisms. (And, in some cases, the ecologists and other professionals going out in the field actually love these arthropods!) Instead, the goal for health and safety officers and project managers is to anticipate and mitigate risk through awareness, planning, and basic precautions.

Knowing what to expect and how to respond is often the most powerful safeguard. The combination of concise risk ratings and detailed biological profiles is intended to empower readers to make informed decisions suited to their unique work environments and health priorities.

EXPLANATION OF THE EXPOSURE AND SEVERITY SCALES

To systematically assess, compare, and communicate risks posed by various arthropods of medical or occupational significance, two standardized scales, an Exposure Scale and a Severity Scale, were developed for use in Part 2. These scales are intended to provide a structured framework to evaluate the likelihood of human contact with the arthropod and the potential consequences of that interaction.

Exposure and severity are also provided for each disease, to provide health and safety managers a realistic view of the risks associated with each disease and not just the entomological agent. The methodology for developing each scale is summarized below.

EXPOSURE SCALE

The Exposure Scale reflects the frequency and likelihood that ecologists, environmental professionals, and even the general public may come into contact with a given arthropod under normal field or occupational conditions within their normal range in North America. If the organism or pathogen can be encountered across most of North America, no map is provided, but if it is geographically limited in its extent, then a map is provided to give distributional context. Dark color indicates regular presence, while light color indicates regular absence, and a middle shade indicates that the agent is regularly present only in border areas or very rarely. An example is the widow spiders (p. 95), which are common in the western United States, less so in the southwest and southeast, and even less so in the northeast into Quebec and Ontario. Although reported once or twice in the past, these spiders are very uncommon in the northern Great Plains and all of Canada except Quebec and Ontario.

The Exposure Scale was informed by the following:

- **Ecological Abundance and Geographic Range**: Species with widespread distributions and high population densities were considered more likely to be encountered
- **Behavior and Habitat Overlap with Humans**: Diurnal, synanthropic, or anthropophilic species were rated as having higher exposure potential
- **Occupational Relevance**: Arthropods common in agriculture, forestry, construction, or field research settings received elevated exposure ratings
- **Historical Case Data and Nuisance Reports**: Existing literature and health department records were reviewed to assess reported contact frequency

The resulting scale is ordinal, ranging from 1 to 5, as described below. For all entries, a range of exposures is included because of extremely disparate biogeographic conditions (i.e., extremely common in certain situations, extremely rare otherwise).

This scale reflects how frequently or easily a human (especially an ecologist, environmental professional, or member of the general public) is likely to come into contact with the arthropod under typical North American conditions.

1. **Rare Encounter**: The arthropod is infrequently encountered by humans. It has a limited distribution, highly specialized habitat, or cryptic habits. Only those working in very specific ecological niches are likely to encounter it
2. **Uncommon Exposure**: The arthropod is present in the environment but is not usually encountered during normal outdoor or occupational activity. Some risk exists for those working in certain seasons, habitats, or specific geographic regions

3. **Moderate Exposure**: The arthropod is occasionally encountered in the course of outdoor work or recreational activities. It may be locally abundant in some areas or habitats, especially under certain conditions (e.g., seasonally active or weather-dependent)
4. **Frequent Exposure**: The arthropod is commonly encountered during fieldwork or in everyday outdoor settings. It is widely distributed, often active during human activity periods, and may be drawn to human habitations or workplaces
5. **Ubiquitous and Persistent Exposure**: The arthropod is very frequently encountered, difficult to avoid, and may be synanthropic or anthropophilic. It is almost guaranteed to be encountered during fieldwork in many regions, posing a constant nuisance or hazard

SEVERITY SCALE

The Severity Scale ranks the medical or logistical impact of an arthropod encounter. This includes direct harm (e.g., bites, envenomation, allergic reactions), indirect effects (e.g., as vectors of pathogens or parasites), psychological effects (e.g., revulsion or delusion), and logistic effects (e.g., creating hazardous conditions for equipment). The scale was informed from the following:

- **Clinical and Toxicological Data**: Case studies, poison control data, and CDC resources were consulted to determine the seriousness of injuries or illnesses caused
- **Pathogen Transmission Potential**: Species capable of spreading significant diseases received higher severity scores
- **Duration and Reversibility of Effects**: Chronic conditions, lasting disability, or fatalities elevated severity ratings
- **Intervention Requirements**: Need for hospitalization, antivenom, or public health response influenced scale placement

Severity was also scored on a 1–5 scale, with 1 indicating mild or negligible impact and 5 indicating high medical or occupational hazard, such as neurotoxic envenomation or vector-borne epidemics. Again, entries reflect a range of severity levels, particularly when the typical case results in mild to no effects, while a not-insignificant number of cases (e.g., neuroinvasive disease, anaphylactic reactions) may result in life-threatening conditions. This scale reflects the potential harm posed by the arthropod, including direct effects (e.g., envenomation, allergic reactions) and indirect effects (e.g., disease transmission, psychological stress, logistic burden).

1. **Minimal or No Harm**: Contact may cause no noticeable effect or only mild, self-limiting irritation (e.g., brief annoyance, minor itch). No medical treatment is typically required. Equipment is not affected
2. **Mild Harm**: Interaction may result in localized discomfort, swelling, or minor allergic reaction. Effects are short-lived and generally not medically serious. Over-the-counter remedies are usually sufficient. Workers

experience mild psychological awareness of the arthropods around them and react defensively. Equipment may require minor attention from large infestations

3. **Moderate Harm**: The arthropod may cause significant local symptoms (e.g., painful bite, rash) or act as a secondary vector of pathogens. Medical attention may be required, especially in sensitive individuals, but recovery is expected without long-term effects. Workers may develop significant psychological issues related to arthropod presence, while equipment suffers reduced operating capacity

4. **Severe Harm**: Exposure can lead to serious medical conditions requiring clinical treatment. Examples include neurotoxic or cytotoxic venom, systemic allergic reactions, or transmission of significant pathogens (e.g., Lyme disease, ehrlichiosis). Equipment may fail due to overwhelming arthropod presence

5. **Life-Threatening or Debilitating Harm**: Contact may result in fatality, permanent disability, or major public health concern. These include vectors of major human diseases (e.g., malaria, plague) or causes of severe envenomation syndromes requiring emergency intervention. Equipment is guaranteed to shut down

Together, these scales and their narratives serve to inform risk management strategies, field safety training, and prioritization in occupational health guidelines. Figure 3.1 provides a color-coded graphical representation of these scales as a risk matrix in which green areas in the bottom left are relatively low-risk and red areas in the top right are relatively high risk under normal circumstances.

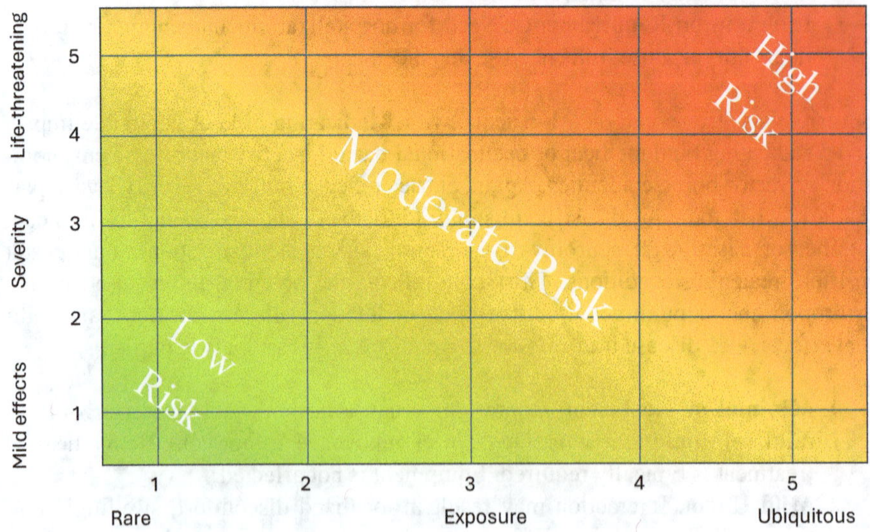

FIGURE 3.1 Graphical representation of exposure and severity scales (Exposure × Severity matrix) for assessing relative risks of entomological threats.

Similar matrices are provided for groups of organisms and/or diseases throughout Part 2 of the guide. Although there is narrative discussion on exposure and severity, utilizing the terminology and associated numeric values defined above, a dark oval is placed on each matrix as a visual reference. It should be remembered that the size of the oval is only indicative of the range of risk; for example, Zika virus has a large oval because its exposure ranges from 1 (rare) to 2 (uncommon) and its range of potential severity extends from 1 (asymptomatic) to 4 (severe), depending on each person's individual situation. A large oval should not be interpreted as a greater risk. Likewise, a small oval simply indicates a more precise level of exposure or severity. Instead, interpretation of each oval should be based on where it falls on the matrix, with placement nearer the upper right corner indicating much higher risk; larger ovals should be interpreted more as a function of greater variability or higher uncertainty. Many ovals also have a shading gradient, with darker shading representing more likely risk regimes of exposure and severity.

Furthermore, exposure × severity matrices are not produced for organisms of Transportation, Equipment, and Operations hazards, since they are entirely incidental. When swarming or causing problems, there will likely be thousands of individuals; otherwise, they will be rare and of minimal consequence.

Many ecologists and environmental professionals may already be aware of the entomological risks that may be encountered in the field. They may know of the biogeographical distributions of various entomological taxa, which ones bite, sting, spread disease or otherwise can cause harm, and which ones will be seasonally active. These professionals can be a great asset for health and safety officers or project managers when assembling health and safety plans (HASPs) and training field crews.

Even though field crews may be briefed on anticipated entomological risks before field deployment – and many ecologists and environmental professionals may know and understand the risks better than health and safety officers or project managers – workers should still be reminded often about the potential risks. It is also helpful if workers note the presence of new or additional entomological hazards in field books or field notes or the on-site copy of the HASP. Notes should be explicit to best inform future risk analysis of repeated field activities. Some example notes:

- "Ticks particularly prevalent in grasses along the access route"
- "Chiggers abundant in the tall rushes"
- "Many sources of standing water so mosquitoes very dense and aggressive at dusk"
- "Don't go near the outcrop; lots of abandoned swallow nests with bugs"

ECOLOGICAL AND ENVIRONMENTAL OCCUPATIONAL ACTIVITIES THAT INCREASE EXPOSURE

Occupational exposure to arthropods is closely tied to the type, timing, and location of field activity. Certain tasks inherently increase the likelihood of encountering medically significant, venomous, or nuisance arthropods, especially when those tasks take place in rural, undeveloped, or ecologically diverse areas. Understanding which work activities elevate entomological risk is critical for anticipating hazards, selecting protective gear, and incorporating reasonable safety measures into job planning.

Vegetation surveys, wildlife tracking, and wetland delineation are among the highest-risk activities in this context. These tasks often require prolonged contact with dense underbrush, tall grasses, forest edges, open standing water, or saturated ground, all of which are prime habitats for ticks, mosquitoes, chiggers, biting flies, and wasps. Technicians conducting transect walks, installing camera traps, or flagging vegetation may brush directly against insect harborages or disturb nesting sites, resulting in bites, stings, or allergic responses. In some regions, these activities may also coincide with heavy emergence periods for black flies, deer flies, or other aggressive biters.

Soil sampling, drilling, and geotechnical assessments pose risks not only from biting arthropods but also from ground-disturbing activities that expose or provoke them. Ground-dwelling ants, spiders, scorpions, or wasps may react defensively when soil is probed or disturbed. Workers kneeling or placing hands near holes, cracks, or debris are at increased risk of contact with arthropods using those microhabitats. Insect-infested soil or decomposing organic matter may also harbor pathogens or allergens, posing additional, often invisible threats.

Stream and aquatic sampling activities carry high risk for mosquito and biting midge exposure, especially in warm months and stagnant water conditions or stream margins. Wet wading into vegetated wetlands, swamps, or riparian zones exposes skin directly to aquatic and semi-aquatic insect communities. Sampling teams may also encounter horse flies, fire ants on floating debris, or stinging insects nesting in overhanging branches or grassy banks. Even brief exposure near water bodies can result in concentrated bites and, in some regions, introduce the potential for vector-borne disease transmission. Some aquatic invertebrates, such as giant water bugs and crayfish, may deliver painful bites or pinches in aquatic environments.

Forestry, logging, and tree-climbing work bring workers into contact with arboreal habitats where bees, wasps, and spiders are more likely to be nesting. Vibrations from chainsaws, hammering, or climbing activity can agitate hidden colonies. Additionally, forest canopy workers face a greater likelihood of brushing against caterpillars with urticating hairs or accidentally contacting wasp nests not visible from below. Tree hollows, under-bark crevices, and accumulated leaf litter also harbor insects capable of delivering defensive bites or stings.

Overnight fieldwork, early morning deployments, or work during dusk and dawn significantly increase the likelihood of arthropod encounters. These time periods correspond with peak activity for many mosquitoes, no-see-ums, and crepuscular insects. Workers setting up tents, launching boats, or preparing gear at these times are often caught off-guard without personal protective equipment (PPE) in place. Insect exposure in sleeping quarters, especially those without sealed enclosures, can lead to cumulative bites, allergic responses, or psychological discomfort over time.

Occupational settings that require artificial lighting at night can inadvertently increase worker exposure to insects. Common work environments include road construction zones, bridge or dam projects, permanent building security installations, remote generator or gage boxes, stream or lake monitoring stations, forested basecamps, and youth or recreational campsites. In these locations, the use of bright lights such as halide floodlights, mercury vapor lamps, vehicle headlights, or portable light-emitting diodes (LEDs) may attract a variety of nocturnal insects, including mayflies, caddisflies, beetles, moths, and mosquitoes. Swarms may impair visibility, create slippery surfaces, clog equipment like radiators or intake vents, and increase the likelihood of insect bites, allergic reactions, or other entomological hazards. Special consideration should also be given to ecological research sites using blacklight (UV) traps, which are intentionally designed to attract insects and may become a nuisance or vector concern if placed near active work or sleeping areas. These light-related activities, though often essential for operations, represent a consistent and often overlooked pathway for increased insect exposure in both developed and remote work settings (Table 3.1).

Structural inspections, cave entry, and confined space evaluations add another dimension to entomological risk. Dark, enclosed, undisturbed spaces provide excellent refugia for spiders, stinging insects, or stored-product pests. Workers performing these inspections may focus on structural or technical aspects and neglect to assess

TABLE 3.1
Insect Attraction Potential for Different Kinds of Lights Commonly Used in Ecology and Environmental Occupation Settings

Type of Light	Insect Attraction	Insects Attracted	Notes
Incandescent	High	Moths, beetles, midges, flies	Strong UV/blue light emissions; very warm light; often attracts the widest range of insects.
Halogen	High	Similar to incandescent	Hot and bright; often used in floodlights, very attractive to many nocturnal insects.
Mercury vapor	Very high	Moths, beetles, aquatic insects	Strong UV component; commonly used in outdoor security lights and stadium lighting. Sometimes used deliberately in traps by entomologists.
Metal halide	High	Various night-flying insects	Bright white light with a high UV component; often used in large construction zones.
Fluorescent (standard)	Moderate	Flies, beetles, some moths	Emits some UV; less attractive than mercury vapor or incandescent.
Blacklight (UV-A)	Extremely high	Moths, lacewings, flies, beetles	Used deliberately in traps by entomologists; not appropriate in areas where insects are a nuisance.
LED (cool white/ blue tint)	Moderate to high	Flies, beetles, some moths	Emits some UV/blue; attraction depends on wavelength and brightness.
LED (warm white)	Low	Few insects	Lower UV/blue emissions; preferred for low insect attraction.
Headlamps/ flashlights (vary in type of light)	Varies	Small flying insects, especially near faces	Especially disruptive when worn on the head or carried close to the body.
Vehicle headlights (vary in type of light)	Moderate to high	Mayflies, caddisflies, midges, beetles	Can cause massive insect swarms, especially near aquatic habitats.

insect activity beforehand. Additionally, PPE intended for mechanical hazards may not always protect against arthropod exposure.

Heavy-equipment operators, linemen, and construction personnel working in natural or overgrown areas face secondary risks when insects interfere with equipment or distract personnel. Wasps nesting in machinery, ants shorting electrical boxes, or swarms of flies reducing visibility on windshields all pose indirect but serious safety threats. Even in jobs not directly involving biological surveys, entomological hazards can arise unexpectedly and should be included in job hazard analyses (JHAs).

Overall, any outdoor occupation that places workers in prolonged or repeated contact with natural or semi-natural environments can lead to increased arthropod exposure. Awareness of seasonal patterns, geographic hotspots, and behavior-specific risks is essential for mitigating these threats and ensuring the health and safety of all field personnel.

ORGANIZATIONAL AND INDIVIDUAL STRATEGIES FOR REDUCING EXPOSURE

INDIVIDUAL AND ORGANIZATIONAL RESPONSIBILITY

Reducing exposure to arthropod hazards requires both personal diligence and corporate planning. At the organizational level, employers can provide policies, supplies, and infrastructure: allocating funds for PPE purchases, stocking approved repellents, maintaining screened facilities when feasible, and offering training on tick checks or bite management. On the individual level, workers must be trained to recognize risks, wear protective gear correctly, and apply repellents responsibly (Werner et al. 2019).

A layered approach, combining engineering controls, repellents, PPE, and targeted pest management, provides the most reliable protection. By embedding these practices into standard operating procedures (SOPs) as described in detail in a later section, ecological and environmental professionals can reduce preventable illness and injury from arthropods in the workplace.

Engineering and Environmental Controls

Engineering and environmental controls form the first line of defense against arthropods of health and safety concern. Whenever possible, modifying the work environment reduces insect contact without relying on chemicals or constant vigilance. In buildings or field stations, air curtains installed at doorways disrupt fly entry. Fine-mesh window and door screens are a standard barrier against mosquitoes and midges. In vehicles, workers should use recirculating air mode to avoid pulling insects inside, especially when driving at dusk in mosquito-dense areas. Maintenance of fleet vehicles, including properly operating lights and tires with appropriate tread, can help when swarming organisms build up around roadways. Around work camps, proper waste management, covered latrines, and elimination of standing water dramatically reduce breeding sites for pest species.

Chemical Repellents

The CDC, the U.S. Environmental Protection Agency (EPA), and the U.S. Department of Defense agree that chemical repellents remain one of the most effective tools when exposure cannot be avoided (Werner et al. 2019). DEET (20%–30%), picaridin (20%), IR3535, and oil of lemon eucalyptus are all supported by evidence as effective personal repellents – see the sidebar for more information. While some workers prefer natural or homeopathic options (citronella, lavender, essential oils), their effectiveness, unfortunately, is often short-lived and far less reliable. Repellents must be applied according to label directions, with reapplication as needed in high-exposure areas. For tick-prone zones, permethrin-treated clothing usually provides lasting protection, killing ticks and mosquitoes on contact (Table 3.2).

TABLE 3.2

Comparison of Common Chemical Arthropod Repellants

Active Ingredient	Typical Concentration	Mean Protection Time	Key Findings	Notes/ Limitations
DEET	20%–30%	4–6 hours (sometimes longer)	Consistently best documented; CPT ~300 minutes at 23.8%	Can damage plastics/ synthetics; greasy feel; safe with decades of use data
Picaridin (Icaridin)	20%	4–6 hours	Comparable to DEET against mosquitoes; better tolerated on skin and materials	Some variability in field performance; less greasy than DEET
IR3535	10%–20%	2–4 hours	Repels mosquitoes, ticks, flies; effective at higher concentrations	Shorter duration than DEET/ picaridin; reapply frequently
Oil of lemon eucalyptus (PMD)	20%–30%	4–6 hours (sometimes up to 11 hours in lab studies)	EPA-registered plant-derived repellent; comparable to DEET under some conditions	Not for children <3 years; availability limited; can cause skin irritation
Citronella oil	5%–10% (varies)	10–30 minutes	Initial repellency >95%, but drops below 60% in 2 hours	Volatile; requires frequent reapplication; short-lived
Lavender, lemon, other essential oils	Variable	<30– 60 minutes	Some initial effect but inconsistent and highly formulation-dependent	Pleasant aroma; not reliable for occupational protection

Sources: Fradin and Day (2002), Trongtokit et al. (2005), Yoon et al. (2015), JAMA (2016), Gouge et al. (2018), and Lee (2018).

The EPA maintains a website, last updated in June 2019, to aid individuals in choosing appropriate chemical repellants: https://www.epa.gov/insect-repellents/find-repellent-right-you. It is worth noting that no repellent is a magic bullet; real-world effectiveness depends on proper application, reapplication, coverage, exposure intensity, and integration with other protective measures, such as clothing, screens, and insect control.

Chemical repellents are excellent tools for reducing arthropod exposure during work, but they are not intended to remain on the skin once exposure risk has ended. After work, it is important to wash repellents off thoroughly because these substances are designed to be biologically active and can irritate the skin with prolonged contact. In rare cases, they may trigger rashes, allergic responses, or exacerbate existing skin conditions if left on overnight. Washing also reduces the chance of transferring repellent residues onto food, bedding, children, or pets once employees leave the field environment.

The most effective method for removal is straightforward: wash with warm water and a mild soap, taking extra care to scrub exposed areas such as the forearms, wrists, face, and ankles where repellent was applied most heavily. For lipids or oil-based repellents, using a gentle, fragrance-free cleanser helps break down residues more completely. Showering soon after returning from the field is best (and looked forward to by many workers!), since it not only removes repellent but also rinses away sweat, dust, or potential allergens and pathogens. Employees should change into freshly laundered clothing, as repellents may also cling to fabrics. In this way, routine post-exposure hygiene not only protects skin health but also complements the protective measures taken in the field, ensuring both immediate comfort and long-term well-being.

Vaccinations

Very few of the arthropod-borne diseases in North America have approved vaccines. There is a vaccine (Ixchiq™), approved by the U.S. Food and Drug Administration in 2023, that can provide protection against chikungunya virus, spread by mosquitoes. For the rare case in which tetanus is acquired after a bite or pinch that broke the skin, a widely available vaccine exists and is frequently part of the standard suite of childhood vaccines.

Vaccines are currently in experimental trials for zika virus, also spread by mosquitoes, and Lyme disease, spread by ticks. There are horse vaccines available for West Nile virus, eastern equine encephalitis, and western equine encephalitis, but none approved for humans. Internationally, vaccines are available for tickborne encephalitis, Japanese encephalitis, and yellow fever, none of which are endemic in North America, but could be encountered during travel.

Unless ecologists or environmental professionals are specifically working in areas in which chikungunya is a high threat, organizational management may not necessarily need to encourage or require vaccination. However, since environmental professionals often work in settings where contamination from soil is possible, current tetanus vaccination is a prudent measure. Since tetanus is a risk for occupational activities beyond entomological threats, workers should be encouraged to stay up to date on their tetanus immunizations anyway, and to seek medical advice if a bite or injury becomes contaminated.

Personal Protective Equipment

Appropriate clothing serves as the first and most reliable layer of personal protection against biting and stinging arthropods (Werner et al. 2019). Workers should wear lightweight, long-sleeved shirts and long pants tucked into socks to reduce mosquito and fly contact and use wide-brimmed hats with netting when insects are abundant. Some military uniforms are factory treated with insecticides and are best utilized when the entire uniform is worn properly; these factory-treated uniforms also do not require field treatment with permethrin.

In areas with high tick activity, booted coveralls or gaiters help prevent ticks from reaching the skin at the ankles. Vinyl or nitrile gloves provide a smooth, non-porous barrier when handling animals, soil, or vegetation that may harbor arthropods or pathogens. In situations where dense swarms of midges or mayflies occur, a handkerchief, dust mask, or other light respiratory covering can limit inhalation or contact. PPE should always be suited to both the environment and the task, offering effective coverage while maintaining comfort and mobility, especially under hot or humid field conditions.

Pest Control Interventions

Where insect populations pose a serious occupational hazard, targeted pest control may be necessary (Werner et al. 2019). This includes residual insecticide sprays in and around buildings, larviciding in water bodies where mosquitoes breed, or fogging for adult mosquitoes during outbreaks. Control measures should be integrated with environmental sanitation. For example, spraying without addressing standing water will yield only short-term relief. Professional pest control services may be warranted for corporate field stations, while smaller-scale ecological projects can often rely on simple but regular interventions such as draining containers and managing refuse.

Strategies That Do Not Work

Not all "folk solutions" or commercial gimmicks are effective. For example, flea or tick collars worn around the ankles provide no meaningful protection and may expose workers to unnecessary pesticide residues. The United States Department of Defense even prohibits service members from donning flea/tick collars, instead promoting their own insect repellant system. Similarly, ultrasonic insect repellents and many "bug-repelling bracelets" have consistently failed under scientific testing. Reliance on such ineffective measures can create a false sense of security, leaving individuals vulnerable to bites and disease. A health and safety program should emphasize evidence-based strategies and clearly communicate which products or practices lack efficacy.

As much as it is important to use PPE and apply repellants in the field, it is equally important not to wear attractants. Dark colored clothing can be attractive to mosquitoes, horse flies, and deer flies by increasing body heat and providing contrast. Bright floral prints (especially in shades of yellow) can visually guide pollinating insects such as bees. Strong perfumes, lotions, sunscreens, and scented hair products, especially floral, fruity, or sugary scents, are strongly attractive and help distinguish workers from the "unscented" environment, also attracting pollinators. Even some shiny or reflective fabrics and jewelry can be attractive to insects looking for places to lay eggs, since they can mimic the reflection of light off of water. Finally, body odor and sweat components like lactic acid, ammonia, and carbon dioxide, are strong attractants for blood-feeding arthropods like mosquitoes and other flies. To minimize potential entomological health and safety hazards, ecologists and environmental professionals should opt for light-colored, matte, tightly woven, fragrance-free, and clean garments, ideally treated with permethrin for added protection

Shared Accountability

Organizations have an obligation to establish policies and provide resources that reduce risk broadly. This is especially true with health conditions or vulnerabilities that cannot reasonably be assumed across all employees. For example, while bee stings are a potential hazard in outdoor work, an organization cannot assume that *every* employee is severely allergic. Instead, it is up to the individual who knows of such a condition to take appropriate measures such as carrying an epinephrine auto-injector, avoiding unnecessary risk, and seeking medical consultation for personalized precautions.

No matter how robust an organization's health and safety policies may be, each individual remains ultimately responsible for his or her own safety in the workplace. This does not absolve the employer of all responsibility, but it places the day-to-day safety decision-making in the hands of the individual, where knowledge of personal health status is clearest.

In general, employees are not required to disclose specific medical conditions, such as allergies to bee stings, to their employer, even when relevant to workplace risks. However, in the United States, disclosure can be helpful, since it allows the organization to make reasonable accommodations under the Americans with Disabilities Act (ADA). For example, an employee with a life-threatening bee sting allergy who informs their employer could request accommodations such as being assigned less frequently to high-risk areas or having a stocked first-aid kit with epinephrine nearby.

If an employee does choose to disclose a medical condition, the organization then has a responsibility to protect that information under HIPAA (Health Insurance Portability and Accountability Act). Health details cannot be disclosed to coworkers or supervisors beyond what is strictly necessary for safety, and only with the employee's consent. Note, however, that the information in this guide is for educational purposes only. It should not be taken as medical or legal advice. Individuals should consult qualified medical professionals for health concerns and licensed legal counsel for workplace policy decisions.

Notifiable Vector-Borne Diseases

In the realm of public health, *notifiable diseases* are conditions that, by law or regulation, must be reported to local, state, or national health authorities upon diagnosis. These reporting requirements exist to facilitate early detection, trend monitoring, and rapid response to emerging outbreaks. Many arthropod-borne diseases fall into this category due to their potential for rapid spread, serious health consequences, or geographic emergence in previously unaffected areas. The list of reportable diseases is not static and may be updated as new pathogens are identified, transmission patterns shift, or changes occur in surveillance priorities.

Most users of this guide will not be concerned with reporting disease; that will be done by attending physicians and medical personnel as a function of their occupation.

But, for ecologists, environmental consultants, field researchers, and others working in outdoor settings, knowledge of reportable vector-borne diseases is a critical component of occupational health and safety through simple awareness. While the likelihood of contracting many of these diseases is low in any single encounter, cumulative risk increases with frequency of exposure, seasonal activity, and geographic range. Field personnel may actually be among the first to notice a pattern, such as unusually high tick densities or clusters of mosquito bites, and, in some cases, may even be the index case for disease detection in a region. (Not that anyone wants that distinction!)

The following list of vector-borne diseases are currently (2025) notifiable at the federal level through the CDC's National Notifiable Disease Surveillance System (NNDSS).

- Anaplasmosis (tickborne)
- Chikungunya virus disease
- Eastern equine encephalitis virus disease
- Powassan virus disease
- St. Louis encephalitis virus disease
- West Nile virus disease
- Western equine encephalitis virus disease
- Babesiosis (tickborne)
- Spotted fever rickettsioses (e.g., Rocky Mountain spotted fever, etc.) (often under "spotted fever rickettsiosis")
- Lyme disease (tickborne) – part of routine national surveillance since 1991
- Tularemia (transmitted by ticks, deer flies, etc.)

All of these, plus some others that are regionally important, are reportable at the state level. The presence or absence of a disease from these lists does not necessarily indicate its risk or relevance to a particular site. Some diseases may be rare but highly consequential, while others are common but underreported. If desired, ecologists and environmental professionals may consult state and local health departments for current, region-specific guidance. Note also that the purpose of these reporting systems is epidemiological; legal and medical questions should be referred to qualified counsel or licensed healthcare professionals.

Practical Application in Fieldwork

For ecological and environmental professions, this means employees should be equipped with the knowledge and autonomy to self-manage personal health risks, while employers provide baseline protections, such as training, access to PPE, first-aid readiness, and vector control measures (Werner et al. 2019). When both sides understand their responsibilities, the workplace is safer, more respectful of privacy, and more compliant with legal requirements.

INCORPORATING ENTOMOLOGY INTO HEALTH AND SAFETY DOCUMENTS

Health and safety documentation such as SOPs, HASPs, and JHAs is critical for mitigating risk during field-based environmental and ecological work.

An SOP is a written protocol that outlines consistent, repeatable methods for managing specific hazards or tasks to ensure worker safety in the field or laboratory. A JHA is a task-based risk assessment tool that breaks down individual work activities, identifies associated hazards, and prescribes control measures to reduce risk. A HASP is a comprehensive, site-specific document that integrates relevant SOPs and JHAs to provide overarching guidance on protecting personnel during project execution; it typically includes emergency procedures, roles and responsibilities, and hazard-specific controls tailored to the project location and scope. These documents are not intended to be exhaustive compendiums of all potential risks. Rather, their strength lies in being broad enough to guide decisions under changing field conditions, while still identifying and addressing significant, foreseeable hazards, especially those related to entomological threats.

Incorporating arthropod-related hazards into these documents is essential for operations involving outdoor fieldwork. Biting, stinging, parasitic, or disease-spreading arthropods, including ticks, mosquitoes, fleas, mites, and certain flies or beetles, can pose risks ranging from nuisance-level distraction to life-threatening allergic or pathogen-related illnesses. Swarming arthropods may pose logistical, mechanical, or transportation hazards that, again, range from a mere nuisance to equipment failure or potential for motor vehicle accidents. While it is neither practical nor advisable to detail every possible species in these documents, planners should ensure that entomological threats are explicitly mentioned in hazard identification, with provisions for training, PPE, repellents, and symptom monitoring.

An example SOP outlining a standardized response to entomological hazards is provided in Appendix A. This template may be adapted to suit specific project types, ecoregions, or agency requirements, or it may remain broad enough for use across the entire continent. It includes guidance on general PPE use, arthropod avoidance strategies, response protocols for stings and bites, and procedures for documenting and reporting exposures.

JHAs should break down each task or exposure category and include brief entries for likely entomological hazards. For example, tasks such as vegetation surveys, soil sampling, or handling animal carcasses should be flagged for potential exposure to ticks, chiggers, biting flies, or urticating caterpillars. The corresponding mitigation may include tick checks, DEET-based repellents, wearing permethrin-treated clothing, and having access to epinephrine for allergic responses. Tasks such as structure inspections should include language pointing out the potential for exposure to spiders, centipedes, or wasps, and the corresponding mitigation may include flashlights, work gloves, and phone numbers for poison control centers in case of bites. Emphasis should be placed on simple, actionable controls rather than encyclopedic detail. An example JHA, examining aquatic ecology/biomonitoring work, is included in Appendix B.

For HASPs in particular, consultation with field ecologists or environmental biologists during plan development is highly recommended. These professionals often possess region-specific knowledge of arthropod biogeography and habitat preferences. Their input can greatly improve the relevance and effectiveness of entomological hazard planning by identifying periods of peak activity, likely species encounters, or regional disease concerns that may not be apparent to health and safety officers or project managers alone. This collaboration helps ensure that the plan is not only compliant but genuinely protective of field personnel – it does not include a cut-and-paste litany of entomological risks that would not occur simply because they do not even occur in the geographic region or ecological context. Instead, a valid HASP addresses real entomological risks.

A selected portion of an example HASP that addresses the entomological health and safety concerns for a fictional aquatic ecology/biomonitoring project on three streams in Pueblo County, Colorado, is included in Appendix C.

Importantly, health and safety documents should be treated as living documents – open to updates based on recent incidents, new regional disease emergence, or post-fieldwork debriefs. Including entomological considerations is not merely a formality; it helps prepare teams for common and uncommon field threats, reduces avoidable illness or lost time, and strengthens the overall culture of safety within environmental work.

By keeping these documents flexible, field-relevant, and biologically informed, project leaders and safety officers can significantly reduce the risk associated with arthropod encounters. Thoughtful integration of entomological hazards into planning documents enhances not only individual safety but also the overall success and continuity of long-term field projects.

REFERENCES

Fradin, MS, Day, JF. 2002. Comparative efficacy of insect repellents against mosquito bites. *New England J. Med.* 347: 13–18.

Gouge DH, Li S, Nair S, Walker K, Bibb C. 2018. Mosquito and Tick Repellents. University of Arizona Cooperative Extension Bulletin AZ1761.

JAMA. 2016. Insect repellents. *JAMA* 316: 766–767.

Lee MY. 2018. Essential oils as repellents against arthropods. *Biomed. Res. Int.* 2018: 6860271.

National Research Council. 1989. *Improving Risk Communication*. National Academies Press, Washington, DC.

Trongtokit Y, Curtis CF, Rongsriyam Y. 2005. Efficacy of repellent products against caged and free flying *Anopheles stephensi* mosquitoes. *Southeast Asian J. Trop. Med. Public Health* 36: 1423–1431.

Werner SL, Banda BK, Burnsides CL, Stuber AJ. 2019. Zoonosis: Update on existing and emerging vector-borne illnesses in the USA. *Curr. Emerg. Hosp. Med. Rep.* 7: 91–106.

Yoon JK, Kim KC, Cho Y, Gwon YD, Cho HS, Heo Y, Park K, Lee YW, Kim M, Oh YK, Kim YB. 2015. Comparison of repellency effect of mosquito repellents for DEET, citronella, and fennel oil. *J. Parasitol. Res.* 2015: 361021.

Part 2

The Arthropods

In Part 2 of this book, entomological hazards are listed as separate entries, first by their hazard type (stings, non-pathogenic bites, potentially pathogenic bites, physical irritants and allergens, potentially pathogenic non-biting contact hazards, and transportation, equipment, and operational hazards). Within each hazard type, organisms are listed taxonomically with arachnids, crustaceans, and myriapods first, and then insects. For pathogen transmission, diseases and syndromes follow the group of organisms responsible as vectors. Panic-inducing entomological agents are not addressed with separate entities, although they may be mentioned.

Each entry for a group of arthropods includes the following:

- **General name of the group**
- Pathologic organism, if applicable
- Ecological status ("entomological parasites," "entomological vectors," or "entomological agents," depending on their ecological status as a parasite, a disease vector, or a non-potentially pathogenic organism that stings, bites, or otherwise irritates) followed by a summary of species, genera, or families involved
- "Exposure and Severity Ratings," with notes on each and an exposure × severity graph. The numeric range of exposure and severity is explained in narrative bullet points, and definitions for the ranges of exposure and severity were provided in Part 1
- A few pertinent "References" and bibliographic citations are included at the end of each chapter
- A few paragraphs are provided to describe and explain the group, as well as provide general guidance on associated risk

DOI: 10.1201/9781003745709-5

- "Symptoms" with bulleted list
- "Occupational Exposure" with bulleted list
- "Prevention" with bulleted list of recommendations
- "What to do if Affected" with bulleted list of recommendations

For diseases associated with potentially pathological bites (ticks, kissing bugs, lice, fleas, mosquitoes, and sand flies) or contacts (dung beetles and filth flies), the taxonomic names of the pathogen and specific vectors are also included with the "Exposure and Severity Ratings," references, and descriptive paragraphs. The rest of the entry is usually truncated to simply the "Symptoms" section, because the other portions of the entry are usually redundant with the vector group. For example, all the diseases associated with mosquitoes have the same occupational exposures to mosquitoes, preventative measures, and recommendations to seek medical treatment if and when symptoms are realized.

Some arthropods have multiple mechanisms for harm, so they could feasibly be placed into multiple categories. In general, they have been placed into categories that are the most likely hazards, real or perceived. For example, fire ants are most often associated with their stings, but it is possible that they can erect a nest in equipment sitting on the ground; they are categorized in "Stings," not "Transportation, Equipment, and Logistics."

There are only two exceptions. Tarantulas can deliver a painful, though rarely dangerous, bite, so they are placed in "Non-Pathogenic Bites," and they commonly wander onto roads in the American Southwest during fall, causing slippery road conditions, so they are also placed in "Transportation, Equipment, and Logistics." Cockroaches are well-known for their attraction to filth (although some, especially in the South, can be found in rather nice buildings!), so they are placed in "Potentially Pathogenic Non-Biting Contact," but they are also documented to harbor potent allergens to a large proportion of the populace and can trigger asthma, so they are also included in "Physical Irritants and Allergens."

4 Stings

ARACHNIDS

SCORPIONS

Entomological Agents: Order Scorpionida: *Centruroides*, *Vaejovis*, and related genera (Figure 4.1)
  Exposure and Severity Ratings (Figure 4.1)

- **Exposure Level: 2–4**
  - Region-specific: frequent (4) and diverse in deserts of the Southwest (e.g., AZ, NM, TX, NV, southern CA), but uncommon (2) elsewhere within their range from northern CA east to KS and MO. Also uncommon (2) along the Gulf Coast to central FL
  - Only tiny populations exist in states like OH, IL, IN, SD, WV, and only in the farthest south and west portions of each state
  - Poison control centers report ~16,000 scorpion exposures/year; of these, ~10,000 originate in AZ, with NV, TX, and FL each reporting ~500–1,000 calls annually
  - Highest exposure rates per capita occur in metropolitan areas, like Las Vegas, Phoenix, Tucson-Nogales, San Antonio, and Roswell (NM)
- **Severity Level: 1–4**
  - Most species: mild (1) localized pain; ~85% of cases
  - Neurotoxic species: moderate (3) harm that requires more advanced medical treatment only for children or sensitive individuals
  - Only one confirmed fatality from 1964 to 2025

References: Abroug et al. (2020), Feola et al. (2020)

Scorpions are nocturnal arachnids found worldwide, with the highest occupational relevance in desert, tropical, and subtropical regions. They are commonly encountered under rocks, logs, debris, or within sleeping quarters, shoes, and clothing. While most of the 90 or so North American species produce painful but non-lethal stings, certain scorpions, particularly in the genus *Centruroides* (e.g., *C. sculpturatus*, the Arizona bark scorpion), possess neurotoxic venom that can cause serious systemic effects, especially in children or elderly adults.

Most scorpions sting defensively, often when accidentally stepped on or trapped against the body.

Symptoms
- Sharp, burning pain at the site of the sting
- Tingling, numbness, or localized swelling

DOI: 10.1201/9781003745709-6

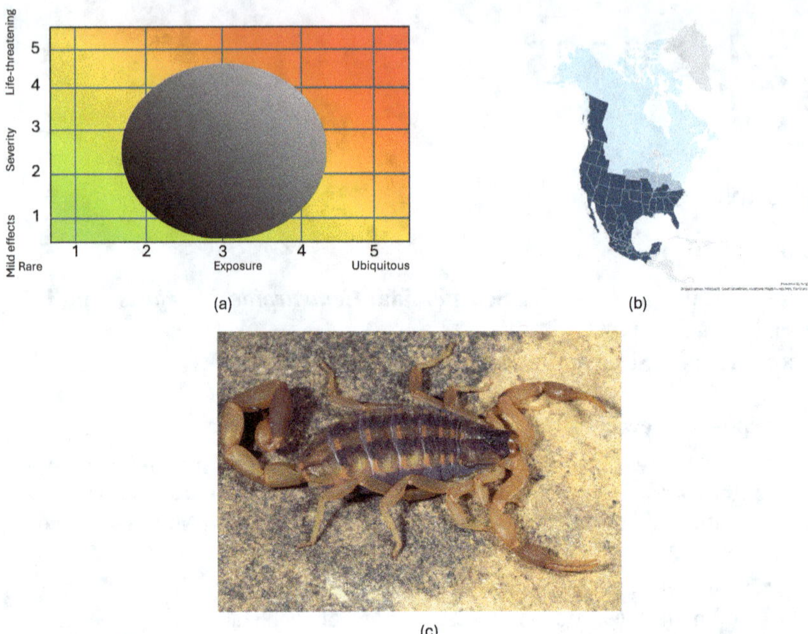

FIGURE 4.1 Scorpions. (a) Exposure × severity matrix; (b) geographic distribution; (c) striped back scorpion, *Centruroides vittatus*.

- In neurotoxic species (especially *Centruroides*):
  - Muscle twitching, restlessness, slurred speech, blurred vision, or difficulty breathing
  - Systemic reactions may include hypertension, vomiting, sweating, or convulsions
  - Severe envenomation is rare in adults but can be life-threatening in children
- Symptoms generally begin within minutes of the sting

U.S. fatalities are extremely rare and mostly associated with *C. sculpturatus* in Arizona.

Occupational Exposure

Scorpions are encountered by ecology and environmental professionals in:

- Southern United States and, extralimitly, Central and South America, North Africa, and parts of Asia
- Rocky field environments, excavation zones, and desert ecology surveys
- Rural and outdoor sleeping areas such as tents, cabins, or floor bedding
- Stored gear, shoes, and clothing left on the ground
- Construction and maintenance involving piles of materials, wood, or debris

Scorpions are most active at night and avoid bright sunlight.

Prevention

Shake out boots, gloves, and clothing before use.

- Do not leave bedding, shoes, or packs on the ground overnight
- Use flashlights or UV lights to inspect sleeping areas, many scorpions fluoresce under UV light
- Wear closed-toe shoes and gloves when working in rocky or debris-laden areas
- Seal entry points in buildings and field stations to prevent scorpion ingress
- Train staff to identify dangerous species, especially in endemic areas

In highly infested areas, elevated cots and netting can reduce risk during overnight stays.

What To Do If Affected

- Clean the sting site with soap and water
- Apply cold packs to reduce pain
- For mild stings:
  - Use oral antihistamines, nonsteroidal anti-inflammatory drugs (NSAIDs), and monitor symptoms
- For neurotoxic reactions:
  - Seek immediate medical attention
  - Administer antivenom (available for *C. sculpturatus* in some regions) if prescribed
  - Keep the patient calm and still to slow venom spread
- Observe children closely even if symptoms appear minor

Prompt recognition and symptom-based care are usually sufficient.

INSECTS

FIRE ANTS

Entomological Agents: Order Hymenoptera, Family Formicidae: *Solenopsis invicta* (red imported fire ant), *S. richteri* (black imported fire ant), and their hybrid – distributed throughout the southern United States – as well as *Myrmica rubra* (European fire ant) – distributed in the Northeastern United States from Maine to Virginia (Figure 4.2). Two native species, *S. xyloni* and *S. geminata*, also occur in the South but are of relatively minor importance

    Exposure and Severity Ratings (Figure 4.2)

- **Exposure Level: 3–4**
  - Moderately (3) common across the southeastern United States, expanding into western and southern states
  - More frequent (4) in disturbed soils than in natural settings

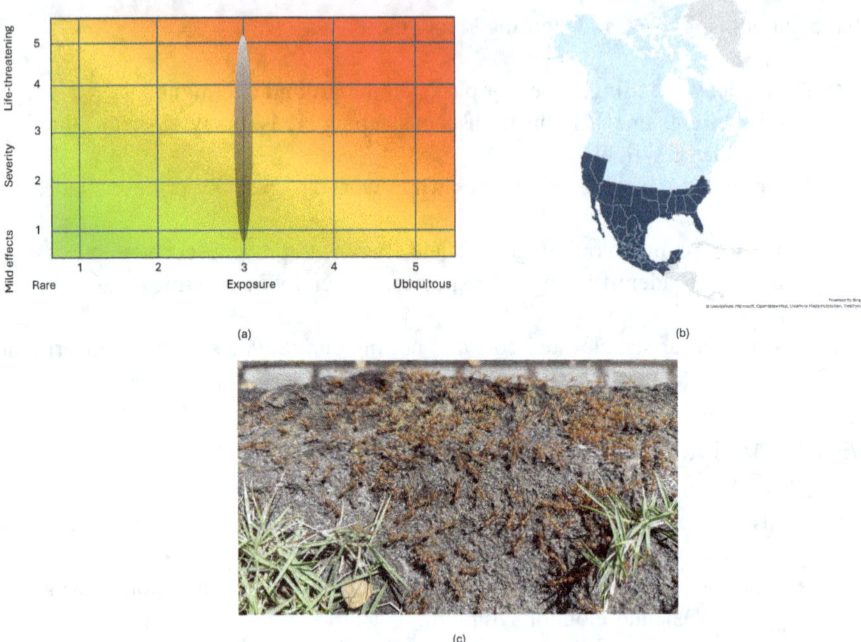

FIGURE 4.2 Fire ants. (a) Exposure × severity matrix; (b) geographic distribution; (c) red imported fire ant, *Solenopsis invicta*.

- **Severity Level: 1–5**
  - Individual stings cause mild (1) pain, pustules, and irritation
  - However, fire ants are known to swarm and sting en masse, resulting in multiple stings, which can increase the severity to severe (4)
  - Rarely, hypersensitive individuals may experience life-threatening (5) anaphylaxis

References: Tschinkel (2013), Schmidt (2016), Wang et al. (2018), Kemp et al. (2000)

Fire ants are aggressive, venomous ants introduced from South America. They establish large mounds in disturbed areas, including agricultural lands, power stations, roadsides, and construction sites. When disturbed, fire ants swarm and sting en masse, injecting venom through a stinger located at the rear of the abdomen. Their sting results in a burning sensation, followed a couple days later by formation of a sterile, white pustule.

Most reactions are localized, but hypersensitive individuals may experience systemic allergic reactions ranging from hives and difficulty breathing to life-threatening anaphylaxis. Because fire ants are common in southern fieldwork settings, they represent a serious occupational hazard, particularly to those unaware of their presence or with known insect sting allergies.

Symptoms

- Burning, stinging sensation
- Formation of itchy white pustules within 24 hours
- Swelling, redness, and pain at the site
- Allergic reactions: hives, dizziness, shortness of breath
- Rarely, **anaphylaxis** requiring emergency care

Occupational Exposure

Ecologists and environmental professionals are exposed to fire ants when:

- Working in fields, pastures, cleared lots, or disturbed soils
- Utility and construction crews near mound habitats
- Surveyors and ecologists operating near water control structures, roadside shoulders, or wetlands
- Crews unknowingly standing or setting up equipment on mounds

Prevention

Visually inspect areas for fire ant mounds before field deployment.

- Wear boots and long pants, and avoid standing near visible mounds
- Use ant bait or contact insecticide around high-risk sites if return work is expected
- Carry epinephrine auto-injectors for personnel with known sting allergies
- Train field crews to recognize fire ants and respond quickly to stings

What To Do If Affected

Wash area with soap and water.

- Apply cold compress and topical antihistamines or steroids
- Avoid scratching to prevent secondary infection
- For systemic reactions, administer epinephrine and seek emergency care
- Monitor for signs of delayed allergic response

OTHER STINGING ANTS

Entomological Agents: Order Hymenoptera, Family Formicidae: *Pseudomyrmex, Myrmecia* **(rare imports),** *Tetramorium*, **and certain native species in** *Pogonomyrmex, Myrmica*, **and** *Paratrechina* **(Figure 4.3)**

    Exposure and Severity Ratings (Figure 4.3)

- **Exposure Level: 2–3**
  - Uncommon (2) presence throughout North America; moderately (3) common in desert, alpine, or imported pest zones
- **Severity Level: 1–3**
  - Stings range from minimal (1) to moderate (3), causing localized swelling
  - Systemic reactions are exceptionally rare

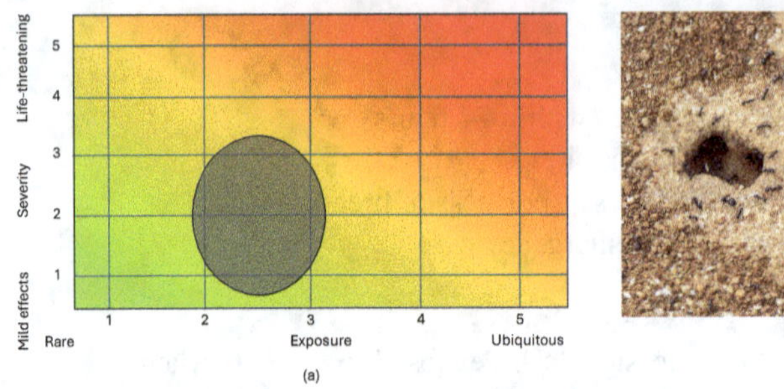

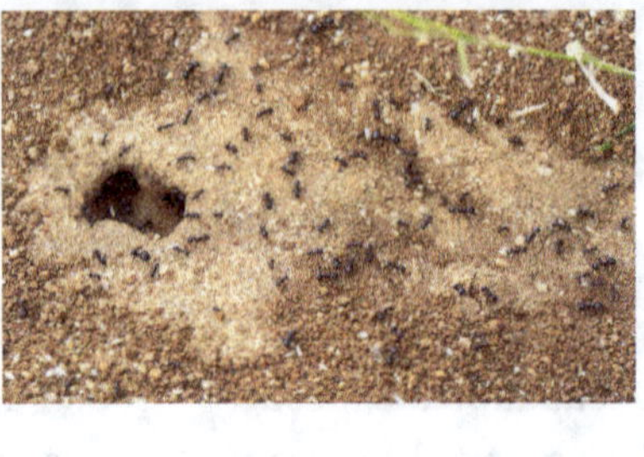

FIGURE 4.3   Other stinging ants. (a) Exposure × severity matrix; (b) Western harvester ant, *Pogonomyrmex occidentalis*.

References: Haddad et al. (2012), Schmidt (2016)

Several species of ants in North America, beyond *Solenopsis*, are capable of stinging. Among them, harvester ants (*Pogonomyrmex* spp.) deliver a potent sting considered more painful than that of fire ants; most species are located in arid and semi-arid environments in the southwestern United States, but *P. badius* is distributed in the southeast into Florida. Among imported species, *Tetramorium immigrans*, the pavement ant, has a milder sting, while *Myrmecia pilosula*, the bulldog ant, packs an even more painful sting. A few native ants in forested or alpine ecosystems also sting, though typically with milder effects.

These ants are generally less aggressive than fire ants and usually sting only when provoked or trapped against the skin. Pain varies by species, but reactions are generally localized and self-limiting. However, allergic responses are possible, especially for repeated exposures among outdoor workers.

Symptoms

- Sharp or burning pain at sting site
- Swelling, redness, or itching
- Mild systemic symptoms in sensitive individuals
- No pustule formation, unlike fire ants

Occupational Exposure

Ecologists and environmental professionals could be exposed to stinging ants when they:

- Work in desert, grassland, or mountainous habitats
- Cause disturbance of nests in soil, under rocks, or at base of plants
- Conduct activities involving digging, rock turning, or equipment setup on infested ground

Prevention

- Survey sites for ant activity prior to work
- Wear gloves and long sleeves when handling soil or debris

- Avoid kneeling or resting hands on ground without inspection
- Educate crews on the appearance and behavior of local stinging ants

What To Do If Affected
- Clean wound and apply ice
- Use antihistamines or topical creams for itching
- Watch for signs of swelling or allergic response
- Report reactions for future risk assessment and first-aid planning

STINGING FLYING WASPS

Entomological agents: Order Hymenoptera, Families Vespidae (yellowjackets, paper wasps, hornets), Pompilidae (spider wasps), and Sphecidae (thread-waisted and digger wasps); a few other families may rarely be implicated (Figure 4.4)
Exposure and Severity Ratings (Figure 4.4)

- **Exposure Level: 2–4**
  - Generally uncommon (2) to frequent (4), depending on habitat
- **Severity Level: 2–4**
  - Most stings are mild (2) to moderate (3), certainly memorable
  - Wasps in enclosed places (buildings, vehicles) can cause moderate (3) concern among occupants
  - Danger of anaphylaxis to hypersensitive individuals is severe (4)

References: Schmidt (2016)

Wasps of the families Vespidae, Pompilidae, and Sphecidae are frequent concerns in ecological and field-based professions due to their ability to sting and, in some cases, aggressively defend nests. These wasps vary in social structure, behavior, and medical relevance:

Vespidae includes social wasps such as yellowjackets (*Vespula*, *Dolichovespula*), paper wasps (*Polistes*), and hornets (*Vespa*), including the so-called "murder hornets" (*Vespa mandarinia*) that are native to East Asia and were found in Vancouver,

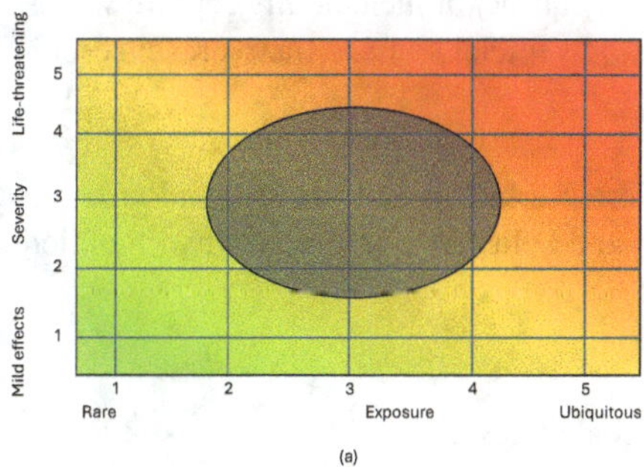

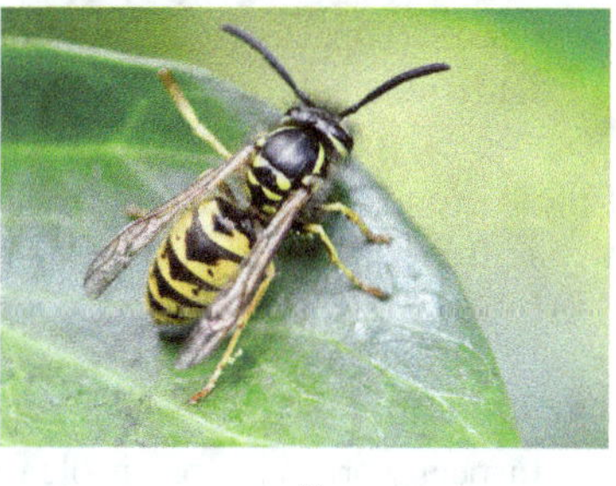

FIGURE 4.4 Flying stinging wasps. (a) Exposure × severity matrix; (b) common yellow-jacket, *Vespula vulgaris*.

BC, and neighboring areas of Washington State from 2019 to 2024. *V. mandarinia* is now considered to be eradicated from North America. All of these wasps live in colonies, are highly defensive of nests, and can deliver multiple stings. Nests may be visible and hanging from trees or manmade structures, or they can be hidden (ground-nesting species); the latter are almost never noticed until they are disturbed and defensive.

Pompilidae are solitary spider wasps, often with very painful stings (e.g., *Pepsis*, the tarantula hawks), but are non-aggressive unless provoked.

Sphecidae are solitary wasps such as mud daubers and thread-waisted wasps. They are non-aggressive, nest in burrows or crevices, and are more of a surprise hazard when disturbed.

While most stings cause localized pain, anaphylaxis is a serious concern in allergic individuals. Vespid wasps, particularly yellowjackets, pose the highest risk of mass stinging incidents.

Symptoms

- Sharp, immediate pain followed by swelling, redness, and itching; some stings are particularly painful
- Multiple stings can result in extensive local reaction or systemic symptoms
- Anaphylaxis: rapid onset of hives, difficulty breathing, hypotension, dizziness, or loss of consciousness
- Severity of reaction varies by sting location, number of stings, and individual sensitivity

Occupational Exposure

These wasps are encountered in:

- Vegetation clearing, landscaping, and trail maintenance
- Field sampling, especially near logs, structures, or flowering plants
- Utility and construction work, where nests may be hidden in walls, underground, or equipment
- Agricultural and ecological research, particularly in late summer and fall when wasps are most defensive
- Entomological field trapping, which may attract or incidentally capture wasps
- Enclosed spaces, such as buildings or vehicles, where their presence can cause much alarm

Of these groups, Vespidae are the most likely to attack seemingly randomly, especially in the fall, or to swarm. Pompilids and sphecids sting only when handled or severely disturbed.

Prevention

- Inspect work sites for visible or concealed nests
- Avoid bright clothing, perfumed products, and rapid movements around foraging wasps
- Keep food and drinks covered during field activities
- Wear protective clothing (long sleeves, gloves) in high-risk areas

- Do not swat wildly at wasps; it is considered offensive and triggers defensive actions
- Workers with venom allergies must carry an epinephrine auto-injector
- For known nesting areas (e.g., inside utility boxes or eaves), schedule pest control removal
- Avoid placing traps or workstations near trash bins or fallen fruit, which attract yellowjackets

What To Do If Affected

- Wash area with soap and water
- Apply ice and oral antihistamines or NSAIDs to reduce swelling
- Do not scratch, to avoid secondary infection
- For anaphylaxis:
  - Administer epinephrine immediately
  - Call emergency services
  - Lie the victim down with legs elevated and monitor breathing
- If multiple stings occur or the sting is near the throat, eyes, or genitals, seek medical care

Teams in remote field sites should have a first-aid protocol and transport plan for allergic reactions.

VELVET ANTS

Entomological Agents: Order Hymenoptera, Family Mutillidae: *Dasymutilla*, *Timulla*, and related genera (Figure 4.5)
Exposure and Severity Ratings (Figure 4.5)

- **Exposure Level: 1–2**
  - Rare (1) or uncommon (2); localized in dry, sandy, open habitats, mostly in the southern and western United States but extending north into Canada
  - Easily avoided with caution

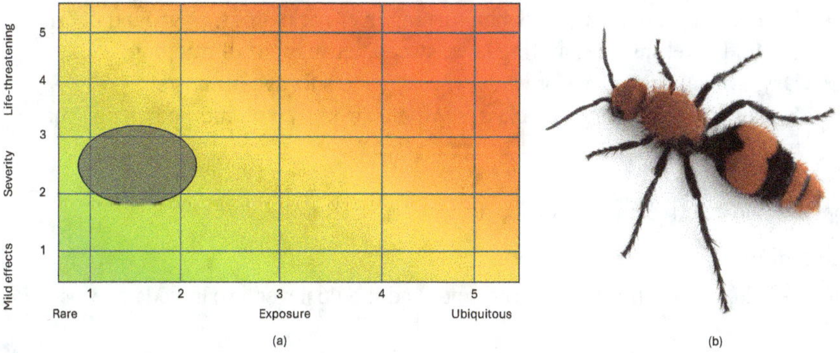

FIGURE 4.5 Velvet ants. (a) Exposure × severity matrix; (b) red velvet ant, *Dasymutilla occidentalis*.

- **Severity Level: 2–3**
  - Sting pain is mild (2) to moderate (3): intense but short-lived
  - Operational disruption can be mild (2) from fear of injury

References: Schmidt (2016), Williams et al. (2023)

Velvet ants are wasps, not true ants. The females are wingless, often brightly colored with dense red, orange, or black setae (hair), and resemble fuzzy ants, which is why they are considered separately from the other stinging wasps in which the females are generally winged. Males are winged and do not sting. Females are solitary parasitoids, laying eggs in the nests of other bees or wasps, and are often encountered wandering on the ground.

Velvet ants are not aggressive, but if handled or stepped on, females can deliver a severe sting, sometimes described as among the most painful insect stings in North America. Their nickname, "cow killer," reflects the pain – not any actual lethality – and only applies to certain large species. *Dasymutilla occidentalis* can occur on sandy beaches along the Great Lakes and could pose a risk to workers in riparian and beach habitats.

While they pose no severe medical risk to most people, their stings are traumatic and can temporarily incapacitate field workers, especially if multiple individuals are disturbed (e.g., during sweep netting or ground surveys).

Symptoms

- Immediate, intense pain at the sting site
- Swelling, redness, and burning sensation lasting up to an hour or more
- Occasionally, localized numbness or bruising
- Rare allergic reactions, but anaphylaxis is extremely uncommon
- Psychological effects (panic, fear) may linger in novice workers

Stings are usually single; velvet ants do not swarm or chase.

Occupational Exposure

Velvet ants are encountered in:

- Sandy or open habitats, especially pine barrens, deserts, and scrublands
- Field surveys, particularly when turning over rocks, logs, or ground debris
- Ground-level insect sampling (e.g., sweep netting, pitfall trapping)
- Dry, undisturbed paths or trails where females forage for hosts
- Ecology and entomology classes, where brightly colored specimens may tempt handling

They are most active during warm, sunny days in summer.

Prevention

Educate field workers that these are not ants, and should never be handled unnecessarily.

- Wear gloves and long pants when working in dry, sandy regions
- Use caution when kneeling or sitting on the ground, especially in open scrub
- Mark areas of high velvet ant density for team awareness

- Train workers to identify brightly colored insects that may sting
- Avoid barefoot or exposed footwear in known habitat zones

Because velvet ants are solitary, infestations or nest removal is not applicable.

What To Do If Affected

- Wash the sting site with soap and water
- Apply ice or a cold compress
- Take oral antihistamines or NSAIDs to manage swelling and pain
- Monitor for signs of allergic reaction, though such responses are rare
- Report the sting to field supervisors, especially in institutional or instructional settings
- Use the event as a teaching opportunity, with safety reminders

There is no antivenom or specific treatment beyond pain relief.

EUROPEAN HONEYBEES

Entomological Agent: Order Hymenoptera, Family Apidae: *Apis mellifera* (honeybee), both managed and feral populations (Figure 4.6)
Exposure and Severity Ratings (Figure 4.6)

- **Exposure Level: 3–4**
  - Moderately (3) common to frequent (4) in areas with flowering vegetation or managed hives
  - Millions of stings occur annually among the general public during outdoor activities; account for ~0.5% of all Emergency Department visits
- **Severity Level: 2–5**
  - Most stings produce mild (2) pain; no danger of multiple stings
  - ~5%–7.5% of the North American population is hypersensitive to honeybee stings, resulting in severe (4) symptoms for which medical treatment is necessary
  - ~3% of the population can experience life-threatening (5) anaphylaxis

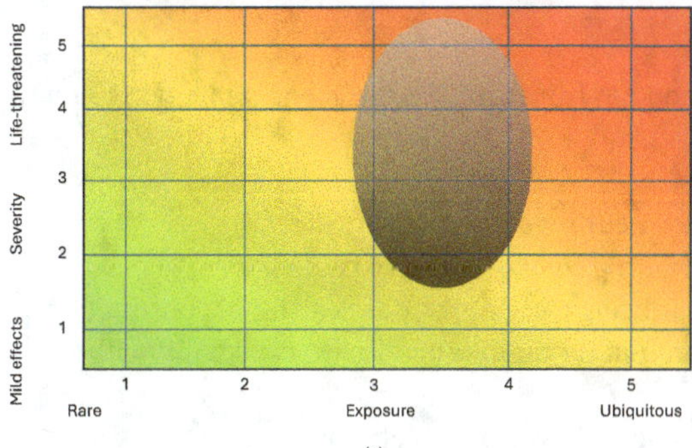

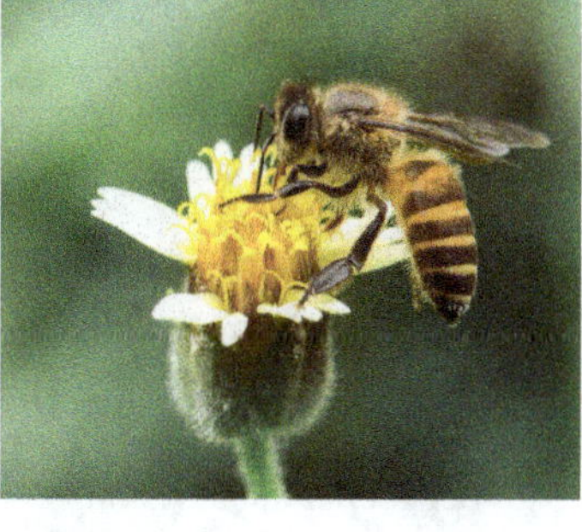

FIGURE 4.6 European honeybees. (a) Exposure × severity matrix; (b) western honeybee, *Apis mellifera.*

References: Schmidt (2016), Stanhope et al. (2017), Carli et al. (2024)

The European honeybee (*Apis mellifera*) is one of the most economically and ecologically significant insects, valued for its role in pollination, honey production, and agricultural productivity. The species has also been domesticated for these purposes, and the strains that have been developed and used in North America are quite gentle. Despite the honeybee's benefits and gentle nature, it also poses health and safety concerns, especially when colonies are disturbed in the field or when individuals with bee venom allergies are exposed.

Honeybees sting in defense of the hive, and unlike wasps or hornets, they typically die after stinging, as their barbed stinger remains embedded in the victim's skin. Though most stings are painful but self-limiting, individuals who are allergic to bee venom may experience severe, even fatal, anaphylaxis.

With the expansion of feral populations, particularly in warmer regions where Africanized honeybee hybrids have established, the risk of aggressive swarming has increased in some environments. Africanized honeybees are addressed separately.

Symptoms

- Immediate pain and burning at the sting site
- The barbed stinger and venom sac may still be attached to the skin, sometimes with muscles still pumping venom
- Redness, swelling, and itching that can persist for several hours or days
- In allergic individuals:
  - Widespread hives, facial swelling, wheezing, hypotension, or loss of consciousness
  - Anaphylactic symptoms typically occur within 15–30 minutes
- In rare cases:
  - Multiple stings can lead to toxic envenomation, kidney damage, or cardiovascular complications

Bee venom contains melittin, phospholipase A_2, and other allergens that often trigger inflammatory and immune responses.

Occupational Exposure

High-risk activities for ecologists and environmental professionals involving honeybee encounters include:

- Pollinator ecology or fieldwork near hives or foraging areas
- Agricultural tasks in orchards, crop fields, or clover pastures
- Accidental disturbance of hives during mowing, brush-clearing, or construction
- Working in proximity to intentionally maintained hives, especially without beekeeper supervision
- Trapping or surveying insects near flowering vegetation

Risk increases during warm, sunny days when foraging activity peaks.

Beekeepers are routinely exposed to honeybees in their occupation (or hobby, for some), so their profession includes specialized protective equipment far beyond what is typically needed by ecological or environmental professionals. Standard beekeeping personal protective equipment (PPE) includes a full bee suit or coveralls, veiled helmets or hoods to protect the head and face, heavy canvas or leather gloves that prevent stings through the fabric, and high-top boots or gaiters that seal pant legs. Some also use smokers to calm bees and thick aprons or reinforced sleeves for additional protection. While these measures are essential for those managing hives or honeybee colonies, most environmental workers only require lightweight, protective clothing and awareness of bee activity; full beekeeping gear is unnecessary outside of direct apiculture work.

Prevention

To avoid bee stings and related hazards:

- Stay aware of hive locations and maintain distance
- Do not wear bright clothing or floral scents in areas with high bee activity
- Remain calm and still if bees are foraging nearby – sudden movements, especially swatting, may provoke stings
- Use protective clothing, including bee suits and veils, when working near managed hives
- Workers with known allergies should carry an epinephrine auto-injector (EpiPen)
- Avoid mowing or disturbing areas with nesting or swarming activity

Education on honeybee behavior and identification can help field workers minimize unnecessary risks.

What To Do If Affected

- Remove the stinger immediately by scraping with a fingernail or dull edge – do not squeeze
- Wash the area with soap and water
- Apply ice packs and take antihistamines or NSAIDs for swelling and discomfort
- Watch for signs of systemic reaction (difficulty breathing, dizziness, hives)
- If symptoms develop, administer epinephrine and seek emergency medical care
- Multiple stings or facial/throat stings should also be evaluated promptly

Prompt and safe removal of the stinger reduces venom delivery and severity.

AFRICANIZED HONEYBEES

Entomological Agent: Order Hymenoptera, Family Apidae: *Apis mellifera mellifera/scutellata* **hybrids (sometimes known as "killer bees")**
    Exposure and Severity Ratings (Figure 4.7)

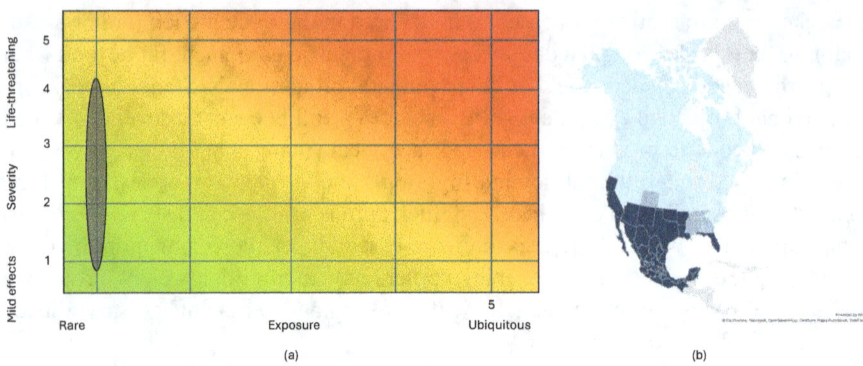

FIGURE 4.7   Africanized honeybees. (a) Exposure × severity matrix; (b) geographic distribution.

- **Exposure Level: 1**
  - Rare (1), mostly restricted to the far southern United States
  - May extend into central and western states during summer in warm years but die back in winter
- **Severity Level: 1–4**
  - A single sting is almost identical to that of the European honeybee, mild (2)
  - These bees tend to swarm, and an attack will often involve multiple stings causing moderate (3) to severe (4) reactions

References: de la Cruz et al. (2025); Schumacher and Egen (2025)

Africanized honeybees are hybrids of two subspecies of the honeybee: African (*Apis mellifera scutellata*) and European (*A. m. mellifera*) honeybees, thus they look virtually identical to the European honeybee (Figure 4.6). They were introduced from Africa into Brazil in the 1950s and spread northward, arriving in Texas by the 1990s. These bees have since spread throughout the southern United States, sometimes displacing gentler strains in some regions.

Although their venom is no more potent than that of European honeybees, Africanized bees pose a far greater threat due to their hyper-defensive behavior, increased swarm size, and persistence in stinging perceived threats. Even small disturbances near a hive may trigger aggressive mass attacks, resulting in hundreds or thousands of stings.

They tend to nest in more exposed locations (e.g., hollow logs, culverts, abandoned vehicles, walls), increasing the likelihood of accidental encounters.

Symptoms

- Multiple simultaneous stings, often targeting head, face, and upper body
- Severe pain, redness, swelling, and potential systemic envenomation
- Victims may suffer:
  - Anaphylaxis, if allergic
  - Toxic reactions from massive venom load: nausea, dizziness, confusion, kidney failure

- Death from asphyxiation, shock, or cardiac arrest, especially in those unable to escape (e.g., elderly, children, or restrained workers)

Survivors of mass stinging events often require hospitalization, IV fluids, and wound management.

Occupational Exposure

Ecologists and environmental professionals most at risk include:

- Field ecologists, wildlife biologists, and agricultural laborers in southern U.S. states
- Utility workers, surveyors, and construction crews near natural or manmade cavities
- People working in culverts, sheds, or old buildings where hives may be hidden
- Outdoor educators or students, especially in rural or semi-urban environments
- Emergency responders in warm-climate urban areas, where colonies can thrive

Africanized bees are active year-round in warm climates and may attack with little warning.

Prevention

- Avoid disturbing cavities or voids in structures, soil, or vegetation
- Maintain at least 100 ft from known hives
- Post warning signs near known infestation zones
- Educate personnel in high-risk regions (e.g., Texas, Arizona, California, Florida)
- Wear protective clothing when exposure is likely, and work in teams with communication plans
- If bees begin to swarm, run away in a straight line and seek shelter in a building or vehicle; do not dive into water
- Individuals with allergies should carry an epinephrine auto-injector

Africanized honeybees will continue pursuit for up to half a kilometer or a quarter-mile, making escape distance and speed critical.

What To Do If Affected

- Run immediately; do not swat or flail, as this is interpreted as offensive and causes the bees to release alarm pheromones
- Cover face and eyes with clothing or arms
- Enter enclosed space (building, car) and close doors/windows
- Once safe, remove stingers quickly by scraping – not squeezing
- For multiple stings or signs of systemic reaction, seek emergency care immediately
- Anaphylactic symptoms require epinephrine administration and hospitalization

Prompt treatment significantly reduces morbidity and mortality from mass stings.

OTHER BEES

Entomological Agents: Order Hymenoptera, Families Apidae: *Bombus* spp. (bumble bees), *Xylocopa* spp. (carpenter bees), Halictidae (sweat bees), and various native solitary bees (Figure 4.8)

Exposure and Severity Ratings (Figure 4.8)

- **Exposure Level: 2–3**
  - Uncommon (2) to moderately (3) common in North America, especially in natural and semi-natural habitats during spring to late summer
- **Severity Level: 1–2**
  - Stings may be minimal (1) to mild (2); generally less painful than honeybee or wasp stings
  - Allergic reactions are possible but less common

Reference: Schmidt (2016)

Many native bees, particularly bumble bees, sweat bees, and carpenter bees, are important pollinators and are typically non-aggressive unless provoked. Most are solitary or form small colonies, and they will only sting if trapped or defending a nest that is actively being assaulted. Unlike honeybees, bumble bees and other bees can sting multiple times without dying.

Sweat bees, though small and often overlooked, are attracted to perspiration and may sting when brushed away. Their sting feels more-or-less like a singed hair. Carpenter bees can appear threatening due to their large size and loud buzzing, but males (which cannot sting) often make a threatening approach, and stings from females are rare. However, disturbance of nests near field sites, structures, or wooden equipment can provoke defensive behavior.

Symptoms

- Immediate burning or stinging pain
- Localized redness, swelling, or itching
- Mild allergic reactions (rash, hives) in sensitive individuals
- Rarely, systemic reactions (especially in those with preexisting allergies)

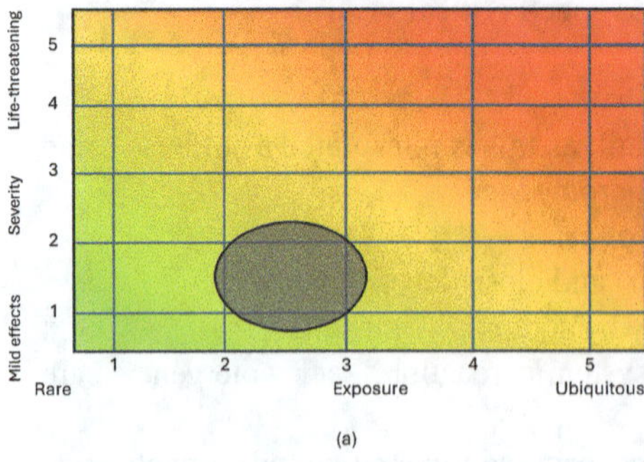

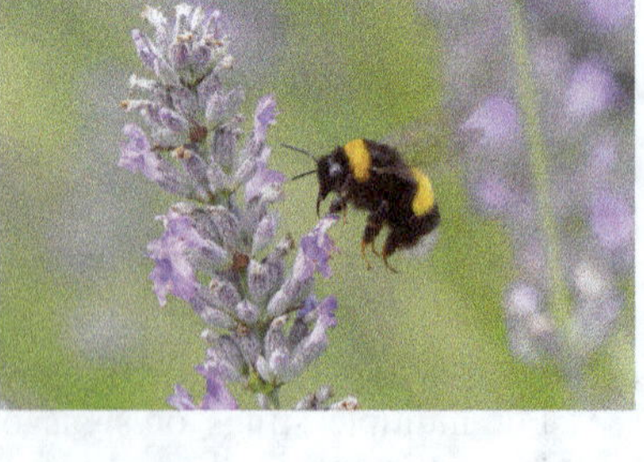

FIGURE 4.8 Other bees. (a) Exposure×severity matrix; (b) buff-tailed bumble bee, *Bombus terrestris*.

Occupational Exposure

Ecologists and environmental professionals may encounter these other bees during:

- Fieldwork in meadows, forest edges, prairies, and gardens during active blooming seasons
- Activities near rotting wood or wooden structures that house carpenter bee nests
- Handling of equipment stored outdoors or near bee foraging areas
- Prolonged activity in pollinator-rich environments such as restoration plots or seed farms

Prevention

- Wear long sleeves and gloves when working near bee habitats
- Avoid swatting at bees; move calmly away from persistent individuals
- Inspect wood structures and field gear for nesting carpenter bees
- Limit use of scented lotions or soaps, which may attract bees
- Educate field personnel on bee behavior and sting avoidance

What To Do If Affected

- Clean the sting site with soap and water
- Apply cold compresses to reduce swelling
- Take oral antihistamines or use topical hydrocortisone for itching
- Monitor for signs of allergic reaction (e.g., swelling beyond the sting site, difficulty breathing)
- In the case of a systemic reaction, seek medical care; a physician may administer epinephrine

Most native bee stings are isolated incidents and pose low medical risk, but repeated exposure or hypersensitivity may elevate concern in sensitive individuals or those working in dense pollinator habitats. Including these risks in pre-deployment briefings is recommended.

REFERENCES

Abroug F, Ouanes-Besbes L, Tilouche N, Elatrous S. 2020. Scorpion envenomation: State of the art. *Intensive Care Med.* 46: 401–410.

Carli T, Locatelli I, Košnik M, Kukec K. 2024. The prevalence of self-reported systemic allergic reaction to Hymenoptera venom in beekeepers worldwide: A systematic literature review and meta-analysis. *Zdr. Varst.* 63: 152–159.

de la Cruz EP, Valencia Dominguez M, Ramos Reyes R, Tofilski A. 2025. Reexamination of honey bee Africanization in Mexico and other regions of the New World. *Sci. Rep.* 15: 16267.

Feola MA, Piscopo A, Casella F, Della Pietra B, Di Mizio G. 2020. Autopsy findings in case of fatal scorpion sting: A systematic review of the literature. *Healthcare* 8: 325.

Haddad V, Costa Cardoso JL, Lupi O, Tyring SK. 2012. Tropical dermatology: Venomous arthropods and human skin: Part I. Insecta. *J. Am. Acad. Dermatol.* 67: 331.e1–331.e14.

Kemp SF, deShazo RD, Moffitt JE, Williams DF, Buhner WA. 2000. Expanding habitat of the imported fire ant (*Solenopsis invicta*): A public health concern. *J. Allergy Clin. Immunol.* 105: 683–691.

Schmidt JO. 2016. *The Sting of the Wild*. Johns Hopkins University Press, Baltimore, MD.

Schumacher MJ, Egen NB. 1995. Significance of Africanized bees for public health: A review. *Arch. Intern. Med.* 155: 2038–2043.

Stanhope J, Carver S, Weinstein P. 2017. Health outcomes of beekeeping: A systematic review. *J. Apicult. Res.* 56: 100–111.

Tschinkel WR. 2013. *The Fire Ants*. Harvard University Press, Cambridge, MA.

Wang L, Lu Y, Li R, Zeng L, Du J, Huang X, Xu Y. 2018. Mental health effects caused by red imported fire ant attacks (*Solenopsis invicta*). *PLoS ONE* 13: e0199424.

Williams K, Pan AD, Wilson JS. 2023. *Velvet Ants of North America*. Princeton University Press, Princeton, NJ.

5 Non-Pathogenic Bites or Pinches

ARACHNIDS

SCABIES MITES

Entomological Parasite: Order Acariformes, Family Sarcoptidae: *Sarcoptes scabiei* var. *hominis* **(human itch mite) (Figure 5.1)**
   Exposure and Severity Ratings (Figure 5.1)

- **Exposure Level: 1**
  - **Rare (1) across North America**: sporadic cases; incidence unknown but estimates range from 0.2% to 2.8% in crowded, institutionalized settings
  - **Frequent (4) globally**: estimated 40,000 cases per million people annually, 2009
- **Severity Level: 1–2**
  - Minimal (1) to mild (2) harm; generally uncomfortable
  - May require medical care if secondary infections occur

References: Emde (1961), Arora et al. (2020)

Scabies is a highly contagious skin infestation caused by the human itch mite, *Sarcoptes scabiei* var. *hominis*. These mites burrow into the outer layers of human skin, triggering intense itching and a rash. Scabies can spread rapidly in crowded or unhygienic conditions, especially in shared housing, shelters, or camps – environments sometimes encountered by ecological and environmental professionals during fieldwork or community studies.

Scabies mites do not survive more than 2–3 days away from human skin, and no animals are known to serve as a reservoir for the human-specific variety.

Symptoms

Symptoms typically begin 2–6 weeks after initial exposure, or within 1–4 days for re-exposures, and include:

- Intense itching, especially at night
- Red, irritated skin with burrow tracks or pimple-like rashes
- Crusting or thickened skin in crusted (Norwegian) scabies, which is highly contagious
- Secondary infections may result from scratching and open lesions

DOI: 10.1201/9781003745709-7

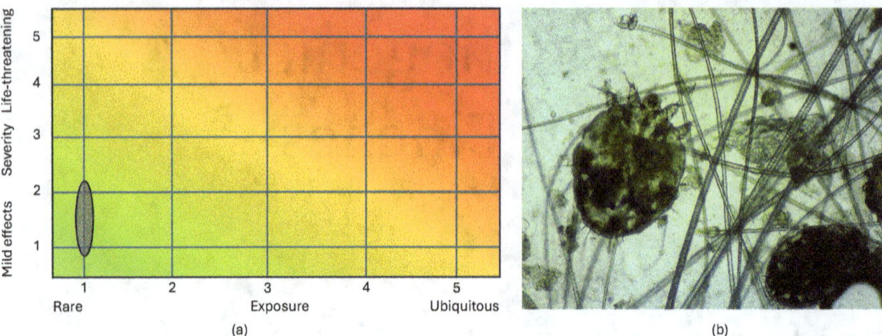

FIGURE 5.1 Scabies mites. (a) Exposure × severity matrix; (b) Scabies mite, *Sarcoptes scabiei* var *hominis*.

- Common sites include the wrists, elbows, armpits, fingers, waist, and buttocks
- Immunocompromised individuals may exhibit more severe symptoms

Occupational Exposure

Though not typically an environmental arthropod, scabies presents a risk when ecology or environmental professionals:

- Work near or within homeless encampments or emergency shelters
- Participate in urban stream or riparian surveys near encampments
- Conduct social-environmental health assessments
- Share bedding, towels, or clothing during field travel or disaster relief deployments
- Come into contact with crusted scabies cases, which can transmit via contaminated materials

Transmission generally requires prolonged skin contact, but crusted scabies may spread more readily through shared items.

Prevention

To avoid infestation:

- Wear protective clothing (long sleeves and pants) in areas of known exposure
- Avoid prolonged physical contact with potentially infested persons
- Bathe regularly and change clothing at least weekly
- Do not share clothing, bedding, or towels with others unless thoroughly washed
- Wash all linens and garments in hot water ($\geq$130°F) for 5–10 minutes
- Consider gloves when entering potentially infested indoor areas

Crusted scabies cases should be treated as highly contagious, requiring stricter isolation measures.

What To Do If Affected

- Seek medical evaluation if itching or rash appears 2–6 weeks after contact
- Diagnosis is usually clinical but may involve skin scrapings
- Treatment includes topical scabicides (e.g., permethrin) and, in some cases, oral ivermectin
- All household or group contacts should be treated simultaneously
- Avoid contact with others until treatment has begun

Prompt treatment effectively eliminates mites, but itching may persist for weeks as a post-infestation reaction.

ZOONOTIC MANGE

Entomological Parasites: Order Acariformes, Family Sarcoptidae: *Sarcoptes scabiei* var. *canis* (sarcoptic mange); Order Trombidiformes, Family Demodecidae: *Demodex* spp. (demodectic mange) (Figure 5.2)

Exposure and Severity Ratings (Figure 5.2)

- **Exposure Level: 1**
  - Rare (1), incidental contact only
- **Severity Level: 1**
  - Usually minimal (1): temporary irritation that resolves spontaneously
  - Animal-borne mange mites cannot live on or reproduce on humans

Reference: Arlian (1989)

Mange is a skin disease caused by mites that infest domestic and wild animals. While these mites are not host-adapted to humans, incidental contact can result in transient infestations or skin irritation. Two main types are encountered occupationally:

- Sarcoptic mange, caused by *Sarcoptes scabiei canis*, is highly contagious among animals and can temporarily affect humans

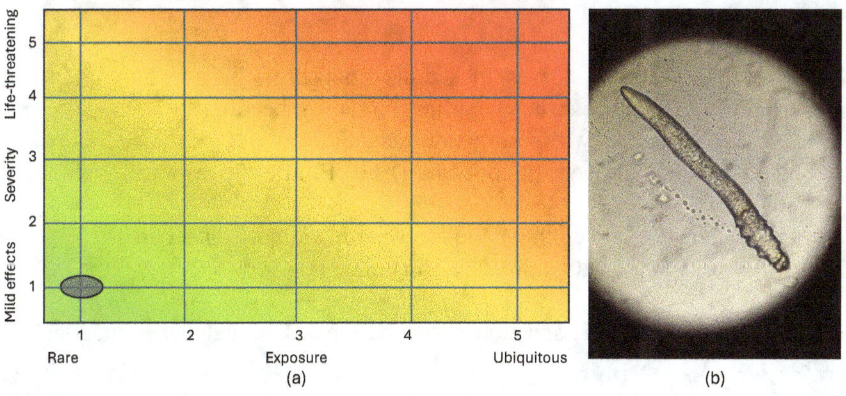

FIGURE 5.2 Zoonotic mange. (a) Exposure × severity matrix; (b) demodectic mange, *Demodex* sp.

- Demodectic mange, caused by *Demodex* spp., is generally less contagious and usually remains localized to individual animals

Mange mites do not complete their life cycle in humans, but their presence on the skin can lead to temporary discomfort and inflammatory reactions.

Symptoms

In humans, symptoms are usually mild and short-lived, appearing within 2–4 days of contact with an infested animal or contaminated bedding:

- Itching and redness, especially on arms, legs, and torso
- Localized rashes or papules
- Sores from scratching, which may become secondarily infected
- In rare cases, hypersensitivity reactions may occur in allergic individuals

Because these mites cannot reproduce on human skin, symptoms often resolve spontaneously once exposure ends.

Occupational Exposure

Risk is elevated for ecology and environmental professionals who:

- Handle wild or domestic animals, including injured or deceased specimens
- Enter dens, burrows, or animal shelters during environmental assessments
- Conduct urban ecology studies or work near homeless encampments where companion animals are present
- Perform structure inspections, particularly in abandoned or rodent-infested buildings

Field biologists, animal control personnel, and environmental health inspectors are among those at elevated risk.

Prevention

To reduce exposure:

- Wear long pants and sleeves, tucked into boots or socks
- Use disposable gloves when handling animals or bedding
- Avoid close contact with visibly infested animals
- Wash clothing and gear in hot water ($\geq$130°F) after fieldwork in high-risk areas
- Use designated field clothing and footwear in animal-contact areas
- Minimize contact with animal bedding or dens

Field workers should report and isolate visibly infested animals when practical and safe to do so.

What To Do If Affected

- Bathe immediately after exposure using soap and water
- Monitor for itching, rash, or irritation

- Most symptoms resolve without treatment, but consult a physician if:
  - Rash persists more than a week
  - Secondary infection develops
  - Hypersensitivity symptoms occur (e.g., severe itching, swelling, or hives)

No specific medical treatment is typically required for mild, transient human cases.

CHIGGERS

Entomological Parasites: Order Trombidiformes, Family Trombiculidae: several species of *Eutrombicula*, especially *E. alfreddugesi* in North America (Figure 5.3)

Exposure and Severity Ratings (Figure 5.3)

- **Exposure Level: 1–4**
  - Southeastern United States: 4 (ubiquitous and common in suitable habitat)
  - Midwest/Northeast: 2
  - Western United States/New England: 1 (generally absent)
- **Severity Level: 1–2**
  - Minimal (1) to mild (2) localized skin irritation
  - Medical treatment rarely required

References: Sasa (1961), Chen et al. (2022)

Chiggers are the larval stage of trombiculid mites, commonly encountered in warm, humid environments throughout the United States. While the chigger stage is nearly microscopic, the adult stage is a fairly large, red, velvety mite – easy to recognize and a warning that larval mites are surely in local vegetation. Contrary to myth, larval chiggers do not burrow into the skin; instead, they inject enzymes into the upper layers of the skin, digesting tissue externally and feeding on the liquefied material. This process triggers the immune system and causes intense itching and dermatitis in humans. Adult trombiculid mites do not bite.

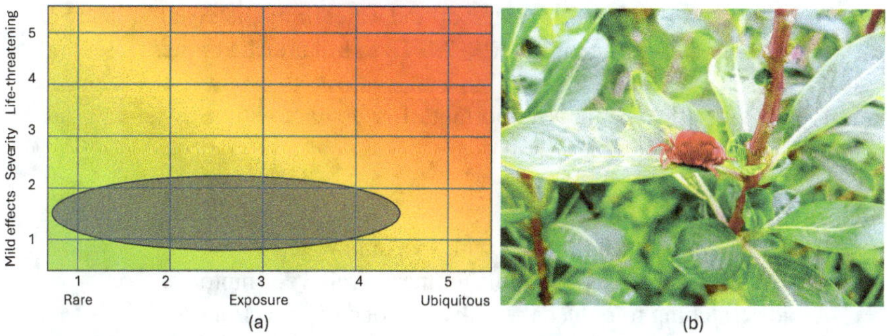

FIGURE 5.3   Chiggers. (a) Exposure × severity matrix; (b) adult trombiculid mite.

Chiggers are most active in late spring through early fall and thrive in dense, wet grass, brush, and edge habitats, including riparian areas, meadows, and forest margins.

Symptoms

Symptoms usually appear within hours to a day after exposure and include:

- Severe itching that may persist for days
- Red, swollen welts or pustules at feeding sites
- Preference for areas in which clothing fits tightly (e.g., waistbands, sock lines, armpits)
- In severe infestations, secondary infections may develop from scratching.
- In rare cases, allergic reactions may occur

While chiggers in North America are not known to transmit disease, some species on other continents can be vectors of scrub typhus.

Occupational Exposure

Ecology and environmental professionals are at risk during:

- Terrestrial field surveys, especially in tall grass or brush
- Wetland delineation and riparian habitat work
- Dam, levee, or structure inspections in natural vegetation
- Monitoring drilling or construction activities in overgrown areas

Exposure is most likely when sitting, kneeling, or walking through infested wet vegetation, particularly in southeastern U.S. states, where chiggers are most abundant.

Prevention

Preventive strategies include:

- Wearing long pants tucked into socks or boots, and long-sleeved shirts
- Applying DEET-based repellents to skin and clothing
- Treating clothing with permethrin, especially around waist and cuffs
- Avoiding sitting or lying directly on the ground in infested areas
- Bathing and scrubbing skin with soap and water immediately after fieldwork
- Laundering clothes in hot water ($\geq 130°F$) to kill attached mites

Preventive hygiene is especially important after contact with grassland or riparian vegetation.

What To Do If Affected

- Wash affected skin thoroughly with soap and water.
- Apply anti-itch creams or antihistamines to relieve symptoms.
- Avoid scratching to reduce the risk of secondary infections.
- If itching or swelling persists for more than a week, consult a physician

Although uncomfortable, chigger bites are not medically serious in most cases and resolve within 7–10 days.

MISCELLANEOUS MITES

Entomological Parasites: Order Mesostigmata, Family Dermanyssidae: *Liponyssoides sanguineus* (house mouse mite), Family Macronyssidae: *Ornithonyssus bacoti* (tropical rat mite), *Ornithonyssus sylviarum* (northern fowl mite); Order Sarcoptiformes, Family Acaridae: *Tyrophagus putrescentiae* (mold mite), and others (Figure 5.4)

Exposure and Severity Ratings (Figure 5.4)

- **Exposure Level: 2**
  - Tend to be uncommon (2), localized depending on environment and habitat disturbance
- **Severity Level: 1–2**
  - Primarily nuisance with minimal (1) to mild (2) symptoms
  - Treatable and self-limiting in most cases

References: Sasa (1961), Chen et al. (2022)

A diverse group of mites outside the typical scabies and dust mite categories can affect environmental and ecological professionals, often through incidental contact with infested animals, abandoned structures, or damp organic materials. These mites include:

- *Liponyssoides sanguineus, Ornithonyssus bacoti* (rodent mites): Parasite of rats and mice that may bite humans after host removal or death
- *Ornithonyssus sylviarum, Dermanyssus gallinae* (poultry mites): found in chicken coops, roosts, or bird nests; may also bite humans
- *Tyrophagus putrescentiae* (mold mite): Thrives in moist, moldy materials or decaying plant matter; does not bite but can cause respiratory irritation if inhaled

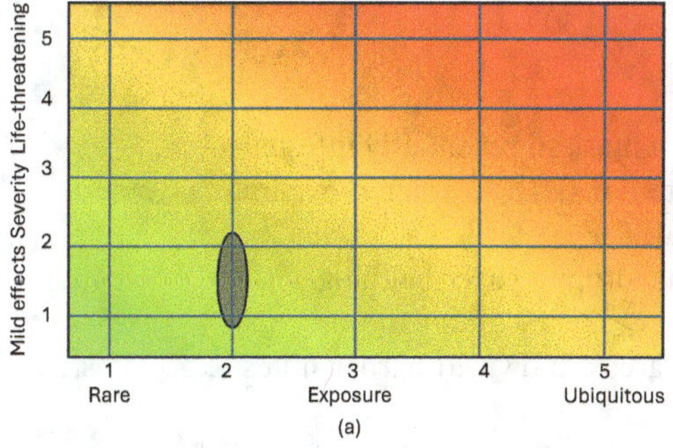

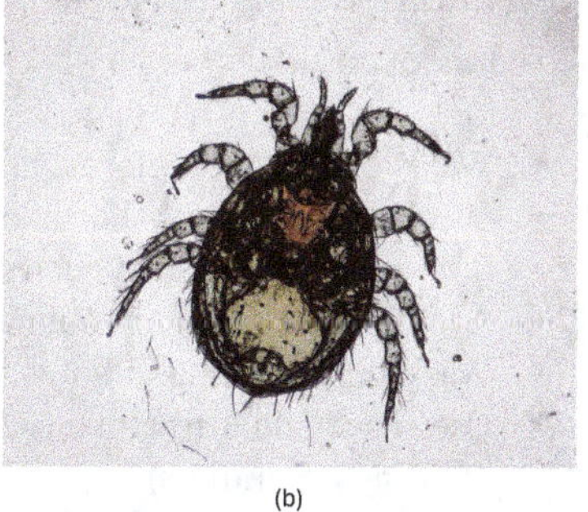

FIGURE 5.4 Miscellaneous mites. (a) Exposure × severity matrix; (b) tropical rat mite, *Ornithonyssus bacoti*.

- Stored product mites (e.g., *Acarus siro*): Can infest grain, flour, and food stores, especially in neglected or humid environments; can likewise cause respiratory irritation if inhaled or ocular irritation if the eye is exposed

While most of these mites do not typically feed on humans, many will bite opportunistically, leaving itchy red welts or causing allergic reactions.

Symptoms

Symptoms depend on the species and exposure type but may include:

- Red, itchy bites, especially on exposed skin
- Localized rashes or papules, often linear or grouped
- Allergic responses such as sneezing, runny nose, or asthma (especially with mold mites)
- Irritation in respiratory tract or skin from airborne mites in infested environments
- Mite dermatitis, particularly in people with frequent exposure to birds or rodents

Because bites may resemble those of bed bugs or fleas, identification of the source is often delayed.

Occupational Exposure

Ecology and environmental professionals may encounter miscellaneous mites during:

- Structure inspections in rodent-infested or derelict buildings
- Fieldwork near abandoned houses, barns, or poultry coops
- Handling of birds, rodents, or animal nests
- Entering crawlspaces, attics, or silos
- Sorting moldy materials, such as compost or food waste
- Long-term storage of botanical or biological samples

Environments with high humidity and organic debris are ideal habitats for many mite species.

Prevention

To reduce exposure:

- Wear long sleeves, gloves, and a mask in potentially infested areas.
- Use High-Efficiency Particulate Air (HEPA)-filtered respirators when disturbing moldy or dusty materials.
- Avoid contact with animal nests, droppings, or bedding.
- Wash field clothing in hot water ($\geq 130°F$) after exposure.
- Use insecticidal treatments in areas known to harbor mites (e.g., infested buildings or trailers).
- Store supplies in dry, sealed containers to prevent infestation.

Minimizing contact with infested animals and environments is the best defense.

What To Do If Affected

- Shower and change clothes immediately after exposure
- Wash clothing, bedding, and gear in hot water
- Apply anti-itch creams or antihistamines for bites or allergic symptoms
- Seek medical attention if symptoms persist, worsen, or bites become infected
- In cases of infestation in structures or trailers, professional pest control may be needed

Most infestations resolve once the environmental source (e.g., rodents or moisture) is eliminated.

WIDOW SPIDERS

Entomological Agents: Order Araneae, Family Theridiidae: *Latrodectus mactans* **(southern black widow),** *L. hesperus* **(western black widow),** *L. geometricus* **(brown widow),** *L. bishopi* **(red widow) (Figure 5.5)**

Exposure and Severity Ratings (Figure 5.5)

- **Exposure Level: 3**
  - Moderately (3) common in field and equipment maintenance settings, especially in southern and western regions

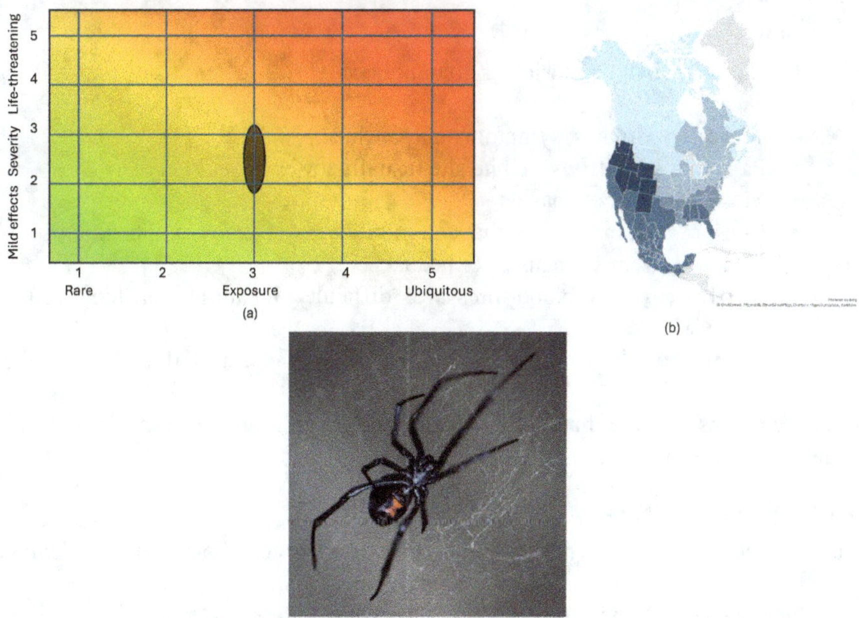

FIGURE 5.5 Widow spiders. (a) Exposure × severity matrix; (b) geographic distribution; (c) black widow spider, *Latrodectus mactans*.

- All 50 states have reported widow spiders, but sometimes imported, and extremely rare in some states
- U.S. poison control centers report ~2,500 cases of black widow envenomations/year
- **Severity Level: 2–3**
  - Bite effects range from mild (2) to moderately (3) painful
  - Mortality exceedingly rare with modern medical treatment: 0 fatalities in 1,015 cases tracked in 2018

References: Diaz (2004), Vetter and Isbister (2008), Vetter (2013), Caruso et al. (2021)

Widow spiders (*Latrodectus* spp.) are medically significant arachnids found throughout North America and many other parts of the world. The black widow is the most famous, known for its glossy black coloration and red hourglass marking, though coloration can vary by species, sex, and age. The brown widow is lighter in color with an orange hourglass, and the red widow is a rare Florida endemic with red legs and a reddish-orange cephalothorax.

Widow spiders are reclusive and non-aggressive, typically found in dark, sheltered environments such as woodpiles, garages, sheds, animal enclosures, electrical boxes, and outhouses. They spin irregular, sticky webs close to the ground or inside cavities. Bites occur when they are accidentally disturbed, often during manual labor or outdoor work.

Their venom contains latrotoxin, which affects nerve terminals, leading to systemic symptoms known as latrodectism.

Symptoms

Initial bite may feel like a pinprick or go unnoticed.

- Within 15–60 minutes, symptoms may include:
  - Pain spreading from the bite site (usually lower extremities)
  - Muscle cramps or spasms
  - Chest or abdominal pain that can mimic a heart attack or appendicitis
  - Sweating, tremors, nausea, or headache
  - Rarely: elevated blood pressure, difficulty breathing, or localized paralysis
- Symptoms typically peak within 1–6 hours and may last for days

Severe reactions are rare, but children, the elderly, and immunocompromised individuals are at greater risk.

Occupational Exposure

Widow spiders are encountered by ecology and environmental professionals during:

- Fieldwork involving firewood, logs, brush, and outdoor debris
- Inspection or repair of equipment stored in sheds, barns, or under buildings
- Handling of camping gear, tarps, or equipment left outside
- Restoration or demolition of older structures

- Agricultural or conservation work in semi-arid or subtropical regions
- Military field training, utility maintenance, or landscaping

They are most common in Southern and Western United States but are found nationwide, especially in warmer months.

Prevention

- Wear heavy gloves when handling brush, firewood, or stored equipment
- Inspect and shake out gloves, boots, or clothing left outdoors
- Store gear off the ground and in sealed containers when possible
- Avoid placing hands into dark crevices or under debris without visibility
- Regularly inspect and clean outdoor storage areas, sheds, and field stations
- Use residual insecticides in known infested areas if necessary

Brown widows tend to be less aggressive and more likely to retreat than black widows but still possess venom.

What To Do If Affected

- Wash bite site with soap and water
- Apply ice to reduce swelling and pain
- Seek medical attention for:
  - Severe pain
  - Systemic symptoms (muscle cramping, sweating, chest pain)
  - Bites in very young, elderly, or immunocompromised individuals
- Antivenom is available but typically reserved for severe cases; most recover without it
- Hospitalization is rare but may be needed for pain control or observation

Early treatment with analgesics and muscle relaxants can reduce the severity of symptoms.

BROWN RECLUSE SPIDER

Entomological Agent: Order Araneae, Family Sicariidae: *Loxosceles reclusa* (brown recluse) (Figure 5.6)

Exposure and Severity Ratings (Figure 5.6)

- **Exposure Level: 1–3**
  - Native range of brown recluse is from southeastern NE, KS, OK, and north/central TX east to southern IN, western KY and TN, and small parts of GA
  - In infested, neglected structures within the native range, these spiders may be moderately (3) abundant
  - Outside of that range, they are rare (1), likely an accidental, non-established introduction
  - Brown recluse does not occur in Mexico or Canada, but Mexico and states from CA to TX have other species of *Loxosceles*

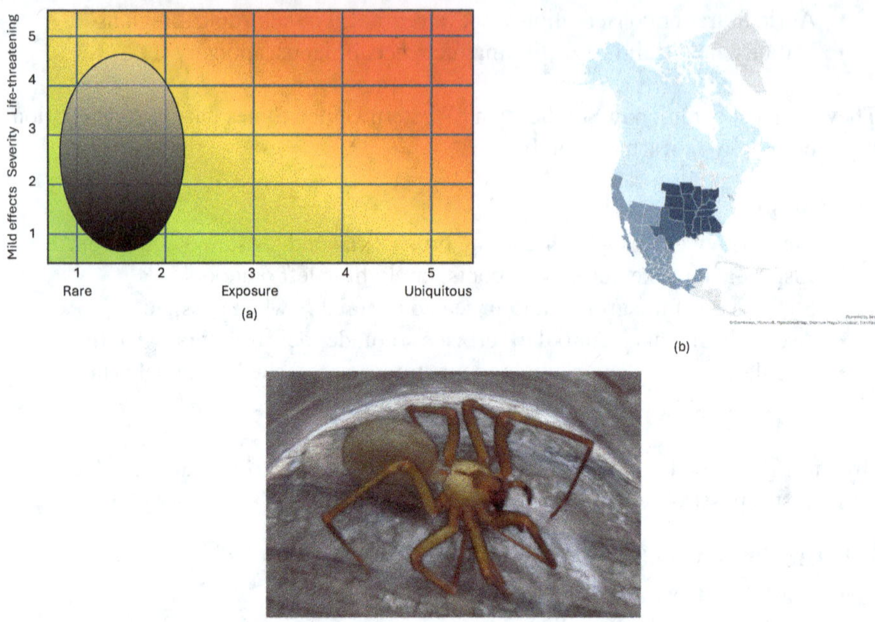

FIGURE 5.6 Brown recluse spider. (a) Exposure × severity matrix; (b) geographic distribution; (c) brown recluse spider, *Loxosceles reclusa*.

- **Severity Level: 1–4**
  - Minimal (1) to mild (2) reaction in most cases
  - Very rare but severe (4) dermonecrosis or systemic effects possible

References: Bennett and Vetter (2004), Diaz (2004), Sandidge and Hopwood (2005), Furbee et al. (2006), Vetter and Isbister (2008), Vetter (2013)

The brown recluse is a small, secretive spider known for its necrotic bite, which has earned it a dangerous reputation – often exaggerated. Native to the southcentral United States, this spider prefers undisturbed indoor areas, such as attics, closets, basements, and storage sheds. It can also be found under rocks, bark, or debris in dry outdoor environments.

Brown recluse spiders are non-aggressive, and bites usually occur when the spider is trapped against the skin (e.g., inside clothing, gloves, or shoes). While many bites are minor or even unnoticed, a small percentage develop serious dermonecrosis. Systemic symptoms are rare but possible.

Due to widespread misidentification, hundreds of brown recluse spider bites are falsely reported every year from across the United States and often blamed for unrelated skin infections. For example, from 1988 to 1996, 66 spider bites were reported as brown recluse out of 246 bites in the Pacific Northwest, where brown recluse spiders are nearly non-existent. Their color pattern with dark brown legs and abdomen and lighter brown cephalothorax is similar to several other spiders, but brown recluse spiders should be easily identified by the violin-shaped marking on their cephalothorax.

Symptoms

Initial bite may be painless or mildly irritating.

- Within 2–8 hours, localized redness, swelling, and blistering may appear
- In some cases:
  - Tissue necrosis, forming an ulcer or eschar (black scab-like encrustation) that may take weeks to heal
  - Secondary infection of open wounds
  - Rare systemic symptoms: fever, chills, nausea, malaise, hemolysis, or kidney dysfunction (most common in children)

Most bites resolve without necrosis; only a minority progress to serious lesions.

Occupational Exposure

Risk to ecology and environmental professionals is elevated in:

- Abandoned or infrequently accessed buildings
- Storage areas, closets, or old equipment lockers
- Warehouses, attics, basements, or supply sheds
- Field work involving old woodpiles, barns, or rural structures
- Handling stored gear, boots, or clothing not used for long periods

They are often accidentally transported in equipment or materials.

Prevention
- Shake out clothing, boots, and gloves before use if stored in suspect areas
- Wear protective gloves when working in dark or cluttered spaces
- Reduce clutter and seal cracks or crevices in buildings
- Use sticky traps and exclusion techniques in indoor environments
- Educate staff on correct spider identification to avoid panic or misdiagnosis
- In endemic areas, inspect cardboard boxes, as they can be attracted to the corrugated surfaces

Do not assume necrotic lesions are brown recluse spider bites unless spider is seen and positively identified.

What To Do If Affected
- Clean the area with soap and water
- Apply cold compresses but avoid excessive pressure
- Do not incise or apply chemicals to the wound
- Seek medical care if:
  - Necrosis develops
  - There is persistent pain or systemic symptoms
  - The wound fails to heal or becomes infected
- Documentation (photographs) of the lesion can help in monitoring progression

Medical professionals may prescribe antibiotics, corticosteroids, or surgical care if needed.

HOBO SPIDER

Entomological Agent: Order Araneae, Family Agelenidae: *Eratigena agrestis* (Hobo spider) (Figure 5.7)
   Exposure and Severity Ratings (Figure 5.7)

- **Exposure Level: 1**
  - Introduced from Europe and now localized to Pacific Northwest (southern BC south to OR and inland to MT, UT, and possibly far western CO)
  - Rare (1) even within its naturalized range due to specific indoor habitats
- **Severity Level: 0–1**
  - Typical case (if any): 0–1
  - Necrosis/systemic symptoms: 0 (now considered unlikely)

References: Baird and Stoltz (2002), Bennett and Vetter (2004), Diaz (2004), Vetter and Isbister (2008), Vetter (2013)

The hobo spider is a non-aggressive, ground-dwelling spider originally native to Europe and now established in the Pacific Northwest and parts of the northern United States. It builds funnel-shaped webs in cracks, basements, rock walls, and other undisturbed spaces, typically near ground level.

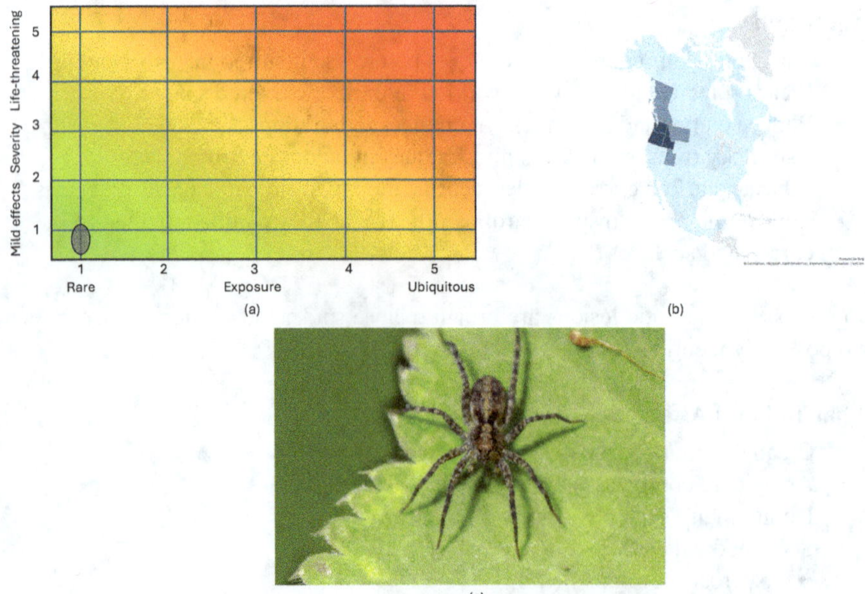

FIGURE 5.7 Hobo spider. (a) Exposure × severity matrix; (b) geographic distribution; (c) hobo spider, *Eratigena agrestis*.

Historically labeled as "medically significant," the hobo spider has been controversially linked to necrotic bites, but current research suggests that it is not a major cause of dermonecrosis in humans. Most bites attributed to hobo spiders are unverified, and the species has been cleared of serious medical concern by many toxicologists.

Still, ecology and environmental professionals in areas with dense populations may encounter these spiders in homes, field structures, or excavation zones, where fear or misidentification (this spider looks like most other species in the Agelenidae family) may disrupt work or cause inappropriate responses.

Symptoms

Rare and poorly documented in confirmed cases

- If bitten, possible localized pain, redness, or mild swelling
- Earlier reports of ulceration or necrosis have not been reliably replicated
- No evidence of systemic envenomation in verified exposures
- Misdiagnosed infections, abscesses, or pressure wounds are commonly mistaken for spider bites

The lack of confirmed serious cases suggests that hobo spider bites are mild or medically insignificant.

Occupational Exposure

Ecology and environmental professionals may encounter hobo spiders in:

- Basements, garages, sheds, and crawlspaces, especially in the Pacific Northwest
- Rock piles, wood stacks, or outbuildings
- Construction, plumbing, or Heating, Ventilation, and Air Conditioning (HVAC) work in older structures
- Field stations, remote cabins, or restoration sites with cluttered storage
- Ecological surveys involving ground debris or pitfall traps

They prefer dry, low-light areas, often near manmade structures.

Prevention
- Wear gloves when working in storage areas or ground-level structures
- Keep clothing and bedding off the floor in spider-prone buildings
- Seal cracks and crevices where spiders may enter
- Use indoor traps for monitoring, not control
- Teach workers to distinguish hobo spiders from recluse and harmless species
- Discourage overreaction — hobo spiders do not chase or seek out humans, and bites are rare
- Routine sanitation is the best deterrent to indoor web-building

What To Do If Affected
- Wash the area with soap and water
- Apply ice or a cold compress for pain or swelling

- Monitor for changes – if a lesion develops, photograph and seek evaluation
- Avoid self-treatment with chemicals or incisions
- Seek medical care for any persistent or worsening wound, regardless of spider involvement
- Report suspected bites in occupational settings, but emphasize the low risk from this species

Documentation helps differentiate spider bites from methicillin-resistant *Staphylococcus aureus* (MRSA) or other skin infections.

SAC SPIDERS

Entomological Agents: Order Araneae, Family Cheiracanthiidae: *Cheiracanthium mildei* **and** *C. inclusum* **(yellow sac spiders) (Figure 5.8)**
  Exposure and Severity Ratings (Figure 5.8)

- **Exposure Level: 2–3**
  - Uncommon (2) to moderate (3) exposure in indoor, field, and agricultural settings, particularly at night
- **Severity Level: 1–2**
  - Minimal (1) bite reaction
  - Rarely, mild (2) necrosis or systemic symptoms

References: Diaz (2004), Vetter et al. (2006), Vetter and Isbister (2008), Vetter (2013)

Sac spiders are small, pale yellow or cream-colored hunting spiders that do not build webs to catch prey. Instead, they construct small silk sacs, often in leaf folds, wall corners, or beneath bark, which serve as resting places during the day. Two species, the introduced *Cheiracanthium mildei* and the native *C. inclusum*, are frequently encountered indoors or in vegetation, especially in agricultural, horticultural, and forested settings.

These spiders are known for occasionally biting humans when trapped against the skin, particularly at night. Their venom is cytotoxic, and while almost all bites are medically minor, a few may cause localized tissue damage.

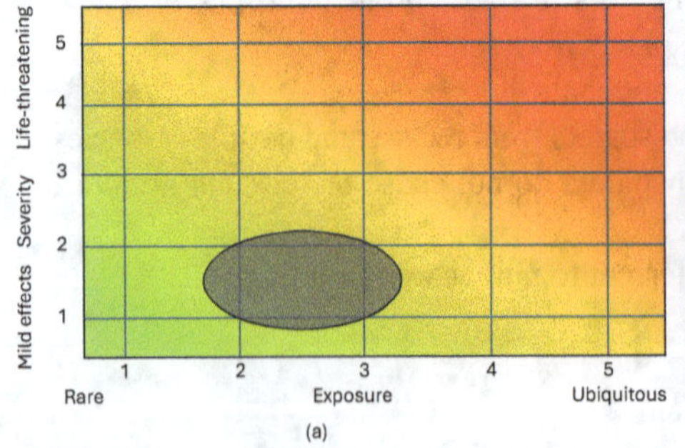

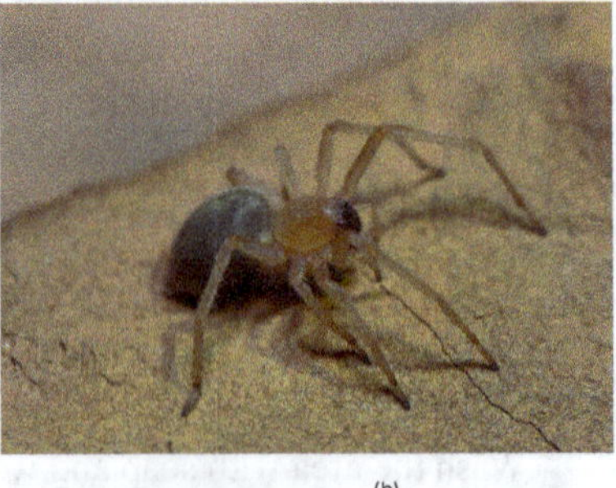

FIGURE 5.8   Sac spiders. (a) Exposure × severity matrix; (b) yellow sac spider, *Cheiracanthium* sp.

Symptoms

Often occur at night, possibly while sleeping or resting

- Sharp, initial pain, followed by redness, swelling, and itching
- In few cases, bites may develop into small ulcers or necrotic lesions (~5–10 mm)
- In rare cases:
  - Secondary infection
  - Mild flu-like symptoms (fatigue, low-grade fever, malaise)
- Bites typically resolve without treatment within 7–10 days.

Bites are usually defensive and not due to aggression.

Occupational Exposure

Sac spiders may be encountered by ecology and environmental professionals in:

- Homes, labs, greenhouses, or storage spaces where they hide in crevices
- Leafy vegetation, rolled leaves, or beneath bark during field surveys
- Overnight stays in cabins, bunkhouses, or field stations
- Horticultural and agricultural settings, especially low shrubs and row crops
- Indoor work in cluttered offices or facilities with poor exclusion or pest control

Bites are most common when workers or students accidentally trap spiders against skin.

Prevention

- Shake out clothing, bedding, gloves, and boots before use, especially in spider-prone areas
- Wear long sleeves and gloves when working in dense vegetation or storage areas
- Seal cracks and crevices indoors to prevent entry
- Reduce clutter and remove unused cardboard, boxes, or leaf litter
- Encourage staff to recognize sac spiders and avoid panic over minor bites
- Avoid letting bed linens or clothes drape onto the floor in field accommodations

Sac spiders are not aggressive and generally try to avoid human contact.

What To Do If Affected

- Clean the area with soap and water
- Apply a cold compress to reduce swelling
- Use antihistamines or nonsteroidal anti-inflammatory drugs (NSAIDs) for itching or pain
- Monitor the bite for ulceration or infection
- Seek medical care if:
  - The lesion enlarges or becomes necrotic
  - Systemic symptoms develop
  - The area does not improve within 5–7 days

In most cases, no advanced treatment is required.

TARANTULAS

Entomological Agents: Order Araneae, Family Theraphosidae: *Aphonopelma*, *Brachypelma*, and related genera (Figure 5.9)
Exposure and Severity Ratings (Figure 5.9)

- **Exposure Level: 1–2**
  - Rare (1) to uncommon (2) in localized desert environments
  - Often used as pets or entomological demonstration animals
- **Severity Level: 1–3**
  - Bite usually results in minimal (1) harm as a minor irritation
  - Urticating hairs can cause mild (1) skin irritation to moderate (3) eye or (rarely) respiratory concerns

Reference: Jalink and Wisse (2021)

Tarantulas are large, hairy, ground-dwelling spiders found primarily in arid and semi-arid environments, especially in the Southwestern United States and Central America. Despite their intimidating appearance, most tarantulas are docile and non-aggressive, and their venom is not medically significant to healthy humans. That said, some tarantula species are somewhat more aggressive than others.

The primary medical risk from tarantulas comes not from their bite but from their urticating hairs – barbed, microscopic bristles that can be released from the abdomen when the spider feels threatened. These hairs can cause skin irritation and eye

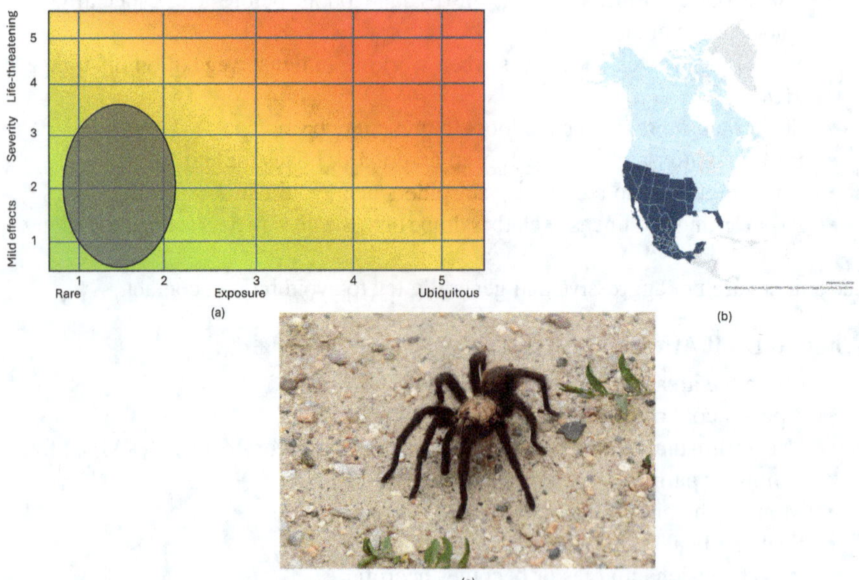

FIGURE 5.9 Tarantulas. (a) Exposure × severity matrix; (b) geographic distribution; (c) Texas brown tarantula, *Aphonopelma hentzi*.

or respiratory inflammation in sensitive individuals, especially in enclosed spaces or after handling.

Tarantulas may wander into field camps or buildings during mating season or be encountered during burrow surveys, rock flipping, or desert work.

In addition to the minor risk from bites, a major transportation and operations risk comes when male tarantulas "migrate" in search of mates during late summer and early fall. This risk is addressed separately below.

Symptoms

- Bite (rare):
  - Mild pain, puncture marks, redness, and localized swelling
  - No significant venom effects in U.S. species
- Urticating hairs:
  - Itchy, red, inflamed skin (contact dermatitis)
  - Eye irritation or conjunctivitis if hairs contact mucous membranes
  - Inhalation can cause sneezing, coughing, or asthma-like symptoms in sensitive individuals
- Severe systemic reactions are extremely rare but possible in allergic individuals

Handling captive tarantulas can also cause sensitization over time.

Occupational Exposure

Tarantulas may be encountered by ecology and environmental professionals in:

- Desert and scrub habitats of the American Southwest
- Burrow and soil sampling, especially during monsoon or mating seasons
- Field stations, cabins, or campsites, particularly at night
- Bioblitzes or educational outreach, where tarantulas may be handled
- Pet trade or lab work involving captive specimens

Male tarantulas are more likely to wander in open areas during the late summer and fall.

Prevention

- Do not handle tarantulas unnecessarily, especially without gloves
- Avoid brushing or disturbing the abdomen, which may trigger urticating hair release
- Wear long sleeves and eye protection when working in dense desert vegetation or burrows
- Keep field accommodations sealed, especially at floor level
- Educate personnel that tarantulas are not dangerous and do not chase or attack
- Handle captive species in well-ventilated areas, and avoid touching eyes or face afterward

Instruct students and workers to treat tarantulas with respect and caution, not fear.

What To Do If Affected

- Bite:
  - Clean with soap and water
  - Apply cold compress for swelling
  - Take analgesics or antihistamines as needed
- Urticating hairs:
  - Gently remove loose hairs with tape or sticky lint roller
  - Rinse eyes or mucous membranes with clean water or saline
  - Seek medical care if respiratory symptoms, eye pain, or persistent rash develops
- Monitor for signs of secondary infection or allergic response

There is no antivenom or specific treatment required in North American cases.

CAMEL/WIND/SUN SPIDERS (SOLIFUGES)

Entomological Agents: Order Solifugae: *Eremobates*, *Galeodes*, and related genera (Figure 5.10)

    Exposure and Severity Ratings (Figure 5.10)

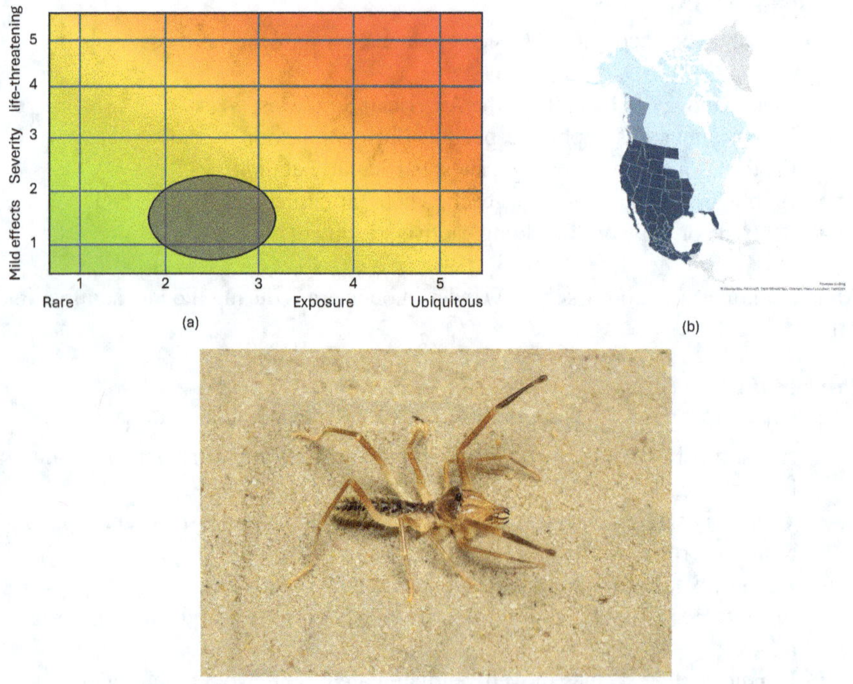

FIGURE 5.10 Solifuges. (a) Exposure×severity matrix; (b) geographic distribution; (c) camel spider, Solifugae.

- **Exposure Level: 2–3**
  - Uncommon (2) to moderately (3) common in arid and semi-arid environments from the CA deserts to TX and CO
  - Rarely encountered outside of this range
- **Severity Level: 1–2**
  - Bites can range from minimal (1) to mild (2) due to pain
  - Non-venomous, but bites can be deep, inducing possibility of secondary infections
  - Mild (2) psychological disruption due to myths and startling appearance

References: Muma (1970), Mullen (2019)

Camel spiders, also called wind scorpions, sun spiders, or solifuges, are fast-moving, non-venomous arachnids found in arid and semi-arid environments worldwide, especially in the Southwestern United States, Middle East, and Africa. Despite sensational myths originating during the Persian Gulf War in 1991, camel spiders do not achieve the size of dinner plates (they are usually less than 30 mm/1.25 in.), do not possess venom, do not chase humans to attack, and cannot kill livestock or people.

However, they are equipped with powerful, pincer-like chelicerae, capable of delivering painful bites if handled or trapped. The bite is mechanical, not venomous, and may result in bleeding, localized swelling, or risk of infection if not cleaned properly.

They are primarily nocturnal predators, emerging at night to hunt insects and small animals, and may seek shelter during the day in cool, shaded areas, including gear, tents, or under rocks.

Symptoms

- Painful mechanical bite, similar to a laceration or pinch
- Redness, localized swelling, possible bruising or bleeding
- Risk of secondary infection if wound is not cleaned
- No venom, no systemic envenomation symptoms
- Psychological effects (fear, anxiety) often exaggerated by myths

Bites are rare, and solifuges usually flee rather than confront humans.

Occupational Exposure

Encounters by ecology and environmental professionals may occur in:

- Desert and scrubland habitats, especially in Southwestern United States and arid international field sites
- Under rocks, logs, tents, or stored equipment
- Nocturnal fieldwork or camping
- Pitfall trapping, burrow studies, or excavation
- Sleeping on the ground, where solifuges may wander into bedding or shoes

They are active at night and avoid bright light.

Prevention

- Shake out boots, sleeping bags, and clothing before use
- Avoid sleeping directly on the ground in arid zones – use cots or tarps
- Wear gloves when working around rocks or debris
- Keep camp gear elevated and zipped closed when not in use
- Educate workers: camel spiders are not venomous and do not pursue people aggressively
- Do not handle solifuges; they can deliver deep, surprising bites

Public perception often exaggerates their threat; training can reduce fear and overreaction.

What To Do If Affected

- Clean the wound thoroughly with soap and water
- Apply a clean bandage and cold compress for swelling
- Use oral pain relievers or antihistamines if needed
- Monitor for signs of infection (increasing redness, warmth, pus)
- Seek medical attention for deep bites, facial wounds, or signs of secondary infection
- Tetanus update may be appropriate for puncture wounds

Since these organisms are not venomous, there is no antivenom – treatment is supportive only.

CRUSTACEANS

CRABS, CRAYFISH, AMPHIPODS, AND ISOPODS

Entomological Agents: Order Decapoda, notably freshwater crayfish in the families Cambaridae and Astacidae, and various shoreline or estuarine crabs; Order Amphipoda, Family Talitridae; and Order Isopoda, Families Armadillidiidae and Porcellionidae; and a few others (Figure 5.11)

Exposure and Severity Ratings (Figure 5.11)

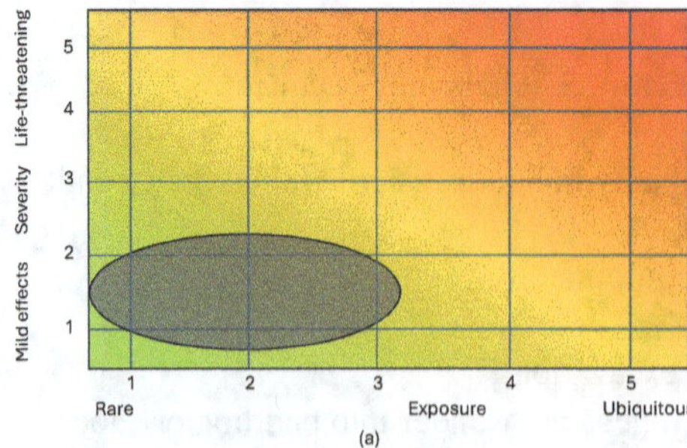

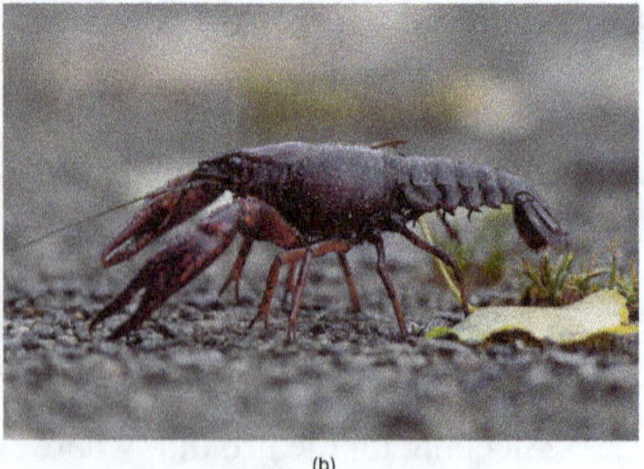

FIGURE 5.11 Crayfish. (a) Exposure × severity matrix; (b) red crayfish, *Procambarus clarkii.*

- **Exposure Level: 1–3**
  - Crayfish and amphipods are common (3) in streams, wetlands, and shallow freshwater bodies throughout North America, a few are estuarine
  - Crabs are more localized (1), found primarily in coastal or brackish environments, salt marshes, and estuaries
  - Isopods are common (3) in damp terrestrial habitats; under logs, leaf litter, stones, or even within manmade structures
- **Severity Level: 1–2**
  - Crayfish and crab pinches range from mild (1) to moderate (2) depending on species size and claw strength
  - Some talitrid amphipods have been known to nibble on exposed human flesh, but the severity is mild (1), at most
  - No venom; risk is primarily mechanical trauma or secondary infection

Reference: Claussen et al. (2007)

Crabs and crayfish are decapod crustaceans with ten legs, including a prominent pair of front claws (chelae) used for feeding, defense, and display. These animals are not aggressive but will defend themselves when threatened. Crayfish are commonly encountered by environmental professionals during freshwater stream sampling, aquatic invertebrate surveys, and hydrological work. Crabs, though less often encountered inland, may be found in coastal estuarine systems, marsh restoration sites, or marine-adjacent environmental zones.

Isopods and amphipods often go unnoticed in health and safety assessments due to their small size and non-aggressive behavior. However, in certain settings, these arthropods may emerge in large numbers or display behaviors (e.g., biting or foul odors) that justify their inclusion in environmental health and safety planning. Talitrid amphipods, often called "beach hoppers" or "sand fleas," are known to inhabit coastal wrack zones, freshwater shores, and damp detritus. While they are mostly scavengers, some species are known to bite exposed human skin, causing minor pinching sensations or small abrasions, especially when field personnel rest on wet sand or wade through wrack lines during night surveys or beach work.

Terrestrial isopods, such as sowbugs and pillbugs, are frequently encountered in damp terrestrial habitats, from logs, leaf litter, and stones, to manmade structures like pump houses, field equipment storage, or moist crawl spaces. While they do not bite, the pungent odor released when disturbed or crushed can make them a minor nuisance.

Most interactions with crustaceans are harmless, but crabs and crayfish are capable of delivering painful pinches if handled carelessly. Large crayfish, in particular, may not release their grip until forcibly removed. While these injuries are not medically serious in most cases, they can break the skin, and care should be taken to avoid secondary infection – especially when working in brackish or stagnant water.

Symptoms
- Mild to moderate pinching pain
- Puncture wounds or abrasions from claw tips
- Swelling, redness, or bruising at the site
- Rare: infection from waterborne bacteria (e.g., *Aeromonas, Pseudomonas*) in open wounds

Occupational Exposure

Crabs, crayfish, and amphipods may be encountered in the following contexts:

- Stream and wetland surveys, while turning rocks, setting traps, or sampling benthic macroinvertebrates
- Estuarine or marsh restoration projects, particularly in tidal or wrack zones
- Hydrological or water quality monitoring, working in shallow bodies of water
- Shoreline inspections, dredging prep, or riparian construction; encounters with shoreline crabs are possible
- Excavations near aquatic habitats, especially if moisture attracts burrowing crayfish
- Isopods are more commonly encountered when
  - Overnight camping or resting on moist ground, sand, or forest floors
  - Working around structures with high humidity or organic decay
  - Storing field gear or clothing in damp environments

Prevention

- Wear sturdy, water-resistant gloves when working in aquatic environments
- Handle crayfish and crabs with care; grasp animals gently but securely on the carapace, out of reach of the claws
- Avoid sticking bare hands into underwater crevices or debris piles
- Educate workers about expected crustacean species and handling precautions
- Clean and disinfect hands and minor injuries promptly after aquatic work
- Avoid resting or sleeping directly on sand or wrack during coastal or freshwater work
- Use ground cloths or tents with sealed bases in known amphipod habitats
- Store gear off the ground in dry, sealed containers
- Inspect clothing, boots, and bedding after working in wet or decaying environments
- Maintain cleanliness in field labs, trailers, or portable structures to reduce attraction

What To Do If Affected

- Gently disengage the animal – do not yank or shake it off, as this may tear skin
- Wash the affected area thoroughly with soap and clean water
- Apply antiseptic and bandage if needed
- Monitor for signs of infection (redness, spreading warmth, pus)
- Seek medical care if wound worsens, becomes infected, or if tetanus vaccination is outdated

Crustaceans are generally harmless, but awareness and respectful handling can prevent unnecessary discomfort or complications.

MYRIAPODS

Centipedes

Entomological Agents: Class Chilopoda: *Scolopendra*, *Lithobius*, *Scutigera*, and other genera (Figure 5.12)
  Exposure and Severity Ratings (Figure 5.12)

- **Exposure Level: 1–4**
  - Present across North America: some species are rare (1), while others may be frequently (4) encountered
  - Common in field settings, especially in warm, damp environments, under logs, rocks, debris
- **Severity Level: 1–3**
  - Most species yield a minimal (1) to mild (2) bite
  - Large *Scolopendra* species can deliver significant, moderate (3) localized pain; however, medical attention is rarely required

References: Kevan (1983), Ombati et al. (2018)

Centipedes are elongated, multi-legged arthropods found worldwide, especially in tropical, subtropical, and temperate environments. While most species are small and harmless, larger tropical or desert centipedes, such as those in the genus *Scolopendra*, are capable of painful envenomation via forcipules, modified front legs that inject venom into prey or perceived threats.

Though centipedes are not aggressive, they will bite in self-defense if handled or accidentally contacted. Their venom is not fatal to humans, but can cause significant pain, localized tissue effects, and occasional systemic symptoms in sensitive individuals.

Centipedes are most active at night and favor dark, damp, or sheltered locations.

Symptoms

- Immediate sharp pain, often described as burning or stabbing
- Redness, swelling, bruising, and occasionally numbness or tingling at the bite site

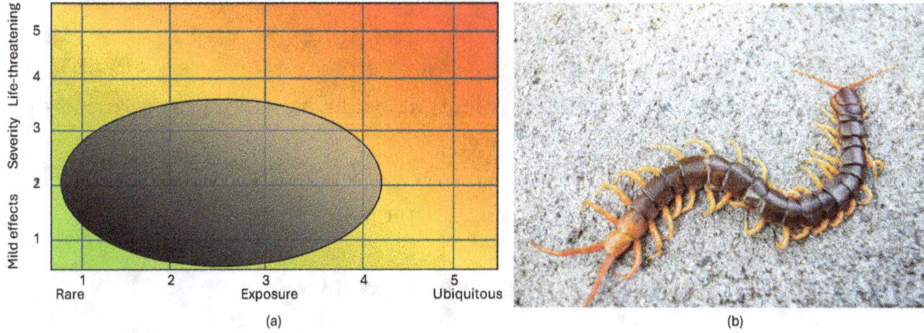

FIGURE 5.12 Centipedes. (a) Exposure × severity matrix; (b) centipede, *Scolopendra* sp.

- Rare symptoms:
  - Headache, nausea, anxiety, dizziness
  - Lymphangitis or cellulitis in severe cases or secondary infection
- Bite marks from forcipules may be visible as paired punctures

While bites are unpleasant, they are not typically dangerous to healthy adults.

Occupational Exposure

Centipedes may be encountered by ecology and environmental professionals in:

- Leaf litter, under logs, rocks, or debris during terrestrial fieldwork
- Field stations, storage sheds, or bunkhouses, particularly in humid or tropical environments
- Excavation, trail maintenance, or soil sampling
- Ecological research involving pitfall traps, ground searches, or leaf litter sampling
- Tents and equipment left on the ground overnight

Certain large species (e.g., *Scolopendra heros*, which attains lengths of 15–20 cm/6–8 in. as adults) are relatively common in Southwestern United States, Mexico, and Central America.

Prevention

- Shake out bedding, gloves, boots, and packs before use
- Wear gloves and long pants when working in debris-rich or ground-level areas
- Avoid placing hands or feet in dark crevices without visual inspection
- Keep living and sleeping areas elevated, dry, and sealed
- Use sticky traps or physical barriers around storage areas in infested regions
- Train personnel in proper identification and avoidance

Emphasize caution when turning over stones or handling leaf litter in warm climates.

What To Do If Affected

- Clean the bite site with soap and water
- Apply cold compresses to reduce pain and swelling
- Take NSAIDs or oral antihistamines as needed
- Monitor for signs of secondary infection, such as spreading redness or warmth
- Seek medical care if:
  - The person experiences systemic symptoms
  - Pain becomes severe or prolonged
  - The bite occurs near the eye, mouth, or genitals

In rare cases, antibiotics or wound care may be required.

INSECTS

AQUATIC TRUE BUGS

Entomological Agents: Oder Hemiptera, Families Belostomatidae (giant water bugs), Notonectidae (backswimmers), and Naucoridae (creeping water bugs) (Figure 5.13)

Exposure and Severity Ratings (Figure 5.13)

- **Exposure Level: 1–2**
  - Locally uncommon (2) in aquatic fieldwork, especially in still or slow waters
  - Rare (1) otherwise
  - May be attracted to streetlights, work lights, and vehicle headlights
- **Severity Level: 1–2**
  - Notonectidae/Naucoridae: bite is minimal (1) to mild (2) with short-term pain
  - Belostomatidae: usually mild (2) due to more painful bite; may impair use of hand briefly

Reference: Haddad et al. (2010)

These aquatic bugs are predatory true bugs adapted to freshwater habitats, often found in ponds, streams, wetlands, and shallow standing water. They have piercing-sucking mouthparts and use proteases, hyaluronidase, phospholipases, nucleases, and other digestive enzymes in their saliva to subdue prey. They bite humans defensively when roughly handled or disturbed.

Belostomatidae (giant water bugs, or "toe-biters") are large, aggressive predators with powerful bites; adults of *Belostoma* spp. are <4 cm while adults of *Lethocerus* spp. can exceed 10 cm. Notonectidae (backswimmers) swim upside down, are often small but quick to bite when captured. Naucoridae (creeping water bugs) resemble smaller belostomatids and often cling to submerged objects.

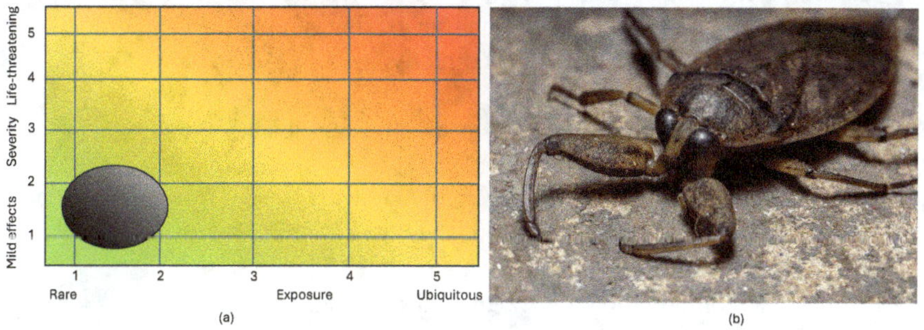

FIGURE 5.13 Aquatic bugs. (a) Exposure × severity matrix; (b) giant water bug, *Lethocerus americanus.*

While these bugs do not seek out humans, accidental contact during aquatic surveys, wading, or netting can result in painful punctures. Bites are not venomous but may be startling and briefly incapacitating due to the digestive enzymes.

Symptoms
- Sudden, sharp pain like a wasp sting
- Swelling, redness, and localized inflammation
- Possible bruising or numbness around the puncture
- Rare reports of:
  - Allergic reaction (itching, hives, mild systemic symptoms)
  - Delayed swelling or blistering
- Most symptoms resolve within 1–3 days

These bugs do not transmit disease in North America.

Occupational Exposure
Exposure risks to ecologists and environmental professionals include:

- Stream sampling, pond netting, or aquatic invertebrate surveys
- Standing in or reaching into shallow water
- Handling leaf packs, submerged debris, or kick-net contents
- Ecological research involving bioassessment, wetland delineation, or amphibian surveys
- Wading, swimming, or placing traps in bug-dense areas

They are particularly common in warm, slow-moving water or during spring/summer field seasons.

Prevention
- Wear protective gloves or waders when conducting aquatic work
- Avoid placing bare hands into nets or leaf litter in water bodies
- Inspect nets and sample trays before handling manually
- Educate field staff about appearance and defensive behavior of water bugs
- Use forceps or sorting spoons when transferring samples
- Avoid handling large aquatic bugs directly

Despite the pain, bites are generally not medically significant.

What To Do If Affected
- Remove the insect gently, if still attached
- Wash the area with soap and water
- Apply cold compress to reduce pain and swelling
- Use NSAIDs or oral antihistamines if necessary
- Monitor for signs of infection or allergic reaction

- Seek medical attention if:
  - Swelling worsens or persists
  - Symptoms spread beyond the bite site
  - Signs of secondary infection appear

No long-term effects are expected.

BED BUGS

Entomological Parasite: Order Hemiptera, Family Cimicidae: *Cimex lectularius* **(common bed bug) (Figure 5.14)**
   Exposure and Severity Ratings (Figure 5.14)

- **Exposure Level: 2**
  - Uncommon (2) in travel or shared accommodations
  - Persistent when a structure is infested and easily transported
- **Severity Level: 2–3**
  - Bites are mild (2), nonlethal, and not disease-transmitting
  - Infestations can be highly irritating and psychologically distressing, resulting in moderate (3) harm when pest control is needed

References: Usinger (1966), Goddard and deShazo (2009), Lai et al. (2016), Akhoundi et al. (2020), Hamlili et al. (2023)

Bed bugs are wingless, blood-feeding insects that hide in cracks, seams, and crevices of beds, furniture, and structures. Active primarily at night, they feed on exposed skin while the host is sleeping. Though they are not known to transmit disease under natural conditions (and exceptionally rarely under laboratory conditions), bed bugs can cause intense itching, allergic reactions, sleep disruption, and mental distress in infested environments.

Bed bug infestations have seen a resurgence worldwide, particularly in hotels, dormitories, shelters, and transportation hubs. Their presence in field housing or

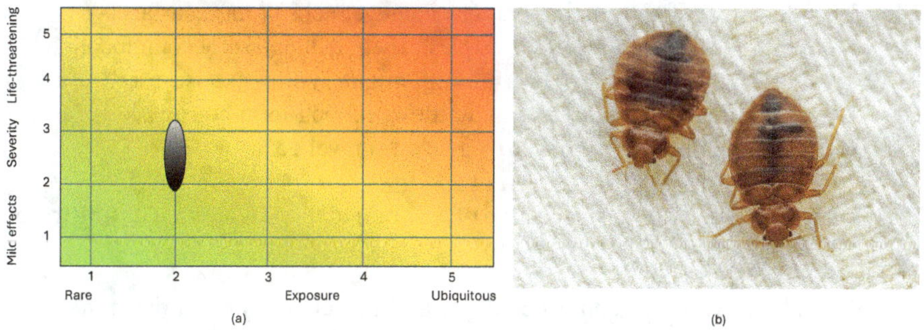

FIGURE 5.14 Bedbugs. (a) Exposure × severity matrix; (b) Bedbug, *Cimex lectularius*.

travel lodging poses a serious nuisance and can lead to unintentional transport to homes or workplaces.

Symptoms

Common signs of bed bug bites and exposure include:

- Red, itchy welts often arranged in lines or clusters (commonly on arms, neck, or legs)
- Localized swelling and inflammation
- Secondary infections from scratching
- Allergic responses, ranging from mild rash to hives
- Anxiety, insomnia, and psychological stress

Bite reactions are highly variable among individuals; some people show no visible signs at all.

Occupational Exposure

Ecological and environmental professionals may encounter bed bugs when:

- Staying in field housing, hotels, bunkhouses, or cabins
- Using public transportation or temporary sleeping quarters
- Conducting inspections of infested buildings
- Working in urban pest surveillance or environmental health
- Reusing shared bedding, sleeping bags, or upholstered gear

Bed bugs are adept hitchhikers and may travel on clothing, backpacks, or equipment.

Prevention

To minimize the risk of infestation or bites:

- Use bed bug apps to identify if hotels have recently had bed bug infestations
- Inspect bedding and mattresses for rust-colored stains, shed skins, or live insects
- Keep luggage off beds and floors; use luggage racks or hard surfaces
- Store clothing and bedding in sealed plastic bags in high-risk accommodations
- Treat or heat-isolate gear ($\geq 120°F$ for 30 minutes) after exposure
- Use encasements on mattresses and pillows in long-term housing
- Consider applying permethrin to luggage or travel gear

Early detection is key; routine inspection of accommodations is advised during travel.

What To Do If Affected

- Wash bites with soap and water; apply anti-itch creams or antihistamines
- Avoid scratching to prevent secondary infection
- If infestation is suspected:
  - Launder clothing and bedding on high heat
  - Vacuum and seal gear
  - Consider professional pest control intervention

- Psychological support may be warranted in cases of severe anxiety or distress

Bed bugs do not transmit disease, but mismanagement of infestations can result in long-term discomfort and social stigma.

SWALLOW BUGS

Entomological Parasites: Order Hemiptera, Family Cimicidae: *Oeciacus vicarius* **(cliff swallow bug) and others**
  Exposure and Severity Ratings (Figure 5.15)

- **Exposure Level: 1**
  - Rare (1); localized to specific bird monitoring or contaminated buildings
- **Severity Level: 1–2**
  - Typical bite reaction is minimal (1) harm
  - Allergic or repeated exposure may have mild (2) effects: itching, discomfort, psychological distress

References: Usinger (1966), Hamlili et al. (2023)
  Swallow bugs are blood-feeding ectoparasites that look very similar to bed bugs (Figure 5.14), but they specialize in feeding on swallows, especially cliff swallows (*Petrochelidon pyrrhonota*) and barn swallows (*Hirundo rustica*). Like bed bugs, they are wingless, flattened, and hide in cracks and crevices near host nesting sites. While they primarily parasitize birds, they will bite humans if nests are disturbed and birds are absent. They are most commonly encountered in ecological work involving bird banding, nest monitoring, or wildlife rehabilitation, as well as any work around structures (barns, eaves, attics, bridges, outcrops) where swallows have

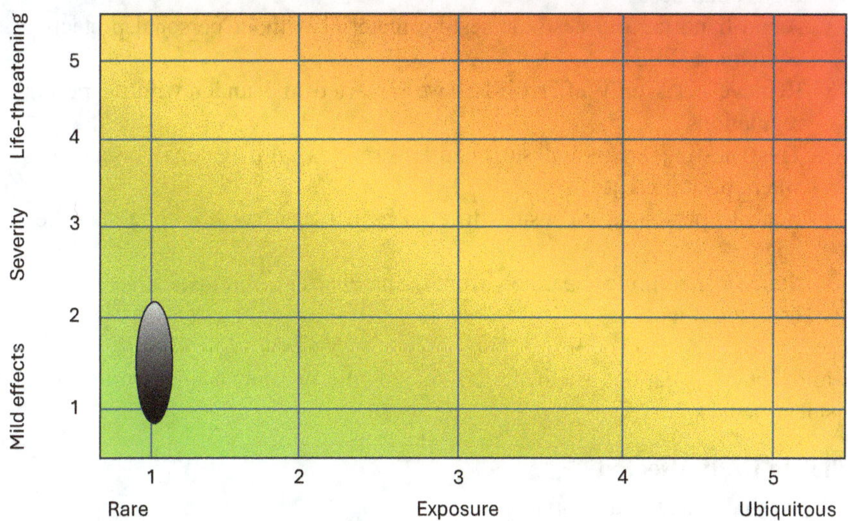

FIGURE 5.15   Swallow bugs. Exposure × severity matrix.

nested. Swallow bugs can survive long periods without feeding and may infest areas long after birds have left.

Though not confirmed as human disease vectors, swallow bugs in the southcentral United States have been found to harbor Buggy Creek virus, a disease of veterinary concern.

Symptoms
- Small, red, itchy welts, similar to bed bug bites
- Multiple bites often appear in linear or clustered patterns
- May cause intense itching, swelling, or allergic reactions in sensitive individuals
- Risk of secondary infection from scratching
- No confirmed transmission of human pathogens

Symptoms may be delayed for hours after exposure and can persist for several days.

Occupational Exposure
Exposure to ecologists and environmental professionals is most likely during:

- Bird banding, nest checks, or cavity surveys
- Handling cliff swallow nests, especially in colonies under eaves or bridges
- Demolition or cleaning of structures previously used by swallows
- Monitoring artificial nest boxes
- Rehabilitation or removal of old barns, silos, or outbuildings

Swallow bugs are resilient and may survive winter conditions or years without hosts.

Prevention
- Wear long sleeves, gloves, and insect-repellent-treated clothing when working around nests
- Avoid handling old nests or nesting material without personal protective equipment (PPE)
- Remove nests only after birds have departed and under wildlife permit regulations
- Treat nesting areas and surrounding crevices with residual insecticides where permitted
- Educate personnel on visual differences between swallow bugs and bed bugs
- Store field clothing separately from living quarters, and inspect gear before bringing it indoors

Swallow bug infestations are distinct from bed bugs but may trigger similar panic if misidentified.

What To Do If Affected
- Wash the area with soap and water
- Apply topical antihistamines or corticosteroids to reduce itching

- Use oral antihistamines if reactions are widespread
- Monitor for signs of secondary infection (e.g., redness, pus, warmth)
- Seek medical attention if:
  - Bites are unusually severe or persist
  - Signs of systemic allergic reaction occur
  - Occupational exposure involves potential virus-positive colonies (research contexts)

Buggy Creek virus is not known to cause human disease.

OTHER BITING TRUE BUGS

Entomological Agents: Order Hemiptera, Families Pentatomidae (stink bugs), Reduviidae (assassin bugs), Coreidae (leaf-footed bugs), Lygaeidae (seed bugs), and Miridae (plant bugs), and others (Figure 5.16)
   Exposure and Severity Ratings (Figure 5.16)

- **Exposure Level: 3–4**
  - Moderately (3) common in most field settings, frequent (4) in flowering and agricultural fields
- **Severity Level: 1–2**
  - Bite is usually minimal (1) to mild (2)
  - Rare allergic response or chemical spray to eyes may induce mild (2) harm

Reference: Schaefer and Panizzi (2000)

The order Hemiptera is highly diverse, encompassing plant-feeding and predatory species, many of which are harmless. However, some true bugs pose occupational health risks through defensive bites, secretion of irritating chemicals, or unintentional contamination of equipment and workspaces.

Aquatic biting true bugs (families Belostomatidae, Naucoridae, and Notonectidae) and the kissing bugs (family Reduviidae: *Triatoma* spp.) are covered separately. Some other hemipterans such as non-triatomine assassin bugs, stink bugs, or plant bugs may

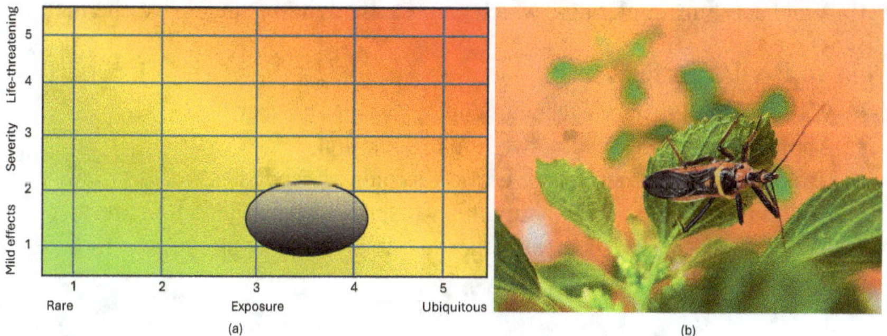

FIGURE 5.16   Other biting bugs. (a) Exposure × severity matrix; (b) assassin bug, *Apiomerus* sp.

also inflict painful defensive bites or cause dermatologic reactions. These interactions are rare but may occur during handling, vegetation surveys, or light trapping.

Some species emit volatile defensive compounds that can irritate eyes, respiratory passages, or skin.

Symptoms

- Localized pain, swelling, or redness at bite site
- Eye irritation, especially if aerosols contact mucous membranes
- Sneezing, wheezing, or nasal congestion in sensitive individuals
- Rare cases of blistering or allergic dermatitis

Bites are typically defensive and not medically serious but may resemble small spider bites.

Occupational Exposure

Ecologists and environmental professionals are most likely to encounter harmful Hemiptera when:

- Sorting or sweeping vegetation during ecological sampling
- Performing nighttime light trapping, especially in warm regions
- Collecting insects by hand for surveys or teaching purposes
- Handling fruit or crops, where stink bugs or predatory bugs may be concealed

Most injuries occur due to accidental contact or mishandling of concealed individuals.

Prevention

To minimize risks:

- Use gloves and forceps when sorting through vegetation or leaf litter
- Do not handle unknown bugs bare-handed
- Avoid rubbing eyes after contact with bug-contaminated surfaces
- When light trapping, wear eye protection to prevent contact with flying insects
- Store swept or shaken vegetation away from workspaces before processing
- Avoid crushing stink bugs, which can release irritating defensive chemicals

What To Do If Affected

- Wash affected skin or eyes with copious water and soap
- Apply cold compresses for swelling or irritation
- Use topical antihistamines or corticosteroids as needed
- Seek medical attention if symptoms worsen or signs of infection appear
- For eye exposures, irrigate eyes thoroughly and consult an eye care provider if pain or blurred vision persists

Most reactions are self-limiting and resolve within hours to a few days.

LARGE ORTHOPTERA

Entomological Agents: Order Orthoptera, Families Acrididae and Romaleidae (Grasshoppers), Gryllidae (Crickets), Tettigoniidae (Katydids), Stenopelmatidae (Jerusalem crickets), and others (Figure 5.17)
Exposure and Severity Ratings (Figure 5.17)

- **Exposure Level: 4**
  - Frequent (4) in active collection work, especially with sweep nets or light traps, and even normal outdoor activity
- **Severity Level: 1–2**
  - Minimal (1) harm from most encounters; may produce a mild (2) skin break from bites or sharp spines
  - Mild (2) startle or psychological reactions are more likely in inexperienced handlers

References: Gangwere (1965), Weihmann et al. (2015), Edel et al. (2024)

Large orthopteran insects, especially robust grasshoppers, katydids, and crickets, are commonly encountered during terrestrial ecological work. While these insects are not venomous and pose no active threat to humans, some species are capable of biting or kicking defensively when captured or handled, particularly large-bodied or predatory forms.

Grasshoppers and katydids have powerful mandibles adapted for chewing tough plant material and may bite painfully if restrained. Crickets (particularly mole crickets and Jerusalem crickets) can also nip skin, though this is uncommon. Most large Orthoptera also have thick, sharp spines along their hind legs that can dig into the skin when attempting to jump.

While these bites are not medically dangerous, they can cause minor lacerations, bruising, and pain, especially in ungloved hands. The Mormon cricket is discussed in more detail in Transportation, Equipment, and Operations Hazards due to its swarming habit and potential to cause road hazards.

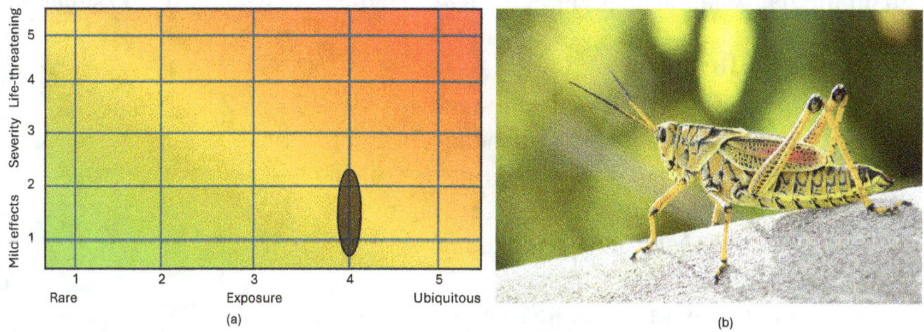

FIGURE 5.17 Large Orthoptera. (a) Exposure×severity matrix; (b) Eastern lubber grasshopper, *Romalea microptera*.

Symptoms

- Painful pinch or bite at site of contact
- Possible bleeding, bruising, or puncture wounds from strong mandibles
- Swelling or redness at the bite site
- Occasional secondary infection if wound is not cleaned
- No venom, no systemic symptoms, and no known disease transmission

The most frequent issue is startled reaction or aversion behavior, especially among untrained personnel.

Occupational Exposure

Encounters with large biting Orthoptera by ecologists and environmental professionals may occur during:

- Sweep netting, beat-sheet sampling, or vegetation transects
- Nocturnal light trapping or fogging samples
- Herbivore monitoring, especially in grassland or savanna ecosystems
- Manual collection or photography of insects in biodiversity work
- Releasing large specimens from containers

Larger orthopterans may be more common in late summer, open field habitats, or tropical regions.

Prevention

- Wear light gloves during sweep netting or when handling large insects
- Instruct field staff not to cup large insects bare-handed, especially mantids and katydids
- Use forceps or aspirators when possible
- Recognize postural threat displays (e.g., katydids spreading wings)
- Educate students and technicians that bites and stabs from leg spines are not harmful but can surprise

With minimal precaution, these insects can be handled safely in most field situations.

What To Do If Affected

- Clean the bite area with soap and water
- Apply antibiotic ointment and bandage, if broken skin
- Use cold compress to reduce swelling or bruising
- Monitor for infection or allergic reaction (rare)
- Medical attention is rarely needed unless:
  - Bite becomes infected
  - Wound is near the eye, fingernail, or joint
  - Patient has compromised immunity or delayed healing

In most cases, no further treatment is required beyond basic wound care.

PRAYING MANTIDS

Entomological Agents: Order Mantodea: *Tenodera sinensis* (Chinese mantid), *Mantis religiosa* (European mantid), *Stagmomantis carolina* (Carolina mantid), *Litaneutria,* and others (Figure 5.18)
  Exposure and Severity Ratings (Figure 5.18)

- **Exposure Level: 1**
  - Rare (1); occasionally encountered in warm, vegetated habitats
  - Exposure is infrequent and incidental
- **Severity Level: 1–2**
  - Larger species are capable of delivering mildly (2) painful bites when handled improperly
  - Most species are incapable of more than minimal (1) harm
  - Mild (2) startle and psychological responses may occur due to surprising movements

Reference: Gangwere (1967)

Mantids (Mantodea), also known as praying mantises, are charismatic predatory insects known for their raptorial forelegs, triangular heads, and large, mobile eyes. They are non-venomous, do not sting, and play a beneficial ecological role by preying on other insects. Though not aggressive toward humans, they can bite defensively if provoked, particularly when captured or handled. Holding on with their strong forelegs and sharp spines, bites from mantids can pierce the skin, occasionally drawing blood, but they do not involve venom or allergenic substances. The largest species include the Chinese mantid (*Tenodera sinensis*, which can attain lengths of 11 cm/4.3 in.) and the European mantid (*Mantis religiosa*, attaining lengths of 7 cm/2.8 in.), both of which can certainly draw blood when biting. Smaller species are also potentially capable of delivering noticeable bites or clinging with their forelegs and sharp spines.

While encounters with mantids are relatively uncommon, ecologists and environmental professionals working in shrublands, meadows, or gardens may occasionally

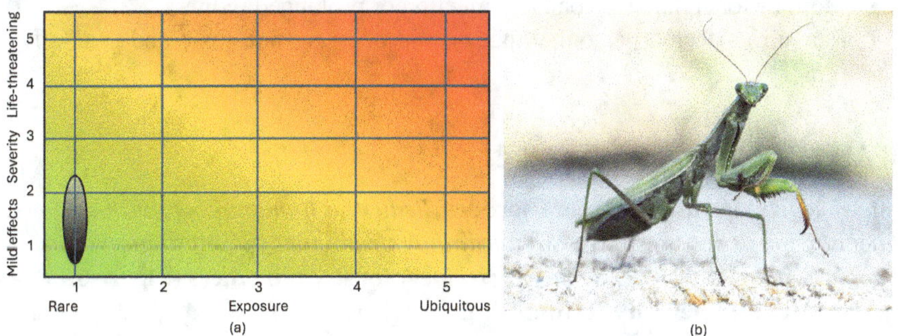

FIGURE 5.18 Praying mantids. (a) Exposure × severity matrix; (b) European mantis, *Mantis religiosa.*

disturb these insects while surveying vegetation or deploying insect traps. Mantids may also be unintentionally brought into contact with humans when clinging to gear, clothing, or vehicles. Although medically insignificant, their size, sudden movement, and strong forelegs may cause startle responses or discomfort, particularly for personnel unfamiliar with insect handling.

Symptoms
- Puncture wounds or scratches from spines on forelegs or defensive bite
- Mild bleeding or bruising at the site of contact
- Rare emotional distress or aversion reaction in insect-sensitive individuals

Occupational Exposure
There is increased likelihood of mantid encounters to ecologists and environmental professionals during:

- Vegetation sampling in fields, meadows, or forest margins during summer and fall
- Deployment of sweep nets, beat sheets, or insect traps
- Nighttime surveys using UV lights or sheet traps near tall vegetation
- Use of mantids in educational or outreach settings involving live arthropods

Prevention
To reduce potential for bites or unexpected encounters:

- Avoid handling mantids, especially with bare hands, if not necessary
- Shake out gloves, clothing, or nets after use in vegetated areas
- Wear lightweight gloves if manually collecting insects or clearing foliage
- Educate field staff that mantids are non-venomous and ecologically beneficial

What To Do If Affected
- Clean the bite area with soap and water
- Apply a disinfectant and cover with a bandage if needed
- Monitor for signs of secondary infection or prolonged redness
- Reassure affected personnel that mantid bites are non-toxic and generally minor

HEAD LICE AND ANIMAL LICE

Entomological Parasites: Order Psocodea, *Pediculus humanus capitis* (head louse), *Haematopinus suis* (hog louse), *Menacanthus stramineus* (poultry louse), *Lipeurus caponis* (wing louse), *Solenopotes ferrisi* (deer louse), and others (Figure 5.19)
   Exposure and Severity Ratings (Figure 5.19)

- **Exposure Level: 2**
  - Generally uncommon (2); head lice may increase in frequency in certain group living or classroom/camp settings

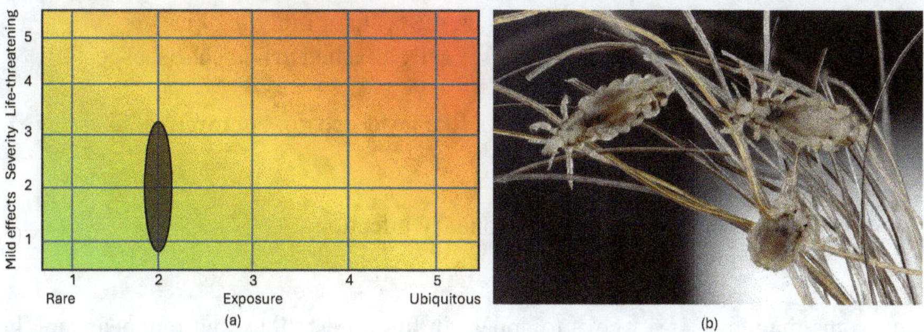

FIGURE 5.19   Head lice and animal lice. (a) Exposure×severity matrix; (b) Human head louse, *Pediculus humanus capitis*.

- Animal lice exposure depends on close contact with infested animals of their bedding
- **Severity Level: 1–3**
  - Mostly minimal (1) to mild (2) discomfort with itching and rash
  - Social/psychological disruption may be moderate (3) due to stigma, isolation, or missed work/school

References: Akhoundi et al. (2020), Fu et al. (2022)

Head lice are obligate ectoparasites that infest the scalp and hair of humans, particularly children but also adults in close-contact environments. These small, wingless insects feed on blood several times per day by piercing the scalp. While head lice do not transmit disease, their bites cause itching, irritation, and potentially secondary bacterial infections from scratching.

Head lice spread primarily through direct head-to-head contact or shared hats, combs, bedding, or headphones. In ecological or educational fieldwork settings, they may spread in tents, dormitories, bunkhouses, or shared transport, especially among students or volunteers.

Animal lice are species-specific ectoparasites that infest livestock, poultry, and wild mammals, occasionally biting humans who work in close contact with infested animals. Though they cannot reproduce on humans, lice such as the hog louse (*Haematopinus suis*), chicken body louse (*Menacanthus stramineus*), or deer louse (*Solenopotes ferrisi*) may cause incidental bites, irritation, or confusion during fieldwork. While not known to transmit disease to humans, animal lice can create discomfort and may be mistaken for more serious ectoparasites like fleas or mites. Exposure risk increases during wildlife handling, animal necropsy, or work in poorly maintained enclosures, barns, or dens.

Though not generally dangerous, lice infestations can be socially disruptive, causing distress and lost time at work or school. Strict hygiene protocols, which are often necessary to prevent spread, often compound time loss.

Symptoms

- Itching of the scalp, particularly at the nape of the neck and behind the ears for head lice

- Red bite marks or scratch wounds on the scalp or other regions
- For head lice, presence of nits (eggs) firmly attached to hair shafts, especially within 1–2 cm of the scalp
- Animal lice cause itchy bite marks like head lice do, but rarely, if ever, lay eggs on humans.
- In severe infestations:
  - Excoriations, crusting, or secondary infection
  - Swollen lymph nodes in the neck

Symptoms may take 4–6 weeks to appear in first infestations, but reappear rapidly upon reinfestation.

Occupational Exposure

Head lice are not associated with poor hygiene, but infestations thrive in close-knit groups. They are most likely to spread to ecologists and environmental professionals in:

- Field courses, summer camps, or residential programs with shared sleeping quarters
- Youth-oriented programs, school trips, or ecological outreach
- Long-duration fieldwork with close quarters and limited hygiene access
- Shared gear or headwear (e.g., binoculars, helmets, headphones)
- Close group transportation, especially vans or buses

Animal lice are typically host-specific, but under certain conditions they may transfer temporarily to humans. Ecologists and environmental professionals are most at risk when:

- Handling or trapping small mammals (e.g., rodents, opossums, squirrels)
- Entering or cleaning abandoned buildings, barns, or wildlife dens
- Performing necropsies or carcass disposal
- Working in animal control, wildlife rehabilitation, or zoonotic disease surveillance
- Camping or storing gear in rodent-infested areas

Prevention

For head lice:

- Instruct participants not to share personal items like hats, brushes, or bedding
- Encourage regular scalp checks in residential settings
- Launder bedding and clothing in hot water and high heat drying if lice are suspected
- Provide individual sleeping gear and label personal items
- In long-term field camps, implement routine cleanliness protocols
- Educate participants that lice are human head treatable and not a sign of uncleanliness

For animal lice:

- Wear gloves and protective clothing when handling wildlife or entering rodent-infested structures
- Use disposable or washable barriers on work surfaces and field gear
- Inspect gear, clothing, and sleeping materials after exposure to known host animals
- Deter rodents and small mammals from storage areas and bunkhouses
- Encourage rodent control and facility hygiene in field stations or wilderness cabins
- Prompt identification and discreet management prevent spread and stigma

What To Do If Affected

- Confirm presence of live lice or nits close to scalp (within ~6 mm)
- Treat with over-the-counter pediculicides (e.g., permethrin) or prescription medications if resistant strain suspected
- Apply topical anti-pruritic creams for minor skin irritation
- Use fine-toothed lice combs daily for 1–2 weeks
- Wash or seal (in plastic bags for 2+ days) clothing, bedding, hats, and soft gear
- Notify other team members or students with discretion and compassion
- Re-treat 7–10 days later to kill newly hatched lice
- There are over 200 "lice clinics" across the United States that can be contacted for lice removal and treatment
- Monitor for signs of rodent infestation, and possible lice infestations, in sleeping quarters or equipment storage
- Report unusual insect activity or recurring bites to supervisors or health authorities
- Medical attention is needed only for severe scratching, skin infections, or treatment-resistant lice

MULTICOLORED ASIAN LADY BEETLE

Entomological Agents: Order Coleoptera, Family Coccinellidae: *Harmonia axyridis* (Asian Multicolored Lady Beetle) (Figure 5.20)
    Exposure and Severity Ratings (Figure 5.20)

- **Exposure Level: 4**
  - Frequent (4) exposure across the United States and southern Canada
  - In some localities, they are displacing native lady bird beetle species
  - As of 2025, AK, MT, and WY are the only states not reporting presence of *Harmonia axyridis*
- **Severity Level: 1–2**
  - Bite reaction: minimal (1) to mild discomfort; usually only a pinch without swelling, but some can break the skin
  - Allergic response or hemolymph contact: rare, but mild (2) and generally among sensitized individuals

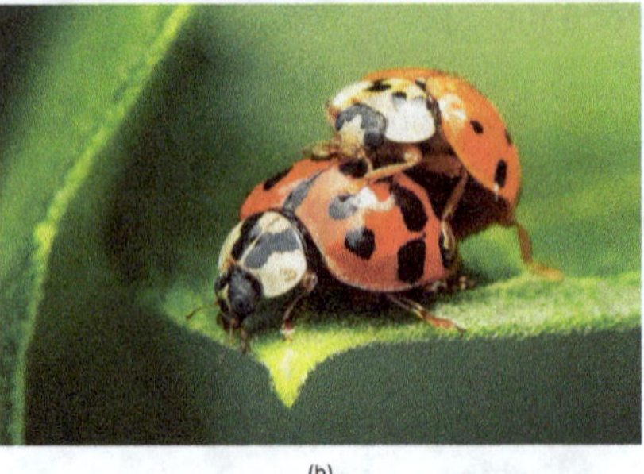

FIGURE 5.20 Multicolored Asian lady beetle. (a) Exposure × severity matrix; (b) multicolored Asian lady beetle, *Harmonia axyridis*.

Reference: Cranshaw (2011)

The multicolored Asian lady beetle (*H. axyridis*) is a non-native, invasive coccinellid introduced in North America for aphid biocontrol. It has become highly abundant in many parts of the United States, particularly in agricultural fields, wooded edges, and urban structures; many localities list it as one of the top nuisance pests in buildings. In the fall, adults aggregate on buildings, including cabins, barns, and field stations, seeking overwintering sites.

H. axyridis is known to bite humans; most lady beetles can bite, but don't. These bites occur when the beetles land on exposed skin, typically during mass flights or swarming. Although not venomous, their mandibles can break skin, causing sharp pain, redness, and mild swelling. Additionally, they can exude a yellow hemolymph when stressed, which stains surfaces and may trigger allergic reactions.

Other coccinellid species, such as *Coccinella septempunctata* (seven-spotted lady beetle) and *Hippodamia convergens* (convergent lady beetle), have also been reported to bite, though much less frequently and far less aggressively than *H. axyridis*.

Symptoms

- Pinching sensation at bite site
- Small red welt or papule, occasionally with mild swelling
- Rare hypersensitivity reactions or contact dermatitis
- Hemolymph exposure may cause burning or staining, and, in sensitized individuals, respiratory or skin allergies

Reactions are generally localized and mild, but repetitive exposure can lead to increased sensitivity.

Occupational Exposure

Bites and nuisance encounters may occur to ecologists and environmental professionals in:

- Fall fieldwork, especially near woodlots, cliffsides, or agriculture-adjacent habitats

- Outdoor construction, biological surveys, or habitat restoration projects in beetle-infested areas
- Entomological trapping or pollinator surveys, especially with yellow pan traps
- Sleeping quarters, labs, or cabins invaded by overwintering aggregations

Exposure risk peaks during autumn overwintering migrations.

Prevention

- Wear long sleeves and gloves when working outdoors in infested areas
- Avoid roughly brushing beetles off bare skin; remove them gently
- Use fine mesh screens on cabins and field stations to exclude beetles
- Avoid yellow or light-colored traps or surfaces that may attract aggregations
- Educate field teams about the difference between native vs. invasive lady beetles
- Be aware of increased risk in riparian zones and ridge lines, where beetles often mass in sunlit areas

In enclosed spaces, vacuuming is preferred over squashing, which can release hemolymph and trigger odor or stains.

What To Do If Affected

- Wash affected skin with soap and water
- Apply cool compresses or topical antihistamines for itching or swelling
- Rinse eyes with sterile eyewash if beetle contact occurs
- Do not rub eyes if hemolymph is present – can cause irritation
- Seek medical attention only if:
  - Symptoms persist >48 hours
  - Signs of infection or allergic reaction appear
  - Multiple bites or respiratory symptoms occur in sensitive individuals

LARGE COLEOPTERA

Entomological Agents: Order Coleoptera, Families Lucanidae (stag beetles), Passalidae (bess beetles), Cerambycidae (longhorn beetles), Tenebrionidae (darkling beetles), Carabidae (ground beetles), and a few others (Figure 5.21)

Exposure and Severity Ratings (Figure 5.21)

- **Exposure Level: 1–3**
  - Rare (1) to moderate (3) exposure
  - Tend to be localized and encountered in wooded areas, under logs, or in pitfall traps
- **Severity Level: 1–2**
  - Minimal (1) to mild (2) non-venomous bites
  - Some can break skin and allow secondary infections
  - Mild (2) startle reaction if handled improperly

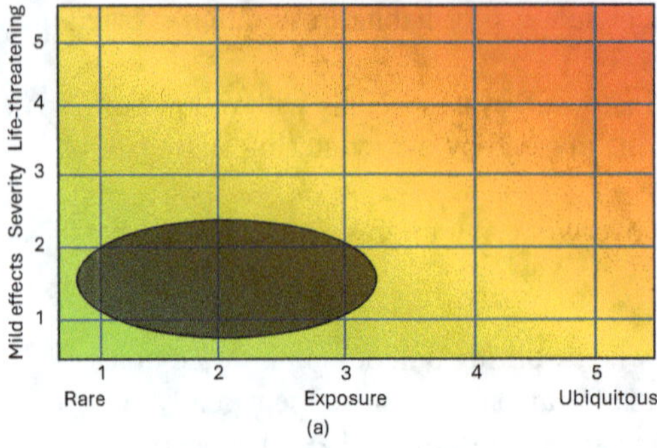

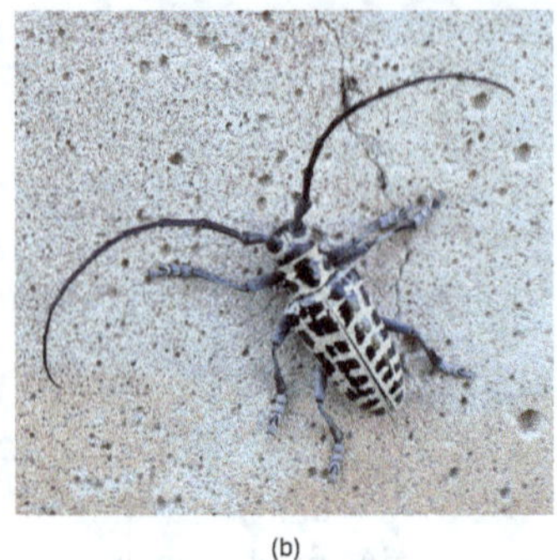

FIGURE 5.21 Large Coleoptera. (a) Exposure × severity matrix; (b) cottonwood borer, *Plectrodera scalator.*

Reference: Krinsky (2019)

While most beetles are harmless and beneficial decomposers or predators, several large-bodied species are capable of delivering strong defensive bites with their mandibles. These bites are not venomous and rarely result in serious injury, but can puncture skin, draw blood, or cause localized pain, particularly if the beetle is mishandled or caught against the skin in gear or clothing.

Notable biting beetle species include stag beetles (Lucanidae) with prominent jaws in males, bess beetles (Passalidae), large ground beetles (Carabidae, such as the genus *Calosoma* and the tiger beetles), and some longhorn beetles (Cerambycidae) in which both sexes may have robust mandibles. While not aggressive, these beetles may bite if restrained, trapped, or inadvertently contacted during field operations. Field biologists, entomologists, and technicians working with pitfall traps, leaf litter, or decaying wood are most likely to encounter these taxa.

Symptoms

- Sharp pinch or bite, potentially breaking the skin
- Localized swelling, bruising, or mild bleeding
- Startle response or reflexive movement, increasing the risk of equipment mishandling or falling
- No venom or toxin; allergic reactions are extremely rare

Occupational Exposure

Increased risk to ecologists and environmental professionals during:

- Forest and woodland surveys, especially under logs, bark, or rotting wood
- Deployment or collection of pitfall traps or light traps
- Manual vegetation or soil sorting, especially in humid or decaying environments
- Entomological sampling, outreach, or educational handling of large beetles

Prevention

- Wear light gloves when handling unknown beetles, especially large-bodied ones

- Avoid placing large beetles in pockets or loose bags without containers
- Educate field staff on common biting beetle families
- Use forceps or collection vials for beetle sampling whenever possible
- Alert staff to the presence of high-density beetle habitats, especially in late spring and summer

What To Do If Affected

- Wash area with soap and water
- Apply cold compress to reduce swelling or pain
- Use topical antiseptic and bandage if skin is broken
- Monitor for infection, though this is rare
- Reassure affected personnel: no venom or systemic hazard is involved

While not a major medical threat, large beetles represent a low-frequency but memorable hazard for field crews, particularly those engaged in active sampling or habitat manipulation. Their bites are best addressed through training, gentle handling, and awareness of beetle families likely to bite if provoked.

DOBSONFLIES

**Entomological Agents: Order Megaloptera, Family Corydalidae (Figure 5.22)
Exposure and Severity Ratings (Figure 5.22)**

- **Exposure Level: 1–2**
  - Rare (1) to moderate (2) exposure
  - Adults may come to lights; larvae are found under rocks along streams
- **Severity Level: 1–2**
  - Minimal (1) to mild (2) non-venomous bites
  - Some can break skin and allow secondary infections
  - Mild (2) startle reaction if handled improperly

References: Contreras-Ramos (1998), Missouri Department of Conservation (2024)

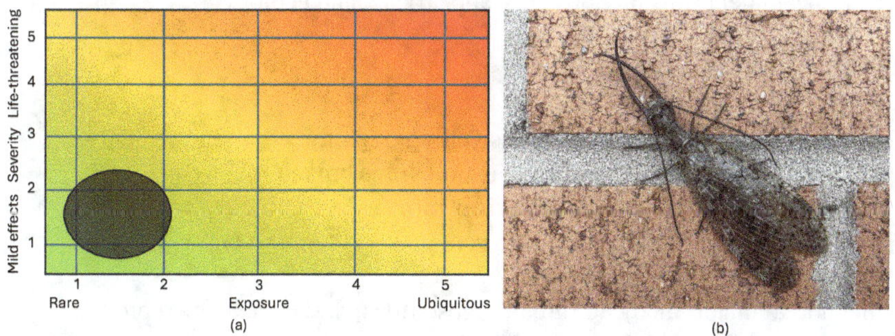

FIGURE 5.22 Dobsonflies. (a) Exposure×severity matrix; (b) dobsonfly, *Corydalus cornutus*.

Dobsonflies are among the largest adult insects in North America, some competing with the large, showy moths for sheer wingspan. Adult males are easily recognized by their outlandishly large mandibles, probably derived from runaway sexual selection in which females prefer males with very large mandibles, so that is what subsequent generations produce. The mandibles themselves are too large to use for feeding or biting; they are only ornamental and for jousting with competitors for mates.

Mandibles on the females are short and stocky and can rarely provide a decent pinch. The immature stages, called hellgrammites, are often found under rocks in edge-waters along streams. They are highly favored as fish-bait for bass, but they can also deliver a surprising bite. They are not venomous.

Because of their large size at lights, the harmless adults are avoided by most people. The larvae are most likely going to be encountered by ecologists and people searching for bait species.

Symptoms
- Sharp pinch or bite, potentially breaking the skin
- Localized swelling, bruising, or mild bleeding
- Traumatic response to these large insects
- Startle response or reflexive movement, increasing the risk of equipment mishandling or falling
- No venom or toxin, some digestive enzymes; allergic reactions are extremely rare

Occupational Exposure
Increased risk to ecologists and environmental professionals during:

- Stream surveys along rocky banks, especially under half-submerged rocks where larvae reside
- Work near lighted roadways along streams
- Deployment or collection of light traps

Prevention
- Wear light gloves when overturning rocks in riparian areas of streams.
- Educate field staff on dobsonfly appearance and ecology

What To Do If Affected
- Wash area with soap and water
- Apply cold compress to reduce swelling or pain
- Use topical antiseptic and bandage if skin is broken
- Monitor for infection, though this is rare
- Reassure affected personnel: no venom or systemic hazard is involved

While not a major medical threat, dobsonflies, large beetles, represent a low-frequency but memorable hazard for field crews, particularly those engaged in active sampling or habitat manipulation. Their bites are best addressed through training, gentle handling, and awareness.

EYE GNATS

Entomological Agents: Order Diptera, Family Chloropidae: *Liohippelates* spp. Exposure and Severity Ratings (Figure 5.23)

- **Exposure Level: 2–4**
  - Uncommon (2); localized to warm, sandy, or disturbed/agricultural areas
  - Distributed across southern United States (CA to SC, north to MO, IL, and IN in the Great Plains and Midwest)
  - Due to frequent (4) abundance, they are reported as a serious nuisance in the Imperial and Coachella Valleys of CA and throughout agricultural areas of FL
- **Severity Level: 1–2**
  - No to minimal (1) medical harm
  - Mild (2) harm as a nuisance
  - May rarely cause secondary bacterial infections

Reference: Klepzig et al. (2022)

Eye gnats, also known as eye flies or grass flies, are tiny, hump-backed flies that do not bite, but swarm around the eyes, nose, mouth, and open wounds to feed on secretions such as tears, sweat, and mucus. Though harmless in terms of stinging or biting, their persistent behavior makes them a serious nuisance to outdoor workers in warm, sandy, or grassy environments.

These flies are most abundant in the southeastern United States and California, particularly during spring and summer, and are frequently associated with agricultural fields, pastures, and disturbed soil. They are implicated in the mechanical transmission of bacterial conjunctivitis (pinkeye) and may also carry enteric pathogens, making them a concern in both human and veterinary contexts.

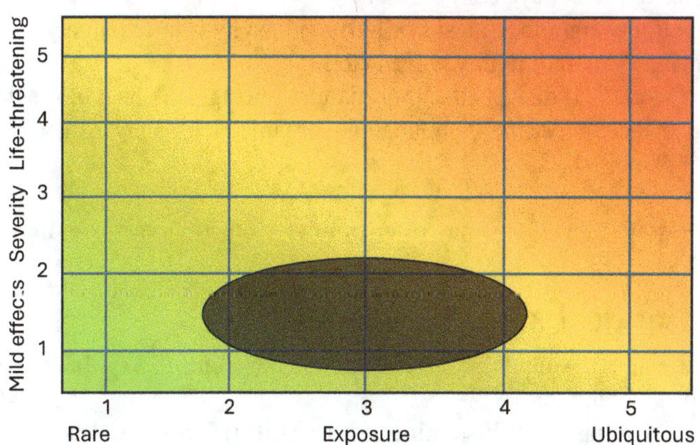

FIGURE 5.23 Eye gnats. Exposure × severity matrix.

Symptoms

While individual flies are small, their behavior can cause:

- Irritation of the eyes, nose, and mouth from repeated landings
- Tearing, redness, or discomfort from eye contact
- Potential introduction of bacterial conjunctivitis (pinkeye) pathogens
- Contamination of small wounds, increasing infection risk
- Psychological stress and distraction during fieldwork due to swarming behavior

They do not pierce the skin, but their persistence and numbers can severely impact work efficiency and comfort.

Occupational Exposure

Eye gnats are commonly encountered by ecologists and environmental professionals during:

- Fieldwork in sandy soils, especially in Florida, Georgia, southern California, and Texas
- Agricultural or ecological surveys in recently tilled or disturbed ground
- Working near livestock pens or animal shelters
- Military exercises or public health operations in tropical or subtropical zones
- Summer work in low-wind environments near weedy fields or roadsides

They are most active in warm, humid weather, especially in areas with organic-rich soil.

Prevention

Because repellents are often ineffective, physical barriers are key:

- Use head nets or face veils during swarming periods, tight-fitting glasses or goggles to protect eyes, if necessary
- Apply lightweight face masks or buffs in heavily infested areas
- Wear light-colored, tightly woven clothing
- Avoid work near disturbed soil or manure during peak heat of the day
- Reduce local breeding by managing organic-rich sandy soil and animal waste

Standard mosquito repellents may offer limited protection, but shielding the face is most effective.

What To Do If Affected

- Rinse eyes or wounds with clean water or saline if flies have contacted mucous membranes
- Use lubricating or antihistamine eye drops if irritation persists
- Monitor for signs of pinkeye: red, itchy, watery eyes with crusting or discharge

- Clean minor wounds and cover with a breathable bandage if flies persist in the area
- If conjunctivitis or infection develops, consult a health care provider for appropriate treatment (typically topical antibiotics)
- Symptoms usually subside quickly once exposure is removed

BITING MIDGES

Entomological Parasites: Order Diptera, Family Ceratopogonidae: *Culicoides* and related genera (Figure 5.24)
   Exposure and Severity Ratings (Figure 5.24)

- **Exposure Level: 3**
  - Moderately (3) common in coastal, marshy, or wetland environments; hard to avoid during peak activity
- **Severity Level: 2–3**
  - Bites are mildly (2) irritating but not medically serious; swarms may produce more moderate (3) irritation
  - Hypersensitivity possible, potentially resulting in moderate (3) harm

References: Akhoundi et al. (2020), Kampen and Werner (2023)

Biting midges, colloquially called "no-see-ums," "punkies," or "sand gnats," are tiny, blood-feeding flies often found in coastal areas, wetlands, and marshes. Although only 1–3 mm long, their bites are disproportionately painful, and their small size allows them to penetrate standard screens and clothing.

In North America, biting midges are primarily a nuisance to humans, and when they swarm, they can be a frustrating nuisance. However, some species of *Culicoides* are known vectors of significant veterinary pathogens such as:

- Bluetongue virus (affects sheep and cattle)
- Epizootic hemorrhagic disease virus (affects deer)

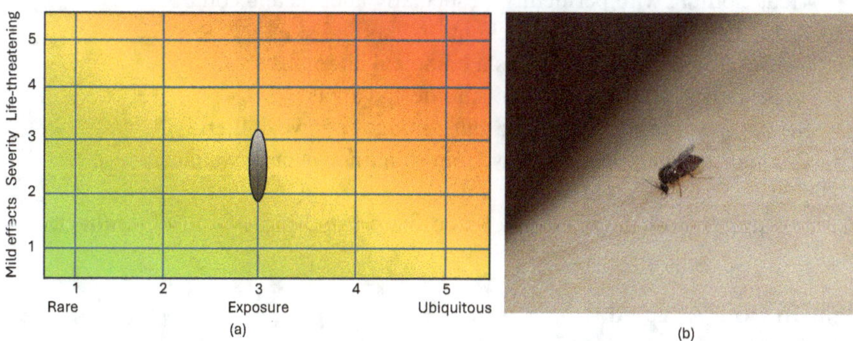

FIGURE 5.24   Biting midges. (a) Exposure × severity matrix; (b) biting midge, Ceratopogonidae.

Though human disease transmission in North America by biting midges is undocumented, some *Culicoides* spp. have been linked to Oropouche virus and filarial parasites in other parts of the world.

Symptoms

Symptoms usually begin within hours of a bite and may include:

- Intensely itchy, red welts or small blisters
- Clusters of bites on exposed skin, especially arms, legs, neck, and face
- Allergic dermatitis or hypersensitivity in some individuals
- Rarely, secondary infections due to scratching

Bite reactions can be more severe than mosquito bites, especially in sensitized individuals or those repeatedly exposed.

Occupational Exposure

Biting midge exposure to ecologists and environmental professionals is likely during:

- Salt marsh or wetland fieldwork, especially near brackish water
- Coastal construction monitoring or vegetation surveys
- Stream and pond monitoring, particularly in low-wind, humid environments
- Camping or working at dusk or dawn, when midges are most active
- Work in southeastern states, Gulf Coast, Caribbean territories, and parts of California and the Pacific Northwest

Their small size and silent flight make them difficult to detect before they bite.

Prevention

Because midges are highly mobile and hard to deter, combine multiple prevention strategies:

- Wear long-sleeved shirts, long pants, and fine mesh head nets
- Treat clothing with permethrin, especially at cuffs and collars
- Apply DEET or picaridin repellents to exposed skin
- Use oil of lemon eucalyptus as a botanical alternative
- Avoid dawn and dusk fieldwork in infested areas
- Set up fans in work shelters or tents; midges are weak fliers
- Camp or store equipment away from standing water or wetland edges

Screens with standard mesh may not stop these small insects – use ultrafine mesh netting.

What To Do If Affected

- Wash affected areas with soap and water
- Apply topical antihistamines or corticosteroids to reduce itching
- Take oral antihistamines for widespread reactions

- Avoid scratching to reduce risk of infection or scarring
- Severe or persistent reactions may require medical evaluation

Reactions can last several days, especially in sensitized individuals with repeated exposure.

BLACK FLIES

Entomological Parasites: Order Diptera, Family Simuliidae: *Simulium*, *Prosimulium*, and other genera (Figure 5.25)
   Exposure and Severity Ratings (Figure 5.25)

- **Exposure Level: 3**
   - Moderately (3) common in coastal, marshy, or wetland environments; hard to avoid during peak activity
   - May be particularly abundant in northern and mountainous regions
- **Severity Level: 2–3**
   - Bites are mildly (2) irritating but not medically serious; swarms may produce more moderate (3) irritation
   - Hypersensitivity possible, potentially resulting in moderate (3) harm

References: Akhoundi et al. (2020), Rivera-Martinez et al. (2025)

Black flies are small, dark-bodied flies with a characteristic humped thorax. They breed in flowing water (streams, rivers, and creeks) and are notorious for their painful, persistent daytime biting, especially in northern and mountainous regions of North America.

While North American species do not transmit disease to humans, their bites can cause intense irritation, allergic reactions, and secondary infections. In Central and West Africa and parts of Latin America, black flies are vectors of *Onchocerca volvulus*, the causative agent of river blindness, a significant global parasitic disease, and *Mansonella*. In veterinary medicine, black flies are vectors for *Onchocerca*, *Dirofilaria*, *Splendidofilaria*, *Trypanosoma*, and *Leucocytozoon* species that do not infect humans.

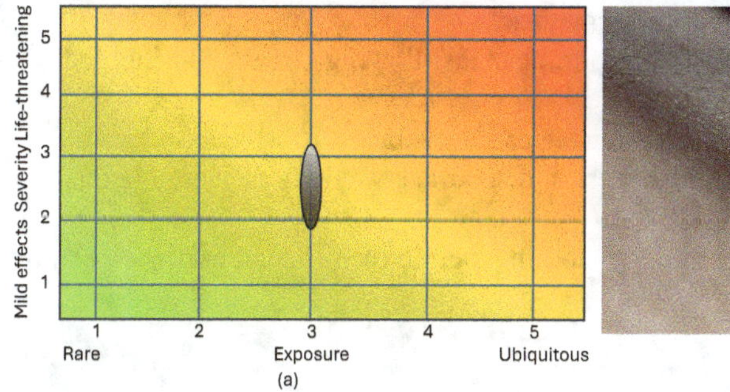

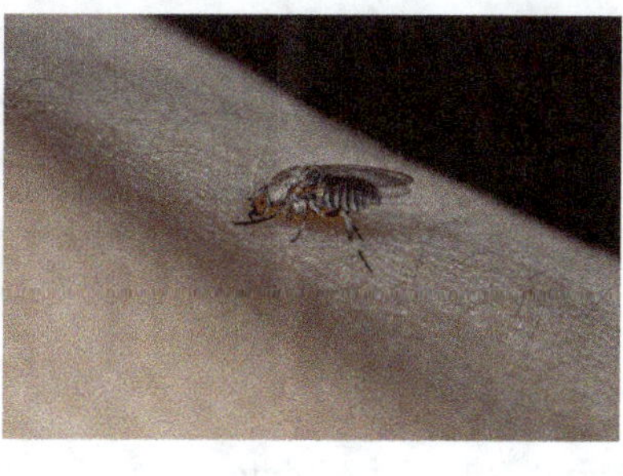

FIGURE 5.25   Black flies. (a) Exposure × severity matrix; (b) Black fly, *Simulium* sp.

Symptoms

Bites usually produce immediate pain followed by:

- Localized swelling, redness, and intense itching
- Formation of small, bleeding punctures or raised welts
- Allergic dermatitis or systemic reactions in sensitive individuals
- Clusters of bites around ears, neck, and scalp, where skin is thin and exposed
- In severe infestations: fever, headache, nausea, or swollen lymph nodes ("black fly fever")
- Scratching may lead to secondary bacterial infections

While not dangerous to most individuals, black fly bites can greatly impact comfort and productivity during fieldwork.

Occupational Exposure

Black flies are most active in late spring and early summer, and exposure is common during:

- Aquatic and riparian ecology work, especially near fast-moving streams
- Trail maintenance, forestry, and camping in northern states and mountainous regions
- Structure inspections or dam work near whitewater or swift currents
- Arctic and boreal region work, where infestations may be severe

They are aggressive daytime feeders, with peak activity in the morning and late afternoon.

Prevention

Prevention requires both repellents and physical barriers:

- Wear long-sleeved shirts, long pants, and head nets
- Tuck pants into boots or socks; wear light-colored clothing
- Use Environmental Protection Agency (EPA)-approved repellents (DEET, picaridin) on exposed skin
- Treat clothing and gear with permethrin
- Avoid areas with heavy vegetation near fast-flowing streams during peak season
- Set up camps away from running water if possible
- Use portable fans in work shelters to discourage weak fliers

Because black flies often bite through clothing, permethrin-treated gear is especially valuable.

What To Do If Affected

- Clean the bite site with soap and water to reduce infection risk
- Apply topical corticosteroids or antihistamines to relieve itching

- Monitor for signs of secondary infection (pus, spreading redness, fever)
- Seek medical attention if symptoms persist or allergic reactions develop

Bite reactions often peak 12–24 hours after exposure and may last for several days.

HORSE FLIES, DEER FLIES, AND YELLOW FLIES

Entomological Parasites and Vectors: Order Diptera, Family Tabanidae: *Tabanus*, *Chrysops*, and *Hybomitra*, and several other genera (Figure 5.26)
  Exposure and Severity Ratings (Figure 5.26)

- **Exposure Level: 3–4**
  - Moderately (3) common, especially in rural areas in summer
  - Frequent (4) activity in suitable habitats and regions
- **Severity Level: 2**
  - Typical bites generally cause moderate (2) pain
  - They are rarely a mechanical vector of some more serious diseases such as tularemia (q.v., severity levels 3–5) or anthrax

References: Krinsky (1976), Akhoundi et al. (2020), Whyte et al. (2020)

Horse and deer flies are medium to large, fast-flying blood-feeding flies known for their painful, slicing bites and relentless pursuit of moving animals and humans. Females feed on blood using scissor-like mouthparts, leaving bleeding wounds that can become infected or allergic in sensitive individuals.

In the United States, they are primarily a nuisance biting species to humans, but deer flies (*Chrysops* spp.) have rarely been implicated in the transmission of *Francisella tularensis* (tularemia). Over 35 viruses, bacteria, protozoans, and helminths (worms) have been reported as spread by tabanid flies to animals. In Africa, tabanid flies mechanically transmit some trypanosome protozoans, *Loa loa* filariasis, and other pathogens to humans.

Horse and deer flies are most active in hot, humid weather, near wetlands, streams, and wooded trails, often during midday hours when other biting insects are less active.

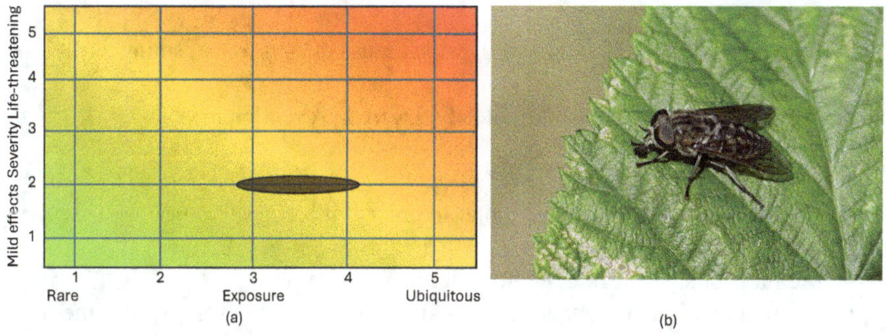

FIGURE 5.26 Horse, deer, and yellow flies. (a) Exposure × severity matrix; (b) Black horse fly, *Tabanus autumnalis*.

Symptoms

- Immediate pain at the bite site
- Bleeding, swelling, and welts
- Clusters of bites, especially on shoulders, back, head, and legs
- Secondary infections due to skin disruption
- Allergic reactions (rash, burning, systemic response in rare cases)
- Risk of tularemia if bitten by an infected deer fly in endemic regions

The persistent, aggressive biting can affect concentration, morale, and safety during outdoor work.

Occupational Exposure

High risk of exposure occurs to ecologists and environmental professionals during:

- Wetland delineation, stream surveys, and trail inspections
- Terrestrial ecology work in lowland forests and marshes
- Dam inspections, levee work, or vegetation monitoring in riparian areas
- Summer fieldwork in humid, forested regions of the Midwest, South, and Northeast
- Working near livestock or wildlife that attract flies in large numbers

Tabanids are visual hunters, attracted to movement, dark colors, and CO_2.

Prevention

Because repellents are only partially effective, combine physical and chemical deterrents:

- Wear light-colored, loose-fitting clothing
- Avoid dark colors (especially black and blue), which attract flies
- Use permethrin-treated clothing for best protection
- Apply DEET, picaridin, or oil of lemon eucalyptus on exposed skin
- Wear broad-brimmed hats and head nets in heavy infestation areas
- Schedule outdoor work for early morning or late afternoon, avoiding peak fly activity
- Avoid disturbing wetlands and livestock areas during warm, sunny days

Horse flies are difficult to deter completely; layered prevention is key.

What To Do If Affected

- Clean bite site with soap and water to prevent infection
- Apply cold compresses and anti-itch creams or antihistamines
- Monitor for signs of infection or allergic reaction
- If bitten in tularemia-endemic areas and fever or ulcer develops, seek medical attention promptly
- In severe allergic cases, a physician may prescribe corticosteroids or epinephrine

While most bites are just painful nuisances, tularemia risk should not be ignored.

LARGE BITING FLIES

Entomological Agents: Order Diptera, Families Asilidae (robber flies), Mydidae (Mydas flies), and rarely Therevidae (stiletto flies), Rhagionidae and Athericidae (snipe flies) (Figure 5.27)
Exposure and Severity Ratings (Figure 5.27)

- **Exposure Level:1–2**
  - Rarely (1) encountered to infrequent (2)
  - Some are more common in arid habitats and others near streams
- **Severity Level: 1–2**
  - Typical bites generally cause mild (1) to moderate (2) pain
  - Larger species bite harder

Reference: Akhoundi et al. (2020)

About the same size as horse and deer flies or larger, these additional families may also inflict painful bites. Normally, these flies prey on smaller insects and only bite in self-defense, and they do not carry any parasites or pathogens to humans.

Robber flies (Asilidae) and the rarer mydas flies (Mydidae) tend to frequent more arid habitats and tend to be longer but less robust than most horse flies. They can produce a surprisingly painful bite if handled carelessly. Stiletto flies (Therevidae) and snipe flies (families Rhagionidae and Athericidae) are smaller and much less frequently encountered. The larvae of snipe flies are aquatic, so they tend to occur around streams. Eastern species of snipe flies do not bite, but some western species do.

Symptoms

- Immediate pain at the bite site
- Bleeding, swelling, and welts

Occupational Exposure

Higher risk of exposure occurs to ecologists and environmental professionals during:

- Terrestrial ecology work in lowland forests, plains, and marshes
- Vegetation monitoring in riparian areas
- Summer fieldwork in semi-arid forested regions

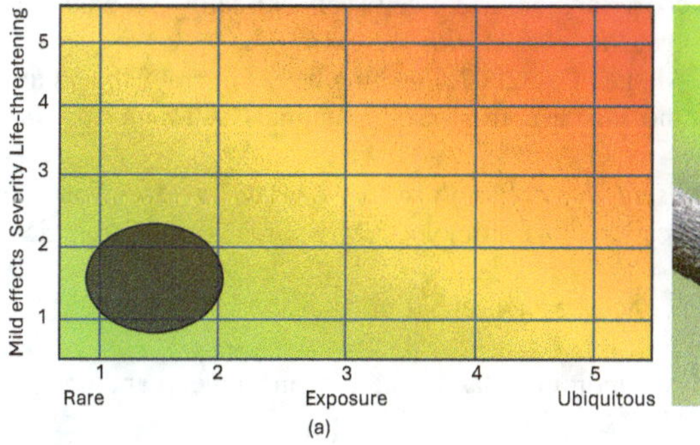

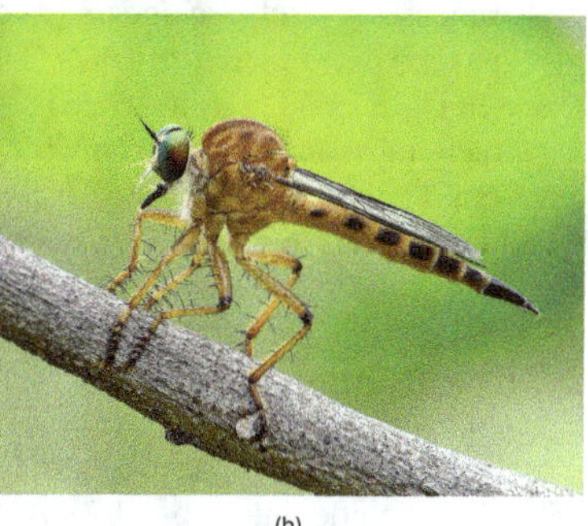

FIGURE 5.27 Large Diptera. (a) Exposure × severity matrix; (b) robber fly, *Efferia* sp.

All of these flies tend to prey on smaller insects and are sometimes captured in nets when targeting other insects.

Prevention

- Wear light gloves when handling large flies, especially large-bodied ones that are actively chasing prey
- Avoid placing large flies in pockets or loose bags
- Educate field staff on common biting fly families
- Use care when removing large flies from insect nets

What To Do If Affected

- Clean bite site with soap and water to prevent infection
- Apply cold compresses and anti-itch creams or antihistamines
- Monitor for signs of infection or allergic reaction

Most bites are just mild to moderately painful nuisances.

REFERENCES

Akhoundi M, Sereno D, Marteau A, Bruel C, Izri A. 2020. Who bites me? A tentative discriminative key to diagnose hematophagous ectoparasites biting using clinical manifestations. *Diagnostics* 10: 308.

Arlian LG. 1989. Biology, host relations, and epidemiology of *Sarcoptes scabei. Ann. Rev. Entomol.* 34: 139–161.

Arora P, Rudnicka L, Sar-Pomian M, Wollina U, Jafferany M, Lotti T, Sadoughifar R, Sitkowska Z, Goldust M. 2020. Scabies: A comprehensive review and current perspectives. *Dermatol. Therapy* 33: e13746.

Baird CR, Stoltz RL. 2002. Range expansion of the hobo spider, *Tegenaria agrestis*, in the northwestern United States (Araneae, Agelenidae). *J. Arachnol.* 30: 201–204.

Bennett RG, Vetter RS. 2004. An approach to spider bites. Erroneous attribution of dermonecrotic lesions to brown recluse or hobo spider bites in Canada. *Can. Family Physician* 50: 1098–1101.

Caruso MB, Sales Lauria PS, Vieira de Souza CM, Casais-e-Silva LL. 2021. Widow spiders in the New World: A review on *Latrodectus* Walckenaer, 1805 (Theridiidae) and latrodectism in the Americas. *J. Venom. Anim. Toxins Trop. Dis.* 27: e20210011.

Chen K, Roe RM, Ponnusamy L. 2022. Biology, systematics, microbiome, pathogen transmission and control of chiggers (Acari: Trombiculidae, Leeuwenhoekiidae) with emphasis on the United States. *Intern. J. Envir. Res. Public Hlth* 19: 15147.

Claussen DL, Gerald GW, Kotcher JE, Miskell CA. 2007. Pinching forces in crayfish and fiddler crabs, and comparison with the closing forces of other animals. *J. Comp. Physiol.* B 178: 333–342.

Contreras-Ramos, A. 1998. *Systematics of the dobsonfly genus Corydalus* (Megaloptera: *Corydalidae*). Thomas Say Publications in Entomology Monographs, Entomological Society of America, Lanham, MD.

Cranshaw W. 2011. A review of nuisance invader household pests of the United States. *Am. Entomol.* 57: 165–169.

Diaz JH. 2004. The global epidemiology, syndromic classification, management, and prevention of spider bites. *Am. J. Trop. Med. Hyg.* 71: 239–250.

Edel C, Rühr PT, Frenzel M, van de Kamp T, Faragó T, Hammel JU, Wilde F, Blanke A. 2024. Bite force transmission and mandible shape in grasshoppers, crickets, and allies is not driven by dietary niches. *Evolution* 78: 1958–1968.

Emde RN. 1961. Sarcoptic mange in the human: A report of an epidemic of 10 cases of infection by *Sarcoptes scabiei*, Variety Canis. *Arch. Dermatol.* 84: 633–636.

Fu YT, Yao C, Deng YP, Elsheikha HM, Shao R, Zhu X-Q, Liu G-H. 2022. Human pediculosis, a global public health problem. *Infect. Dis. Poverty* 11: 58.

Furbee RB, Kao LW, Ibrahim D. 2006. Brown recluse spider envenomation. *Clinics Lab. Med.* 26: 211–226.

Gangwere SK. 1965. The structural adaptations of mouthparts of Orthoptera and allies. *Eos, Rev. Esp. Entomol.* 41: 67–85.

Goddard J, deShazo R. 2009. Bed bugs (*Cimex lectularius*) and clinical consequences of their bites. *JAMA.* 301: 1358–1366.

Haddad V, Schwartz EF, Carvalho LN. 2010. Bites caused by giant water bugs belonging to Belostomatidae family (Hemiptera, Heteroptera) in humans: A report of seven cases. *Wilderness Envir. Med.* 21: 130–133.

Hamllll FZ, Bérenger JM, Parola P. 2023. Cimicids of medical and veterinary importance. *Insects* 14: 392.

Jalink MB, Wisse RPL. 2021. On the dangers of tropical spiders as a pet: A review of ocular symptoms caused by tarantula hairs. *Am. J. Trop. Med. Hyg.* 105: 1795–1797.

Kampen H, Werner D. 2023. Biting midges (Diptera: Ceratopogonidae) as vectors of viruses. *Microorganisms* 11: 2706.

Kevan DKMc E. 1983. A preliminary survey of known and potentially Canadian and Alaskan centipedes (Chilopoda). *Can. J. Zool.* 61: 2938–2955.

Klepzig KD, Hartshorn JA, Tsalickis A, Sheehan TN. 2022. Eye Gnat (*Liohippelates*, Diptera: Chloropidae) biology, ecology, and management: Past, present, and future. *J. Integr. Pest Manage.* 13: 19.

Krinsky WL. 1976. Animal disease agents transmitted by horse flies and deer flies (Diptera: Tabanidae). *J. Med. Entomol.* 13: 225–275.

Krinsky WL 2019. Beetles (Coleoptera). Ch. 9 in: Mullen GR, Durden LA (eds.) *Medical and Veterinary Entomology*. Academic Press, Cambridge, MA.

Lai O, Ho D, Glick S, Jagdeo J. 2016. Bed bugs and possible transmission of human pathogens: A systematic review. *Arch. Dermatol. Res.* 308: 531–538.

Missouri Department of Conservation. 2024. Hellgrammite. MDOC Field Guides.

Mullen GR. 2019. Solpugids (Solifugae). Ch. 24 in: Mullen GR, Durden LA (eds.) *Medical and Veterinary Entomology*. Academic Press, Cambridge, MA.

Muma MH. 1970. *A Synoptic Review of North American, Central American, and West Indian Solpugida (Arthropoda: Arachnida)*. Arthropods of Florida and Neighboring Land Areas, No. 5, Florida Department of Agriculture and Consumer Sciences, Gainesville, FL.

Ombati R, Luo L, Yang S, Lai R. 2018. Centipede envenomation: Clinical importance and the underlying molecular mechanisms. *Toxicon* 154: 60–68.

Rivera-Martínez A, Laredo-Tiscareño SV, Adame-Gallegos JR, de Luna-Santillana EJ, Rodríguez-Alarcón CA, García-Rejón JE, Casas-Martínez M, Garza-Hernández JA. 2025. Viruses in simuliidae: An updated systematic review of arboviral diversity and vector potential. *Life* 15: 807.

Sandidge JS, Hopwood JL. 2005. Brown recluse spiders: A review of biology, life history and pest management. *Trans. Kans. Acad. Sci.* 108: 99–108.

Sasa M. 1961. Biology of chiggers. *Ann. Rev. Entomol.* 6: 221–244.

Schaefer CW, Panizzi AR. 2000. Adventitious biters: "Nuisance" bugs. Ch. 19. Pp. 553–560 in: Schaefer CW, Panizzi AR. (eds.) *Heteroptera of Economic Importance*. CRC Press, Boca Raton, FL.

Theis J, Lavoipierre MM, LaPerriere R, Kroese H. 1981. Tropical rat mite dermatitis: Report of six cases and review of other mite infestations. *Arch. Dermatol.* 117: 341–343.

Usinger RL. 1966. *Monograph of Cimicidae (Hemiptera – Heteroptera)*. Thomas Say Foundation, Baltimore, MD.

Vetter RS. 2013. Spider envenomation in North America. *Critical Care Nurs. Clinics* 25: 205–223.

Vetter, RS, Isbister GK. 2008. Medical aspects of spider bites. *Ann. Rev. Entomol.* 53: 409–429.

Vetter RS, Isbister GK, Bush SP, Boutin LJ. 2006. Verified bites by yellow sac spiders (genus *Cheiracanthium*) in the United States and Australia: Where is the necrosis? *Am. J. Trop. Med. Hyg.* 74: 1043–1048.

Weihmann T, Reinhardt L, Weißing K, Siebert T, Wipfler B. 2015. Fast and powerful: Biomechanics and bite forces of the mandibles in the American Cockroach *Periplaneta americana. PLoS ONE* 10: e0141226.

Whyte AF, Popescu FD, Carlson J. 2020. Tabanidae insect (horsefly and deerfly) allergy in humans: A review of the literature. *Clin. Exper. Allergy* 50: 886–893.

6 Potentially Pathogenic Bites

ARACHNIDS

TICKS

Entomological Parasites: Order Ixodida, Families Ixodidae (hard ticks), Argasidae (soft ticks) (Figure 6.1)
   Exposure and Severity Ratings (Figure 6.1)

- **Exposure Level: 2–4**
  - Uncommon (2) in most urban environments
  - Widespread and frequent (4) in rural habitats, especially during outdoor activities
- **Severity Level: 1**
  - Typical bite causes minimal harm (1)
  - Vector-borne diseases discussed separately

References: Castelli et al. (2008), Haddad et al. (2018), Akhoundi et al. (2020)

Ticks are blood-feeding arachnids that parasitize mammals, birds, reptiles, and amphibians. They are divided into two main families:

- Ixodidae (hard ticks) – include *Ixodes*, *Amblyomma*, *Dermacentor*, and *Rhipicephalus* species
- Argasidae (soft ticks) – include *Ornithodoros* and related genera

Ticks are among the most important vectors of human and animal disease in the United States, capable of transmitting bacteria, viruses, and protozoa. Tick bites also pose risks of local skin reactions, secondary infections, and, in rare cases, tick paralysis, a neurotoxic condition caused by certain female ticks.

Tick activity is typically seasonal, with peaks in spring and summer, though some species remain active year-round in warmer climates.

Symptoms
- Painless or mildly irritating bite
- Localized swelling or redness
- Possible itching, burning, or bruising at the site
- If tick remains attached for extended periods:
  - Greater likelihood of pathogen transmission
  - Larger feeding lesion or granuloma

Bite sites often go unnoticed unless carefully inspected.

DOI: 10.1201/9781003745709-8

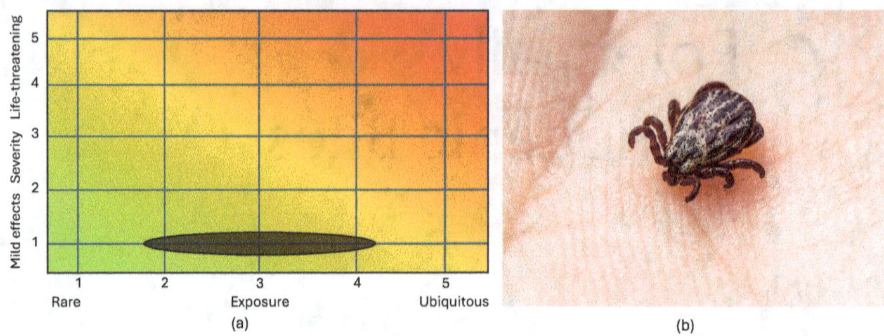

FIGURE 6.1 Tick bites. (a) Exposure × severity matrix; (b) Rocky Mountain wood tick, *Dermacentor andersoni.*

Occupational Exposure

Tick exposure is common for ecologists and environmental professionals engaging in the following activities:

- Conduct fieldwork in tick-endemic regions (e.g., wooded, brushy, or grassy habitats)
- Ecologists, foresters, wildlife biologists, and environmental workers
- Hunters, trappers, and agricultural workers
- Park rangers and outdoor recreationists in the southeastern and midwestern United States
- Forestry, field biology, wildlife handling, and agricultural work
- Trail maintenance and land surveying, particularly in grassy, brushy, or wooded areas
- Monitoring construction or infrastructure projects in rural, wooded areas
- Ecological surveys in rural or suburban environments
- Inspection of animal burrows, nests, or dens
- Engage in activities requiring overnight camping or prolonged immobility, increasing the chance for undetected tick attachment
- Camping, hiking, or sleeping outdoors in endemic regions

Exposure risk increases with:

- Frequent tick encounters
- Inadequate tick prevention practices (e.g., lack of repellents, protective clothing)

It should be noted that handling of live or dead animals rarely involves transmission of ticks because most hard ticks (Ixodidae) feed only once per life stage (larva, nymph, adult), and they may stay attached for days while engorging. The majority of ticks feeding on that animal are firmly embedded and unlikely to abandon the host during brief handling. Once replete, they usually drop off the host to molt or lay eggs. After molting or laying eggs, tick engage in an activity called "questing" in which they crawl onto vegetation and wave their legs in the air to sense their next host passing by. Because of this pattern, ticks are *not* typically moving from one host to another directly; instead, after detachment, they spend time sequestered in the environment before questing for a new host.

That said, there are circumstances where handling infested animals *does* increase risk. Larvae, nymphs, or adults that are still questing or recently moving on the host's fur, feathers, or skin (but have not yet embedded their mouthparts) may crawl onto a handler. When an animal is being restrained or examined, it is possible that restrained ticks may be rubbed loose and end up on the handler's hands, arms, or clothing. Also, handling not only the animal but also its bedding or fur debris may expose workers to ticks that have recently dropped off and are awaiting a new host. This is particularly relevant for domestic animals (dogs, livestock), which can carry high tick burdens and move between humans and tick habitats. This is also the case with recently deceased animals: ticks may have abandoned the dead host and may begin questing in the grass and brush in the vicinity, waiting for a new host. Therefore, veterinary and regular wildlife workers are at somewhat higher risk than, say, ecologists who briefly observe wild animals without restraint.

A few tick groups are especially notable. The brown dog tick (*Rhipicephalus sanguineus*) thrives in kennels and indoor environments, so handling infested dogs is a significant risk, as ticks often wander and quest inside human dwellings. The lone star tick (*Amblyomma americanum*) is aggressive and numerous in parts of the southeastern United States; larvae can occur in "seed tick" clusters and latch onto humans during close animal or habitat contact. Furthermore, some soft ticks (Argasidae) feed more briefly than hard ticks (ranging from minutes to hours). Some soft ticks (e.g., *Ornithodoros* spp.) live in their host's nests or burrows, so disturbing or handling nest-dwelling animals can expose workers to large numbers of ticks in a short time.

Prevention

Preventive measures should be multifaceted:

- Wear light-colored clothing to spot ticks easily
- Use gloves that may allow visibility of ticks or present an intractable surface for them
- Tuck pants into socks, wear long sleeves and permethrin-treated clothing
- Apply Environmental Protection Agency (EPA)-approved repellents (5%–10% DEET, picaridin) to exposed skin
- Perform full-body tick checks after fieldwork – See Box 2.1
- Shower promptly (within 2 hours) to wash off unattached ticks
- After field work, launder field clothing at >130°F for at least 10 minutes so they are fresh for the next use
- Examine gear and pets that may carry ticks indoors
- Use tick-free campsites and work areas when possible

Remember, ticks often attach in hidden areas – early detection is crucial.

What To Do If Affected

- See Box 2.2 on how to remove ticks
- Remove the tick promptly with fine-tipped tweezers
  - Grasp close to the skin and pull upward with steady pressure
  - Do not twist, crush, or burn the tick
- Wash area with soap and water, then apply antiseptic
- Save the tick in alcohol or sealed container for possible identification
- Monitor for symptoms of illness (fever, rash, fatigue, joint pain) or tick paralysis over the next several weeks
- As described for each disease below, if symptoms occur, seek medical attention immediately since early treatment is often best for controlling or eliminating the diseases
- Some tick-borne pathogens can be transmitted during blood transfusions, so it would be prudent to avoid blood donation for 6 months after potentially pathogenic bites

Prophylactic antibiotics may be prescribed after certain high-risk bites (e.g., *Ixodes scapularis* in Lyme-endemic areas).

TICK-BORNE DISEASES AND SYNDROMES

After entries for alpha-gal syndrome and tick paralysis, which are not pathogenic from a microbiological standpoint, the rest of the entries for 13 tick-borne diseases in North America are listed in order of highest risk to lowest risk considering both exposure risk and potential severity (Table 6.1).

For each disease or syndrome, it is best to consult a physician for proper medical diagnosis and treatment and not rely solely on the information provided here. Some

---

TABLE 6.1

Ranking of 13 Tick-Borne Diseases in North America, Considering Both Exposure Risk and Severity

Rank	Disease	Reason for Ranking
1	Lyme Disease	Extremely common in northeastern, mid-Atlantic, upper Midwest, and expanding in range; rarely fatal but can lead to serious chronic complications
2	Rocky Mountain Spotted Fever (RMSF)	Less common than Lyme, but potentially fatal if untreated; more prevalent in southeastern United States, parts of Mexico, and incidence is increasing
3	Ehrlichiosis	Moderate frequency in south-central and southeastern United States; symptoms can be severe but usually treatable
4	Anaplasmosis	Expanding distribution in the Northeast and upper Midwest; severity is moderate, occasionally severe
5	Babesiosis	Increasingly common in Northeast; mild in healthy individuals, but severe in immunocompromised

(Continued)

TABLE 6.1 (*Continued*)
Ranking of 13 Tick-Borne Diseases in North America, Considering Both Exposure Risk and Severity

Rank	Disease	Reason for Ranking
6	Tularemia	Regionally common in central United States; severity can be high, especially in pneumonic form; multiple transmission routes
7	Tick-Borne Relapsing Fever (TBRF)	Regional (western United States in caves or cabins); symptoms can be severe if untreated
8	Powassan Virus	Rare, but extremely serious (10% fatality, high neurological damage); expanding presence in Northeast and Midwest
9	Heartland Virus	Rare but emerging; limited geographic range (central United States); symptoms potentially severe
10	Bourbon Virus	Extremely rare but often severe and sometimes fatal
11	Colorado Tick Fever	Mild to moderate symptoms; limited to Rocky Mountains
12	Other Spotted Fevers	Regional, usually milder relatives of RMSF
13	Southern Tick-Associated Rash Illness (STARI)	Looks like Lyme but is mild and not known to be deadly

diseases or syndromes require immediate medical care upon notice of symptoms. Remember to check for ticks and bring them to the appointment, if possible.

Alpha-Gal Syndrome

Entomological Vectors: Order Ixodida, Family Ixodidae: *Amblyomma americanum* (Lone star tick); occasionally other tick species in localized contexts
   Exposure and Severity Ratings (Figure 6.2)

- **Exposure Level: 2**
  - Uncommon (2); currently appears to be regional with risk localized primarily in the southeastern and midwestern United States
  - However, it appears to be spreading with recent cases in MN, NJ, and NY
- **Severity Level: 4**
  - Activation of alpha-gal syndrome can cause severe (4) harm, requiring long-term dietary management and medical attention

References: Werner et al. (2019), Peterson et al. (2025)

Alpha-gal syndrome is a tick-induced allergic condition triggered by the carbohydrate galactose-α-1,3-galactose (alpha-gal), found in most mammalian (non-primate) meat. The condition develops after bites from certain ticks, most notably the lone star tick (*A. americanum*), which introduce alpha-gal into the human host, sensitizing the immune system.

The mechanism that is thought to occur in this syndrome is that the tick had previously fed on a non-primate mammal and ingested alpha-gal. When the tick

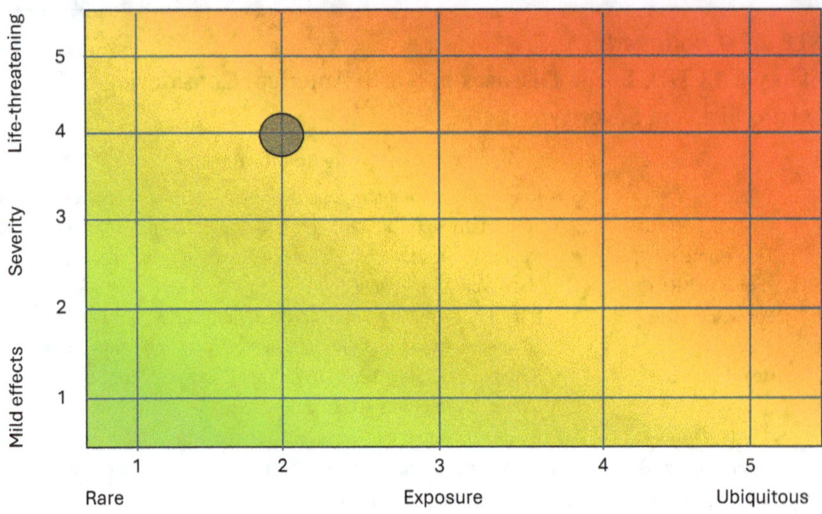

FIGURE 6.2 Alpha-gal syndrome. Exposure × severity matrix.

subsequently bites a human, the alpha-gal is transferred to the human on the tick's mouthparts or in its saliva. Later, consumption of red meat (e.g., beef, pork, lamb, venison) triggers a food allergy. Unlike traditional food allergies, however, which cause immediate reactions, alpha-gal reactions are delayed, typically occurring 3–6 hours after consuming red meat. In sensitized individuals, subsequent exposure to alpha-gal can provoke symptoms ranging from hives and gastrointestinal distress to anaphylaxis, sometimes severe and life-threatening. The condition may persist for months or years, especially with repeated tick exposure.

The syndrome appears to have originated in Australia and is now emerging in incidence and geographic range, particularly in the south, southeast, and lower Midwest United States, mirroring the expanding range of the lone star tick. Cases have also been reported in parts of New York, New Jersey, and Minnesota, and similar syndromes have been noted globally with other tick species.

Symptoms

Reactions vary in severity and timing:

- Typical symptoms (3–6 hours post-ingestion):
  - Hives, itching, and flushing
  - Nausea, abdominal pain, or diarrhea
  - Swelling of lips, throat, or tongue
- Severe symptoms:
  - Respiratory distress
  - Hypotension
  - Anaphylaxis

Symptoms may also be triggered by gelatin, dairy, or pharmaceuticals containing animal-derived ingredients, including some vaccines or monoclonal antibodies.

Tick Paralysis

Entomological Agents: Order Ixodida, Family Ixodidae: *Dermacentor variabilis* (American dog tick), *Dermacentor andersoni* (Rocky Mountain wood tick), and occasionally *Amblyomma*, *Ixodes*, or *Rhipicephalus* species (females only)
  Exposure and Severity Ratings (Figure 6.3)

- **Exposure Level: 1–2**
  - Rare (1) but widespread distribution throughout much of North America (2)
  - Risk is seasonal and primarily in areas with high tick activity in spring and early summer
- **Severity Level: 4–5**
  - Potentially life-threatening if respiratory paralysis develops; rapid improvement with tick removal

Reference: Edlow and McGillicuddy (2008)

Tick paralysis is a neurotoxic condition caused by prolonged attachment and feeding of certain female hard ticks, most notably the American dog tick (*Dermacentor variabilis*) and the Rocky Mountain wood tick (*Dermacentor andersoni*). The condition arises from a salivary neurotoxin secreted during feeding, which can interfere with motor nerve function. While the condition is not caused by a pathogen, its effects can be severe or fatal if unrecognized.

Most cases occur in young children and pets, though adults may also be affected. Risk is highest in the spring and early summer, during peak adult tick activity. Prolonged attachment – often 4–7 days – is required for sufficient toxin accumulation. This condition is frequently misdiagnosed as Guillain-Barré syndrome, botulism, or other neuromuscular disorders.

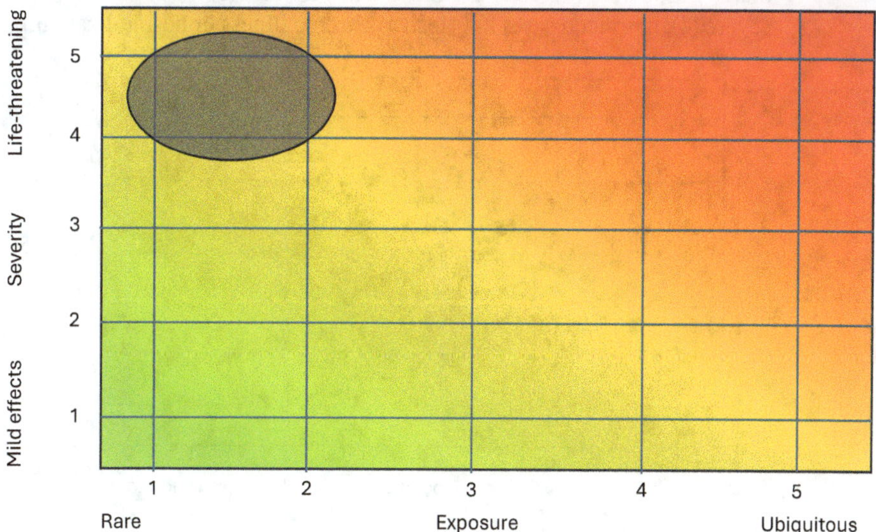

FIGURE 6.3 Tick paralysis. Exposure × severity matrix.

Symptoms

Signs typically begin with vague neurological symptoms and progress over hours to days:

- Fatigue and irritability
- Incoordination and unsteady gait
- Ascending flaccid paralysis (starting in legs and moving upward)
- Slurred speech or facial weakness
- Difficulty swallowing
- In severe cases, respiratory paralysis and death may occur

Symptoms typically resolve within 24–48 hours after tick removal.

Lyme Disease

Pathogen: Order Spirochaetales, Family Borreliaceae: *Borrelia burgdorferi*
   Entomological Vectors: Order Ixodida, Family Ixodidae: *Ixodes scapularis* (deer tick), ***I. pacificus* (western black-legged tick)**
   Exposure and Severity Ratings (Figure 6.4)

- **Exposure Level: 2–4**
    - **USA overall**: uncommon (2): ~8 cases per million; U.S. Centers for Disease Control and Protection (CDC) reports ~30,000 new incidence/ year, with total of 476,000 diagnosed cases
    - **Focal states (e.g., NY and New England)**: frequent (4): 36–88 cases per million
- **Severity Level: 2–4**
    - Many cases mild (2); no certainty as to what triggers more severe symptoms
    - Usually moderate (3): early treatment leads to full recovery
    - Severe (4), untreated cases may lead to chronic illness or hospitalization

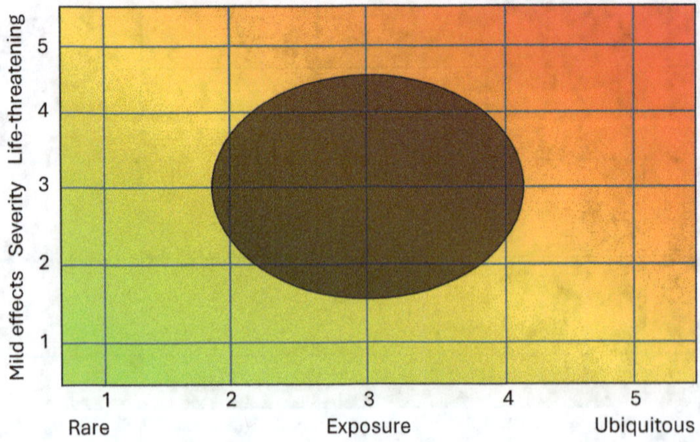

FIGURE 6.4 Lyme disease. Exposure × severity matrix.

References: Borchers et al. (2013), Mead (2015), Eisen et al. (2017), Richardson et al. (2019), Werner et al. (2019), Radolf et al. (2021)

Lyme disease is the most commonly reported vector-borne disease in the United States. Caused by the spirochete *Borrelia burgdorferi*, it is transmitted primarily through the bite of infected *Ixodes* ticks. It is most prevalent in the northeastern, Upper Midwestern, and Pacific coastal states, and is especially concentrated in the New England, Mid-Atlantic, and Upper Great Lakes regions. Although ticks can be active year-round, most human cases occur during the late spring and summer months when immature nymphal ticks are most active and likely to go unnoticed.

Symptoms

Initial signs of Lyme disease may begin 3–30 days after a tick bite and include:

- A red, expanding rash, often forming a characteristic "bullseye" pattern (in ~70%–80% of cases)
- Fever, chills, and fatigue
- Headache, muscle and joint aches
- Swollen lymph nodes

If untreated, the infection can spread to joints, the nervous system, and the heart, leading to:

- Facial palsy and meningitis
- Heart palpitations and dizziness
- Arthritis, especially in large joints
- Numbness, cognitive difficulties, and long-term neurological problems

While most patients respond well to early antibiotic treatment, 10%–20% may experience persistent symptoms lasting months or even years.

Ticks usually must be attached for 36–48 hours before the bacterium is transmitted, so early removal is critical. Monitor for symptoms for 1–4 weeks, and if symptoms appear, seek medical attention immediately. Most early-stage Lyme disease is effectively treated with oral antibiotics such as doxycycline. Delayed treatment can lead to long-term complications, including chronic joint inflammation and neurological effects. This disease is nationally reportable in the United States. Reporting is handled by medical and public health professionals; environmental personnel and their organizations are *not* responsible for direct case reporting.

Rocky Mountain Spotted Fever

Pathogen: Order Rickettsiales, Family Rickettsiaceae: *Rickettsia rickettsii*

Entomological Vectors: Order Ixodida, Family Ixodidae: *Dermacentor variabilis* (American dog tick), *D. andersoni* (Rocky Mountain wood tick), *Rhipicephalus sanguineus* (brown dog tick); possibly others

Exposure and Severity Ratings (Figure 6.5)

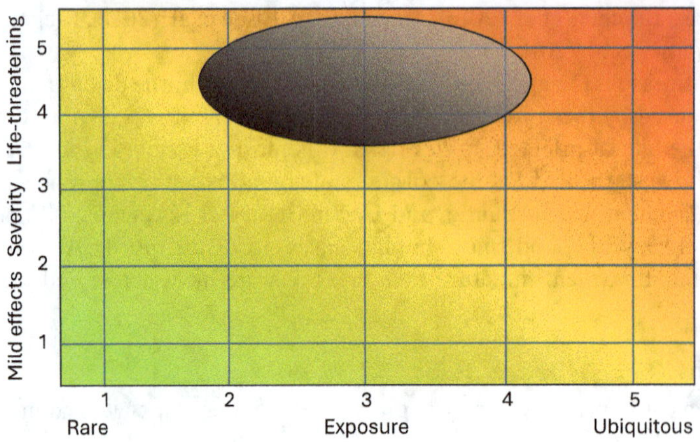

FIGURE 6.5 Rocky Mountain spotted fever. Exposure × severity matrix.

- **Exposure Level: 2–4**
  - Nationwide uncommon (2): 1.9–8.4 cases per million
  - Focal states (e.g., AR, MO, NC, OK, TN) frequent (4): 19–63 cases per million
- **Severity Level: 4–5**
  - Severe (4): requires early treatment; delayed treatment may result in hospitalization
  - Can be life-threatening (5): mortality rate ~0.5% with prompt treatment; rate higher without treatment

References: Eisen et al. (2017), Werner et al. (2019), Foley et al. (2025)

Rocky Mountain Spotted Fever (RMSF) is a serious and potentially fatal bacterial infection caused by *Rickettsia rickettsii*, a pathogen that infects the lining of blood vessels. RMSF is transmitted by several species of hard ticks, with geographic distribution throughout the United States, though it is less commonly reported in the Pacific Northwest and Upper Midwest. Despite its name suggesting presence in the Rocky Mountain cordillera in western North America, the disease is more common in the southeast and south-central states. Most cases occur in the summer months (May to August), though southern regions may experience extended seasons.

Symptoms

RMSF typically manifests 2–5 days after a tick bite, with early symptoms resembling other febrile illnesses:

- Sudden onset of fever, headache, muscle pain, and nausea
- Abdominal pain, vomiting, and loss of appetite
- Conjunctivitis, rash, or bleeding (may not appear until day 5–6)
- Vasculitis may cause tissue and organ damage
- Advanced symptoms: circulatory loss, neurological deficits, internal organ failure, and death

The hallmark rash begins as small, flat, pink, non-itchy spots on the wrists and ankles and may spread to the trunk. The rash appears in ~90% of cases, but it can be absent early on, making early diagnosis challenging – in this case you should rely on the presence of fever and headache as symptoms.

Monitor for symptoms for up to a week. If symptoms appear, seek medical attention immediately, since delay in treatment significantly increases the risk of hospitalization, complications, and death. Treatment, often with doxycycline, is usually started within 5 days of symptom onset because untreated RMSF can be fatal within 8 days.

This disease is nationally reportable in the United States. Reporting is handled by medical and public health professionals; environmental personnel and their organizations are *not* responsible for direct case reporting.

Ehrlichiosis

Pathogens: Order Rickettsiales, Family Ehrlichiaceae: *Ehrlichia chaffeensis*, *E. ewingii*, *E. muris*-like

Entomological Vector: Order Ixodida, Family Ixodidae: *Amblyomma americanum* (Lone star tick); possibly others

Exposure and Severity Ratings (Figure 6.6)

- **Exposure Level: 2**
  - Uncommon (2); found throughout United States but most prevalent east of the Mississippi River and in the Ozarks
  - Reported at <1–3.4 cases per million people nationwide; higher in endemic zones

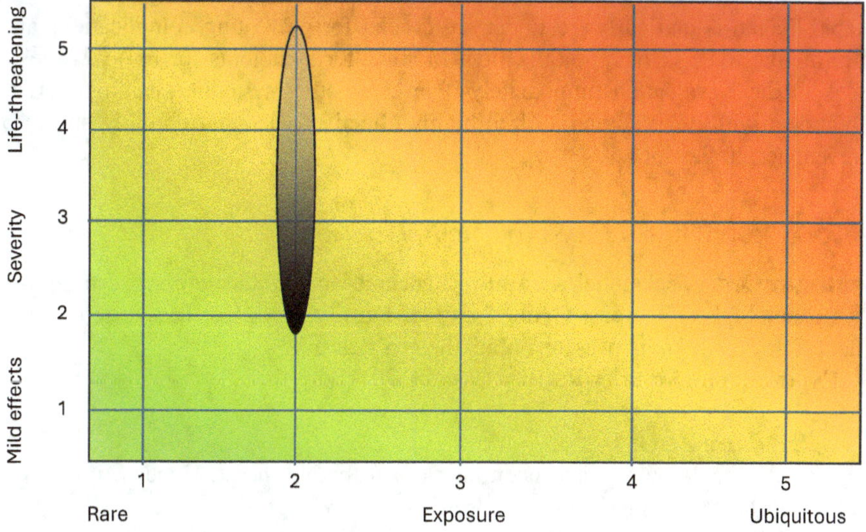

FIGURE 6.6 Ehrlichiosis. Exposure × severity matrix.

- **Severity Level: 2–5**
  - Some people experience mild (2) symptoms, while hospitalization frequently required due to severe (4) harm
  - Can be life-threatening (5), with case fatality rates up to ~3.6%

References: Goddard and Varela-Stokes (2009), Eisen et al. (2017), Werner et al. (2019), Gygax et al. (2025)

Ehrlichiosis is a tick-borne bacterial infection caused by several species of *Ehrlichia*, which invade white blood cells and disrupt normal immune responses. It is most commonly transmitted by the lone star tick (*A. americanum*), although other ticks may also serve as vectors. The disease is found throughout the United States but is most prevalent in states east of the Mississippi River and particularly in the Ozark region. Infections occur year-round but peak during late spring and summer.

Symptoms

Ehrlichiosis typically presents 1–2 weeks after a tick bite. Symptoms may range from mild to severe and include:

- Fever and chills
- Headache and malaise
- Muscle pain, nausea, and vomiting
- Diarrhea and abdominal discomfort
- Conjunctivitis
- Confusion or altered mental state
- Rash (in >60% of children, <30% of adults)
- Difficulty breathing, bleeding, or organ dysfunction
- In severe cases, death (mortality ~1.8%)

Rapid diagnosis and early treatment are crucial for preventing complications and minimizing the risk of hospitalization. Monitor for symptoms for up to 2 weeks. Seek medical evaluation immediately if fever or other systemic symptoms arise. Treatment with doxycycline is often highly effective when started early and may prevent hospitalization.

ANAPLASMOSIS (HUMAN GRANULOCYTIC ANAPLASMOSIS)

Pathogen: Order Rickettsiales, Family Ehrlichiaceae: *Anaplasma phagocytophilum*
    Entomological Vectors: Order Ixodida, Family Ixodidae: *Ixodes scapularis* **(deer tick),** *I. pacificus* **(western black-legged tick)**
    Exposure and Severity Ratings (Figure 6.7)

- **Exposure Level: 1–2**
  - Variable by region: uncommon (2) in the Northeast, Upper Midwest, and Mid-Atlantic; rare (1) elsewhere
  - ~6,500 cases reported nationwide in 2021; case numbers have been rising slowly since 1994

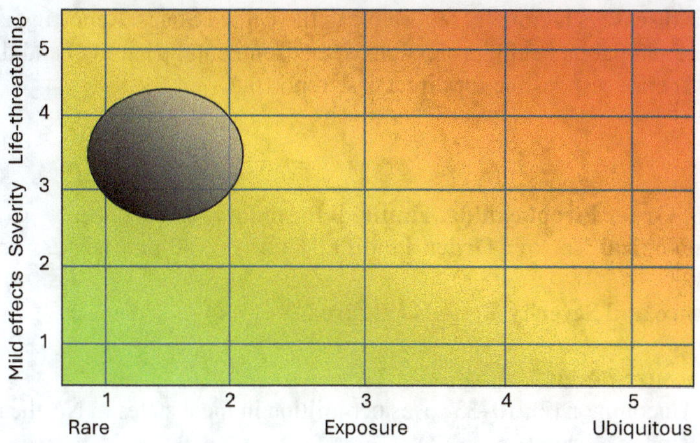

FIGURE 6.7 Anaplasmosis. Exposure × severity matrix.

- **Severity Level: 3–4**
  - Most cases moderate (3) and require treatment, and some severe (4) leading to hospitalization
  - Mortality rare and primarily when severe cases go completely untreated

References: Eisen et al. (2017), Werner et al. (2019), Schudel et al. (2024), Acosta-España (2025)

Anaplasmosis is a tick-borne bacterial infection caused by *Anaplasma phagocytophilum*, an obligate intracellular bacterium that targets neutrophils. This disease is endemic in the northeastern, upper midwestern, and Pacific coastal regions of the United States. The risk is highest during late spring and summer, when tick activity and human outdoor exposure peak.

Symptoms

Symptoms typically begin 1–2 weeks after a tick bite and range from mild to life-threatening depending on the host's immune status. Common manifestations include:

- Fever, chills, and headache
- Muscle aches and malaise
- Nausea and abdominal pain
- Cough and confusion
- Rare complications: rash, hemorrhaging, renal failure, and neurological symptoms
- Mortality rate is low (<1%), but hospitalization is common in severe cases

If untreated, symptoms can escalate, particularly in the elderly or immunocompromised. Monitor for symptoms for at least 2 weeks. If symptoms appear, consult a physician immediately; treatment with doxycycline is usually effective when administered early. This disease is nationally reportable in the United States. Reporting is handled by medical and public health professionals; environmental personnel and their organizations are *not* responsible for direct case reporting.

BABESIOSIS

Pathogen: Order Piroplasmida, Family Babesiidae: *Babesia* spp.

Entomological Vector: Order Ixodida, Family Ixodidae: *Ixodes scapularis* (deer tick)

Exposure and Severity Ratings (Figure 6.8)

- **Exposure Level: 2**
  - Uncommon (2): 10–33 cases per million in focal states in Northeast and Upper Midwest
  - Cases appear to be increasing ~9%/year (based on 2015–2022) in endemic areas
- **Severity Level: 3–4**
  - Often moderate (3)
  - Can be severe (4), with ~44% of symptomatic cases requiring hospitalization

References: Ord and Lobo (2015), Eisen et al. (2017), Werner et al. (2019), Waked and Krause (2022)

Babesiosis is a malaria-like parasitic infection caused by protozoa in the genus *Babesia*, which infect red blood cells. It is primarily transmitted by the deer tick (*I. scapularis*), often in the same regions and seasons as Lyme disease and anaplasmosis. The disease is most prevalent in the northeastern and Upper Midwestern United States,

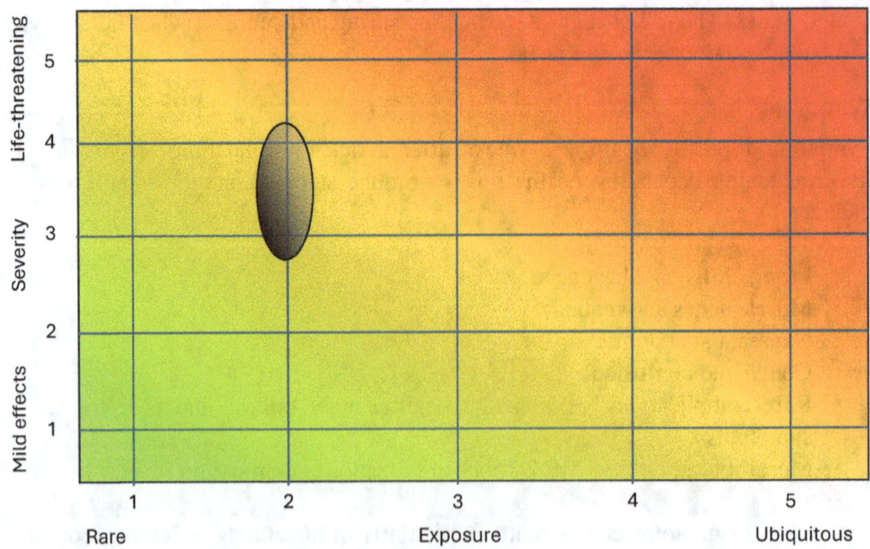

FIGURE 6.8 Babesiosis. Exposure × severity matrix.

especially in New England, New York, New Jersey, Wisconsin, and Minnesota. Most infections occur in the summer months, coinciding with peak nymphal tick activity.

Symptoms

Symptoms typically begin 1–2 weeks after a tick bite and can range from asymptomatic to severe. In symptomatic cases, patients may experience:

- Fever and chills
- Headache and body aches
- Fatigue and loss of appetite
- Nausea and sweats
- Hemolytic anemia and low platelet counts
- Malfunction of kidneys, lungs, or liver
- Blood clots, internal bleeding
- In severe cases, death, particularly in the elderly, immunocompromised, or those without a spleen

Babesiosis can also be transmitted through blood transfusion or congenitally (from mother to child in utero or perinatally).

If bitten by deer ticks, monitor for symptoms for about 2 weeks. If symptoms occur, seek medical attention immediately. Diagnosis typically involves blood smear or polymerase chain reaction (PCR) testing, and treatment includes antimicrobial medications such as atovaquone and azithromycin. This disease is nationally reportable in the United States. Reporting is handled by medical and public health professionals; environmental personnel and their organizations are *not* responsible for direct case reporting.

Tularemia

Pathogen: Order Thiotrichales, Family Francisellaceae: *Francisella tularensis*
   Entomological Vectors: Order Ixodida, Family Ixodidae: *Dermacentor variabilis* (American dog tick), *D. andersoni* (Rocky Mountain wood tick), *Amblyomma americanum* (Lone star tick); also transmitted by *Chrysops* spp. (deer flies) and direct contact with infected animals, water, or aerosols
   Exposure and Severity Ratings (Figure 6.9)

- **Exposure Level: 1–2**
  - Rare (1) across North America: ~0.6 cases per million people annually
  - Slightly higher but still uncommon (2) in central U.S. states
- **Severity Level: 3–5**
  - Most patients experience moderate (3) harm and recover fully with treatment
  - Severe (4) if untreated or exposure route is inhalation; usually requires hospitalization
  - Can be life-threatening (5): mortality <2% and usually due to untreated severe complications

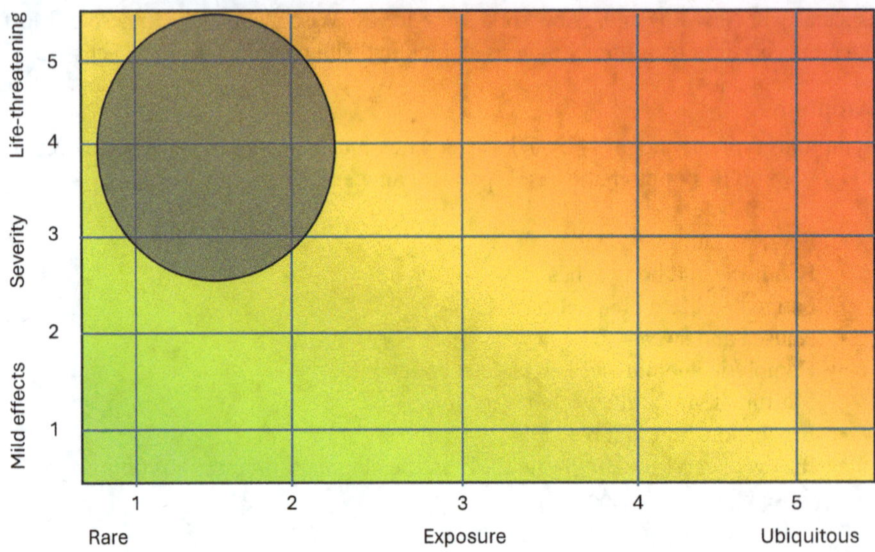

FIGURE 6.9 Tularemia. Exposure × severity matrix.

References: Dennis et al. (2001), Goddard and Varela-Stokes (2009), Eisen et al. (2017), Werner et al. (2019), Yeni et al. (2021), Nelson et al. (2024)

Tularemia is a potentially serious zoonotic disease caused by the bacterium *Francisella tularensis*. It is highly infectious – as few as ten organisms can cause disease – and it can be transmitted in multiple ways, including tick or deer fly bites, handling infected animal tissue, inhalation of contaminated dust or aerosols, or ingestion of contaminated water. The disease is widespread in the United States, occurring in all states except Hawaii, but is most commonly reported in Arkansas, Kansas, North Dakota, and South Dakota. Tularemia is classified as a Category A bioterrorism agent due to its high infectivity, severity, and potential for aerosol dissemination.

Symptoms

Symptoms vary based on the route of exposure but generally develop within 1–14 days of infection. Clinical forms include:

- Ulceroglandular (most common):
  - Skin ulcer at the site of the bite or exposure
  - Swollen and painful lymph nodes
- Glandular:
  - Lymphadenopathy without an ulcer
- Oculoglandular:
  - Eye irritation, swelling, pain
  - Inflammation from rubbing eyes with contaminated fingers
- Oropharyngeal:
  - Sore throat, mouth ulcers, tonsillitis
  - Gastrointestinal symptoms if ingested

- Pneumonic (inhalation):
  - Cough, chest pain, difficulty breathing
- Typhoidal (systemic):
  - High fever, weakness, weight loss, and organ failure

Untreated tularemia can result in severe illness or death, especially in the pneumonic and typhoidal forms. This disease is nationally reportable in the United States. Reporting is handled by medical and public health professionals; environmental personnel and their organizations are *not* responsible for direct case reporting.

Exposure may occur even in the absence of a visible bite or wound. Because of the potential for dust-borne infection, it may be necessary to use respiratory protection, such as an N95 mask, and gloves in dusty environments or when handling potentially contaminated soils. Dust from rodent nests and rabbit burrows is particularly prone to harboring the tularemia bacterium.

If potentially exposed, monitor for symptoms for up to 3 weeks, and if symptoms are even suspected, seek medical treatment immediately. Diagnosis may require serology or culture, but tularemia is generally treated with antibiotics such as streptomycin, doxycycline, and ciprofloxacin. Most patients recover completely with early and appropriate therapy.

Tick-Borne Relapsing Fever

Pathogens: Order Spirochaetales, Family Borreliaceae: *Borrelia hermsii*, *B. parkeri*, *B. turicatae*, and related species

Entomological Vectors: Order Ixodida, Family Argasidae: *Ornithodoros hermsi*, *O. parkeri*, *O. turicata*

Exposure and Severity Ratings (Figure 6.10)

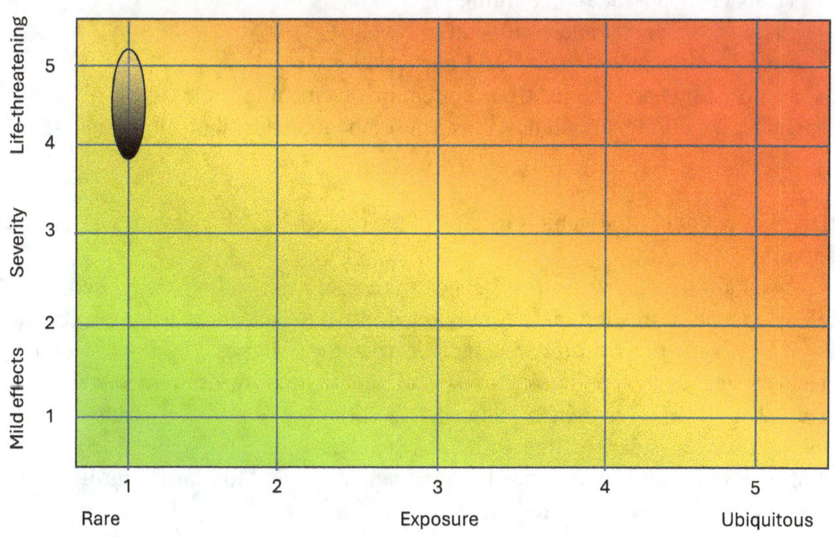

FIGURE 6.10 Tick-borne relapsing fever. Exposure × severity matrix.

- **Exposure Level: 1**
  - Rare (1): <1 case per million persons annually, primarily in the western United States
- **Severity Level: 4–5**
  - Tends to be severe (4), usually requiring hospitalization
  - Repeated fevers, potential for pregnancy-related complications
  - Can be life-threatening (5): mortality <2% and usually due to untreated severe complications

References: Morshed et al. (2017), Eisen et al. (2017), Talagrand-Reboul et al. (2018), Werner et al. (2019), Jakab et al. (2022)

Tick-borne relapsing fever (TBRF) is a bacterial infection caused by various *Borrelia* species and transmitted by soft-bodied ticks of the genus *Ornithodoros*. Unlike hard ticks, *Ornithodoros* ticks feed quickly – often within 30 minutes – and tend to live in rodent-infested rustic cabins, caves, or other secluded dwellings. TBRF is primarily reported in the western United States, including the Pacific Coast, Rocky Mountains, and parts of Texas.

The term "relapsing" reflects the infection's distinctive episodic fever pattern, which can recur several times if untreated.

Symptoms

Symptoms typically begin 4–18 days after exposure and include:

- High fever episodes lasting 3 days, followed by a symptom-free interval of ~7 days
- Each fever episode ends with a "crisis," sometimes reaching 106.7°F
- Body aches, muscle and joint pain
- Headache, nausea, and vomiting
- Fatigue, dizziness, and confusion
- Rash, neck pain, eye pain, and light sensitivity
- Neuropathy and other nervous system involvement in some cases
- Infection during pregnancy may cause spontaneous abortion or neonatal death

Relapses occur due to antigenic variation of the spirochete, which evades the immune response.

Unlike hard ticks, *Ornithodoros* species are nocturnal and typically feed quickly while a person is resting or sleeping, making the exposure insidious. Because the normal hosts of *Ornithodoros* include rodents, it is best to avoid sleeping in rodent-infested cabins or bunkhouses, and to use insecticide-treated bedding or sleeping bags when overnight stays in such facilities are required. If rustic lodging is regularly used, consider treating with a residual acaricide.

Soft tick bites may go unnoticed, so awareness is key. Monitor for flu-like symptoms for up to 3 weeks and seek medical attention immediately if symptoms occur. Diagnosis is often confirmed with blood smears or PCR. Treatment typically involves tetracyclines such as doxycycline, but these drugs must be administered cautiously to avoid Jarisch-Herxheimer reaction, a rapid inflammatory response to spirochaete die-off in the bloodstream. Most patients recover with appropriate antibiotic therapy, though hospitalization is often required.

POWASSAN VIRUS

Pathogen: Order Amarillovirales, Family Flaviviridae: *Orthoflavivirus powassanense*

Entomological Vectors: Order Ixodida, Family Ixodidae: *Ixodes scapularis* **(deer tick),** *I. cookei, I. marxi*

Exposure and Severity Ratings (Figure 6.11)

- **Exposure Level: 1**
  - Rare (1): ~60 cases reported in the United States from 2004 to 2013
  - Numbers appear to be increasing (~1 case/year pre-2005, now up to 20–50 cases per year from 2018 to 2023)
  - Focal in Northeast, Upper Midwest, and mid-Atlantic regions
- **Severity Level: 2–5**
  - Rapid transmission from tick to host
  - Symptoms vary widely, from mild (2) to life-threatening (5)
  - Up to 10% fatality rate in neuroinvasive cases; ~50% of survivors experience permanent neurological deficits

References: Pastula et al. (2016), Eisen et al. (2017), Werner et al. (2019), Campbell and Krause (2020), Hassett and Thangamani (2021)

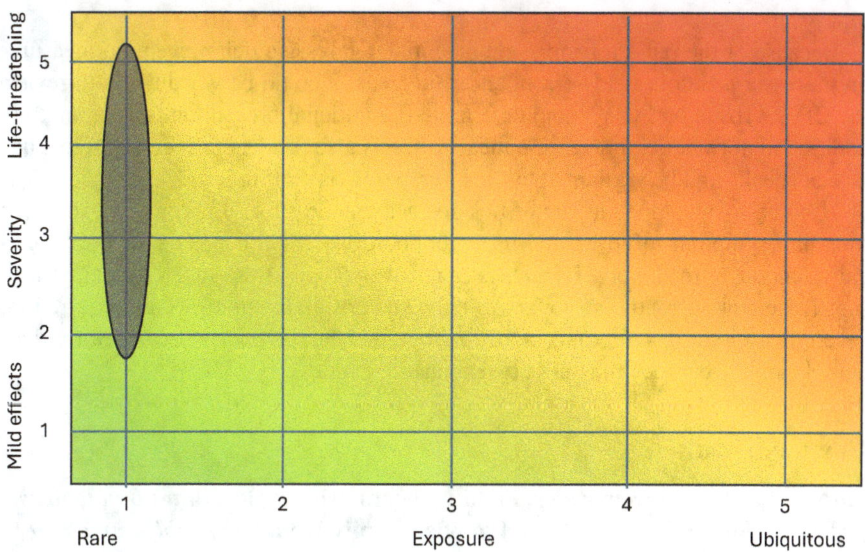

FIGURE 6.11   Powassan virus. Exposure × severity matrix.

Powassan virus (POWV) is a rare but potentially fatal tick-borne flavivirus that causes encephalitis and other neurological complications. Unlike most tick-borne pathogens, POWV can be transmitted within 15 minutes of tick attachment. It is primarily found in the Northeastern United States, Upper Midwest, and parts of the Mid-Atlantic, particularly in Connecticut, New York, Massachusetts, Minnesota, and Wisconsin, but cases have been documented as far south as Virginia.

Although infection is infrequent, the severity of illness and potential for long-term neurological damage make it a growing concern for ecology and environmental professionals in endemic areas.

Symptoms

Symptoms typically appear 1–4 weeks after a tick bite and vary widely, ranging from asymptomatic to life-threatening. Common signs include:

- Fever and headache
- Vomiting and generalized weakness
- Confusion, memory loss, and seizures
- Loss of coordination, speech difficulties
- Encephalitis and meningitis
- Recurrent headaches, muscle wasting, or long-term neurological impairment
- Approximately 10% of symptomatic cases are fatal, and 50% of survivors have permanent neurological damage

Due to its rarity and severity, POWV is often misdiagnosed as other viral or bacterial infections early in illness. This disease is nationally reportable in the United States. Reporting is handled by medical and public health professionals; environmental personnel and their organizations are *not* responsible for direct case reporting.

Because of the rapid transmission potential, aggressive tick prevention measures are necessary. Before fieldwork in endemic areas, it could be worthwhile to review the CDC website on POWV and determine if additional precaution is warranted. In addition to normal tick prevention measures, it is also prudent to increase frequency of tick checks and be vigilant about ticks crawling on clothing.

If bitten by a competent vector tick species, monitor for symptoms for at least a month. If symptoms of fever, confusion, or coordination problems occur, seek medical attention immediately. Diagnosis may involve spinal tap and serological testing. Treatment currently is supportive only, and hospitalization is often required for severe neurological symptoms. Early recognition and supportive care can reduce complications, but they may not prevent lasting damage.

Heartland Virus

Pathogen: Order Hareavirales, Family Phenuiviridae: Heartland *Bandavirus*

Entomological Vector: Order Ixodida, Family Ixodidae: *Amblyomma americanum* (Lone star tick)

Exposure and Severity Ratings (Figure 6.12)

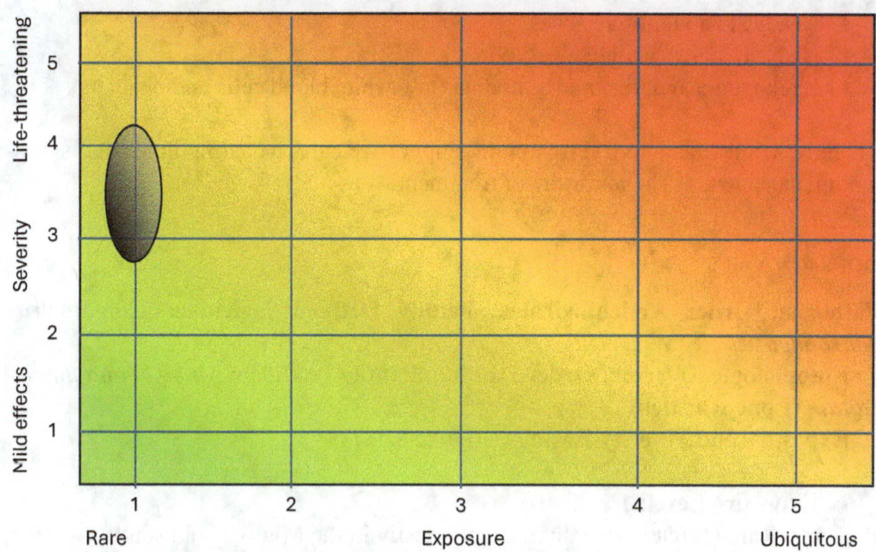

FIGURE 6.12 Heartland virus. Exposure × severity matrix.

- **Exposure Level: 1**
  - Rare (1); 60 cases from its discovery in 2009 to 2022
  - Endemic to the central and southeastern United States (MO, AR, TN, KY, OK)
  - More recently spread to mid-Atlantic (MD, VA, GA)
- **Severity Level: 3–4**
  - Most cases moderate (3) and require medical care; often serious (4) and requiring hospitalization
  - Fatalities rare and limited to older, immunocompromised individuals

References: Eisen et al. (2017), Brault et al. (2018), Werner et al. (2019), Mantlo and Haley (2023)

Heartland virus is an emerging tick-borne pathogen first identified in Missouri in 2009. It is a phlebovirus transmitted by the lone star tick (*A. americanum*), a widely distributed species across the southeastern and central United States. Since its discovery, cases have been reported in multiple states including Missouri, Arkansas, Tennessee, Kentucky, Oklahoma, and Georgia.

The virus causes a non-specific febrile illness that can resemble other tick-borne diseases such as ehrlichiosis. Symptoms typically appear 1–2 weeks after a tick bite and include fever, fatigue, headaches, nausea, diarrhea, and low blood cell counts. Some patients require hospitalization, and fatalities have occurred in older or immunocompromised individuals.

Symptoms

- Fever
- Fatigue and weakness

- Headache and muscle aches
- Nausea, diarrhea, and appetite loss
- Leukopenia and thrombocytopenia (low white blood cells and platelets)

There is no specific antiviral treatment. Supportive care, including fluids and symptom management, is the mainstay of treatment.

BOURBON VIRUS

Pathogen: Order Articulavirales, Family Orthomyxoviridae: *Thogotovirus bourbonense*

Entomological Vector: Order Ixodida, Family Ixodidae: *Amblyomma americanum* **(Lone star tick)**

Exposure and Severity Ratings (Figure 6.13)

- **Exposure Level: 1**
  - Rare (1) but regionally present; mostly in the Midwest and south
  - Eight confirmed cases
- **Severity Level: 3–4**
  - Can result in moderate (3) to severe (4) illness
  - Fatalities have apparently occurred, but rate is unclear due to low number of cases

References: Eisen et al. (2017), Werner et al. (2019), Roe et al. (2023)

Bourbon virus is a thogotovirus first identified in Bourbon County, Kansas, in 2014. It is believed to be transmitted by lone star ticks (*A. americanum*), though its

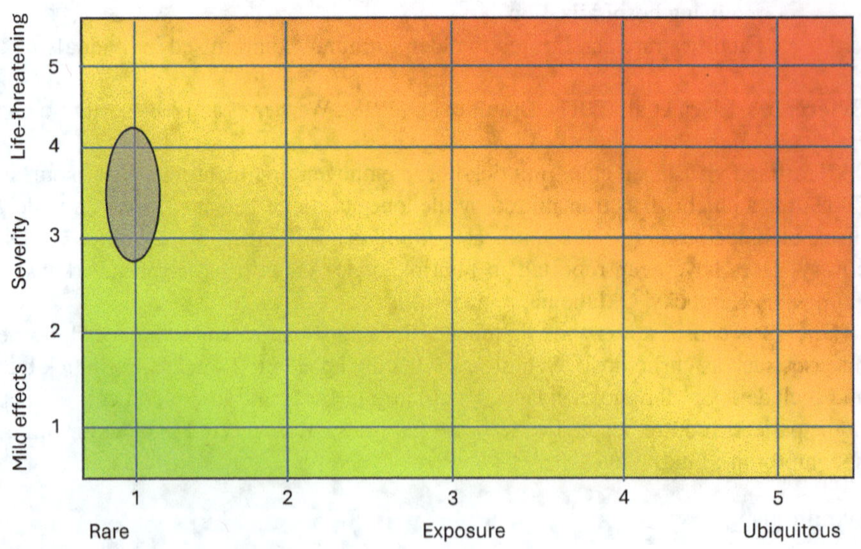

FIGURE 6.13 Bourbon virus. Exposure × severity matrix.

full ecological cycle remains under investigation. Confirmed cases remain very rare, but have been reported in Kansas, Missouri, Oklahoma, and other nearby states.

Symptoms develop within a week or two of a tick bite and resemble other tick-borne illnesses, including sudden fever, fatigue, rash, nausea, and low blood counts. Some patients have developed multi-organ failure. The case fatality rate is unclear due to the small number of confirmed cases, but several deaths have occurred, mostly in older adults.

Symptoms

- Fever and fatigue
- Rash
- Loss of appetite
- Headache and body aches
- Low white blood cells and platelets
- Elevated liver enzymes

There is currently no targeted treatment for Bourbon virus. Patients are treated supportively with fluids and hospitalization if needed. Diagnosis is confirmed by PCR or antibody testing in specialized labs.

COLORADO TICK FEVER

Pathogen: Order Reovirales, Family Spinareoviridae: *Coltivirus dermacentoris*
   Entomological Vector: Order Ixodida, Family Ixodidae: *Dermacentor andersoni* **(Rocky Mountain wood tick)**
   Exposure and Severity Ratings (Figure 6.14)

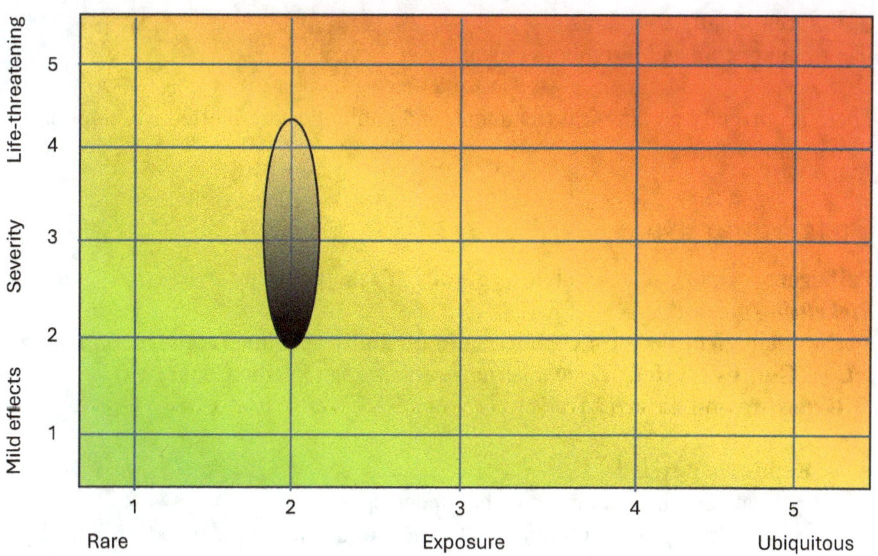

FIGURE 6.14   Colorado tick fever. Exposure × severity matrix.

- **Exposure Level: 2**
  - Uncommon (2), with regional distribution in United States and Canada between 1,200 and 3,000 m (4,000–10,000 ft) in elevation
  - From 2003 to 2023, CDC reported 223 cases, corresponding to ~11 cases/year
- **Severity Level: 2–4**
  - Can be mild (2) and self-limiting, but hospitalization required in ~30% of cases
  - Severe (4) neural involvement, with fatalities extremely rare

References: Yendell et al. (2015), Eisen et al. (2017), Harris et al. (2023)

Colorado tick fever is a viral disease caused by a coltivirus and transmitted by the Rocky Mountain wood tick (*D. andersoni*). It occurs primarily in the Rocky Mountain region, including Colorado, Wyoming, Montana, Idaho, and Utah, with cases concentrated between elevations of 4,000 and 10,000 ft. It typically affects individuals exposed to ticks during spring and early summer.

Symptoms usually begin 3–6 days after a tick bite and include sudden fever, chills, headache, muscle aches, and fatigue. A biphasic fever pattern (initial symptoms followed by a second fever phase) is characteristic in about half of patients. Although most cases are mild, fatigue can persist for weeks. Rare complications include meningoencephalitis or prolonged blood abnormalities.

Symptoms

- Sudden high fever (often biphasic)
- Headache and myalgia
- Fatigue
- Nausea or vomiting
- Occasionally a mild rash
- Leukopenia and thrombocytopenia

There is currently no antiviral treatment, and antibiotics are ineffective. Supportive care usually suffices.

Other Spotted Fevers

Pathogens: Order Rickettsiales, Family Rickettsiaceae: *Rickettsia parkeri*, *Rickettsia* sp. 364D

Entomological Vectors: Order Ixodida, Family Ixodidae: *Amblyomma maculatum* (Gulf Coast tick), *Dermacentor occidentalis* (Pacific Coast tick)

Exposure and Severity Ratings (Figure 6.15)

- **Exposure Level: 2**
  - Data are limited and probably underreported
  - Incidence and uncommon (2) exposure are inferred, based on RMSF rates and regional case reports

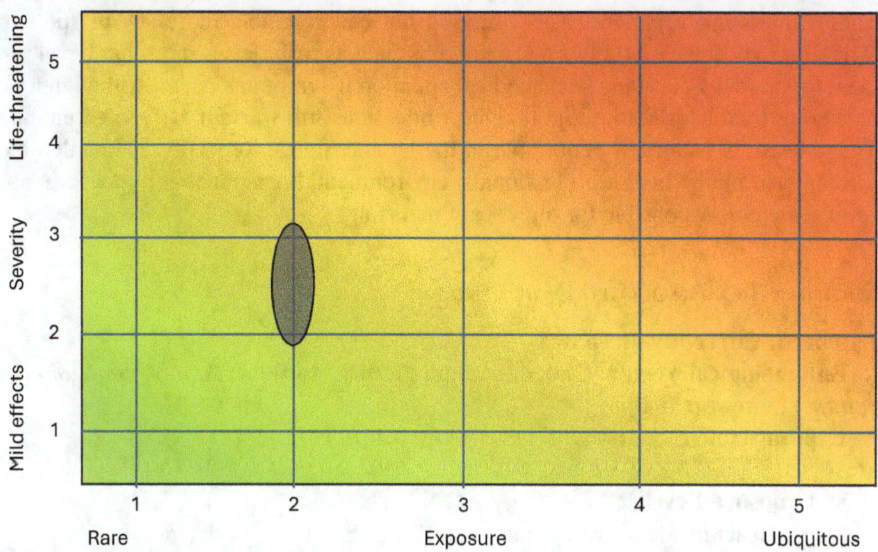

FIGURE 6.15   Other spotted fevers. Exposure × severity matrix.

- **Severity Level: 2–3**
  - Usually self-limiting or mild (2)
  - Hospitalization due to moderate (3) harm rarely needed, but early treatment is advisable

References: Eisen et al. (2017), Allerdice et al. (2019)

In addition to RMSF, other rickettsial infections – caused by *Rickettsia parkeri* and related species – have emerged as less severe, but clinically important tick-borne illnesses in the United States. These "other spotted fevers" occur primarily in the eastern and southern United States, especially along the Gulf and Atlantic coasts, and in parts of northern and central California. They may also occur in international travelers exposed abroad.

Although these diseases are less severe than RMSF, they can still result in significant discomfort, and accurate diagnosis is important to distinguish them from more serious conditions.

Symptoms

Symptoms typically develop within 1–2 weeks of a tick bite and include:

- Fever and headache
- Rash (commonly early in illness)
- Fatigue and malaise
- Eschar (black, crusted scab at the site of the tick bite), a feature more common in *R. parkeri* infections
- Rarely, severe complications such as neurological effects or organ involvement

These illnesses are generally self-limiting but can resemble more severe spotted fevers in early stages. Monitor for symptoms such as rash, fever, or eschar development for up to 2 weeks and seek medical attention if symptoms occur. Although less dangerous than RMSF, these spotted fever infections still warrant early intervention. This disease is nationally reportable in the United States. Reporting is handled by medical and public health professionals; environmental personnel and their organizations are *not* responsible for direct case reporting.

SOUTHERN TICK-ASSOCIATED RASH ILLNESS

Pathogen: Currently unknown

Entomological Vector: Order Ixodida, Family Ixodidae: *Amblyomma americanum* (Lone star tick)

Exposure and Severity Ratings (Figure 6.16)

- **Exposure Level: 2**
  - Exact incidence rate is unclear
  - Uncommon (2) rating inferred from tick distribution and clinical case reports
- **Severity Level: 2**
  - Generally mild (2) symptoms
  - Most cases resolve fully but resemble more serious tick-borne diseases

References: Nicholson et al. (2009), Eisen et al. (2017), Werner et al. (2019)

STARI (Southern Tick-Associated Rash Illness) is an emerging tick-borne condition with clinical similarities to early-stage Lyme disease, but caused by a

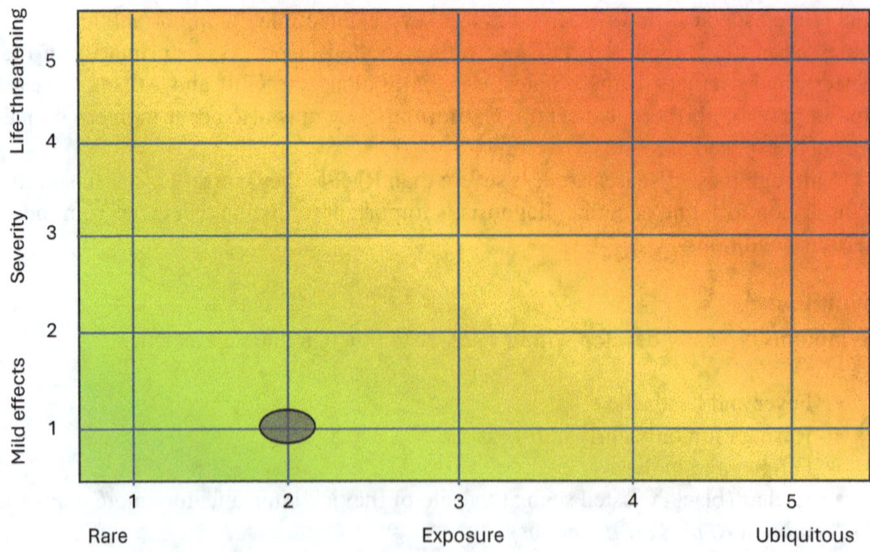

FIGURE 6.16 Southern tick-associated rash illness (STARI). Exposure × severity matrix.

still-uncertain pathogen. The disease is primarily associated with the lone star tick (*A. americanum*) and occurs in a broad swath of the eastern United States, including the Ozarks, Gulf Coast, Atlantic Coast, and as far north as New England.

Despite its similarity to Lyme disease, STARI has not been linked to long-term complications or the chronic symptoms seen in untreated Lyme cases.

Symptoms

Symptoms typically appear within 3–30 days after a tick bite and may include:

- Bullseye-like rash (similar in appearance to erythema migrans)
- Fatigue and headache
- Fever and chills
- Muscle aches

Unlike Lyme disease, STARI has not been definitively linked to joint, neurological, or cardiac complications. Most patients recover fully with or without antibiotic treatment.

Because the identity of the causative agent is uncertain, prevention remains the best defense. However, if bitten, monitor for symptoms as for Lyme disease (up to 4 weeks), and if symptoms such as a bullseye rash or flu-like symptoms develop, seek medical attention. Although STARI appears to be generally mild and self-limiting, it is indistinguishable from early Lyme disease without laboratory testing.

INSECTS

KISSING BUGS

Entomological Parasites: Order Hemiptera, Family Reduviidae: *Triatoma sanguisuga*, *T. gerstaeckeri*, and *T. protracta*; rarely other genera (Figure 6.17)
   Exposure and Severity Ratings (Figure 6.17)

- **Exposure Level: 1–2**
    - Locally rare (1) to uncommon (2) throughout the southern United States (from AZ to SC) in rural field settings
    - Throughout Central and South America, kissing bugs may be frequently (4) encountered, especially in poor housing
- **Severity Level: 1–4**
    - Typical bites result in minimal (1) harm due to nuisance
    - Moderate (3) allergic reactions have been reported in <10% of bite victims in AZ and NM; in repeated exposures, sensitization may result in severe (4) anaphylaxis
    - Chagas disease (addressed separately) increases severity

References: Moffitt et al. (2003), Klotz et al. (2010, 2014a, 2014b), Akhoundi et al. (2020)

Kissing bugs are large, nocturnal blood-feeding insects that get their name from their habit of biting humans around the lips or face while they sleep. Native to the

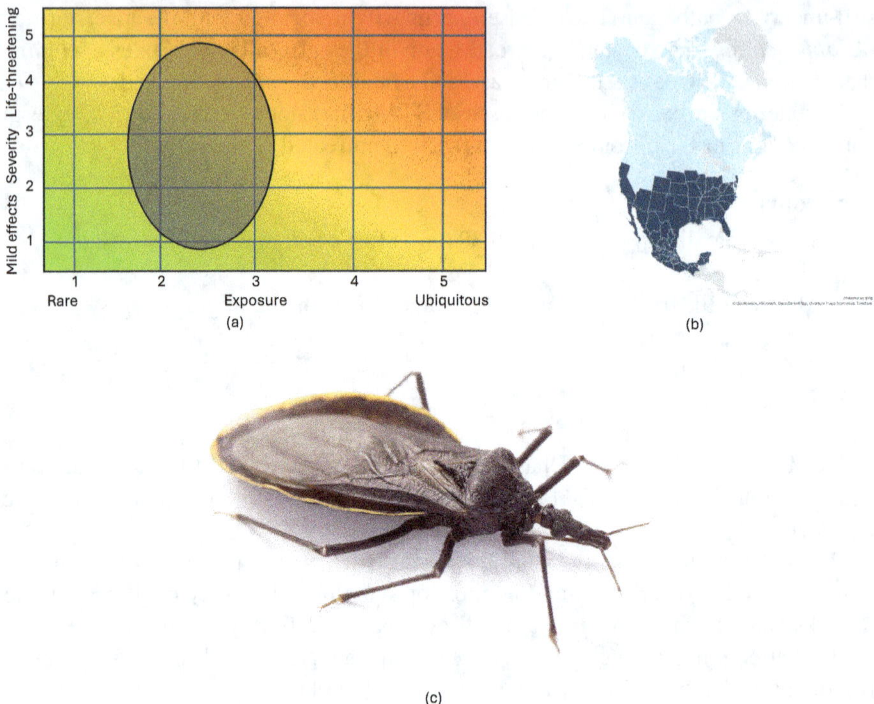

FIGURE 6.17 Kissing bugs. (a) Exposure × severity matrix; (b) geographic distribution; (c) Kissing bug, *Triatoma* sp.

southern United States, Mexico, and Central and South America, these insects are members of the assassin bug family (Reduviidae). While most U.S. exposures result in nuisance bites, some tropical species can transmit the protozoan *Trypanosoma cruzi*, which causes Chagas disease.

Transmission of *T. cruzi* typically occurs when an infected bug defecates while feeding, and the feces contaminate the bite site or mucous membranes when the host scratches his/her face. Although Chagas disease is rare in the United States, both autochthonous transmission and imported cases occur, especially in Texas, Arizona, and California. In the southeastern United States (TN and GA to the Gulf Coast), *Triatoma sanguisuga* has tested positive for *T. cruzi*, but there have been few to no reports of transmission to humans.

Kissing bugs are also associated with severe allergic reactions, including anaphylaxis in sensitized individuals.

Symptoms

Exposure may lead to:

- Painless bite, often unrecognized during sleep
- Redness, swelling, or itchy welts, often on the face, neck, or arms

- In allergic individuals:
  - Severe swelling, hives, difficulty breathing, or anaphylaxis
- In cases of Chagas disease:
  - Acute phase (rarely diagnosed): fever, fatigue, rash, swollen eyelid (Romaña's sign)
  - Chronic phase: may develop years later with cardiac or gastrointestinal complications, including arrhythmias, cardiomyopathy, or megacolon

The risk of Chagas transmission is currently low in the United States, but the public health concern is rising due to vector presence and growing awareness.

Occupational Exposure

Kissing bugs are encountered by ecologists and environmental professionals during:

- Fieldwork in the southern United States, especially rural or semi-rural forested areas
- Sleeping in rustic cabins, bunkhouses, sheds, or tents near woodpiles or animal housing
- Ecological surveys involving rocky outcrops, woodpiles, or rodent nests
- Working in abandoned buildings, under porches, or near dog kennels
- Exposure to dogs and wildlife reservoirs (e.g., raccoons, opossums, armadillos)
- Wildlife handling or necropsy work
- Work around outdoor lighting or camping structures, where kissing bugs may congregate
- International fieldwork in endemic regions of Central and South America

Kissing bugs are attracted to CO_2 and body heat, and they enter dwellings or shelters seeking blood meals.

Prevention

To avoid kissing bug bites:

- Reinforce sleeping areas: patch screens, seal cracks, use bed nets when camping or in rustic housing
- Elevate sleeping cots off the ground and away from walls
- Reduce light use around lodging areas (attracts kissing bugs)
- Use permethrin-treated clothing and gear
- Apply DEET or picaridin before sleeping in exposed environments
- Avoid storing gear or sleeping near wood piles, rodent nests, or pet bedding
- Inspect sleeping quarters in high-risk areas for signs of kissing bugs
- Wear gloves when handling wildlife or carcasses in endemic areas

What To Do If Affected
- Clean the bite site and monitor for swelling or allergic reaction
- If allergic symptoms occur (e.g., facial swelling, wheezing), seek emergency care immediately

- If *T. cruzi* transmission is suspected (especially in endemic countries), consult a travel medicine specialist
- Consider PCR testing or serologic screening if at risk of Chagas exposure
- In confirmed cases of Chagas, antiparasitic treatment (e.g., nifurtimox or benznidazole) may be prescribed

Early treatment reduces the risk of long-term complications from *T. cruzi* infection.

KISSING BUG-BORNE DISEASES

CHAGAS DISEASE

Pathogen: Order Trypanosomatida, Family Trypanosomatidae: *Trypanosoma cruzi*

Entomological Vectors: Order Hemiptera: Family Reduviidae: *Triatoma sanguisuga*, *T. gerstaeckeri*, *T. protracta*, and others (Figure 6.18)

Exposure and Severity Ratings (Figure 6.18)

- **Exposure Level: 1**
  - Autochthonous transmission is rare (1), with highest frequency in TX and CA
  - AZ, LA, and TN have each reported at least one case
  - Infected vectors and animal reservoirs have been found uncommonly (2) in AL, GA, and FL, and less often in 18 other states
  - Most cases in North America are imported from Latin America

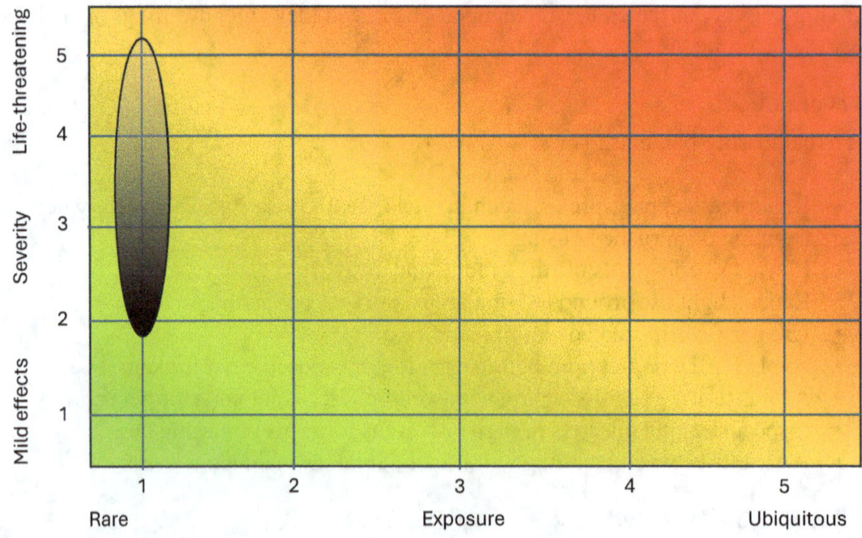

FIGURE 6.18 Chagas disease. Exposure × severity matrix.

- **Severity Level: 2–5**
  - May be asymptomatic or with mild (2) symptoms until chronic effects emerge
  - Severe (4) chronic cardiac and gastrointestinal disease in ~30% of cases
  - May be life-threatening (5) as sudden cardiac death is possible in long-term infections

References: Garcia et al. (2015, 2016), Tian et al. (2024)

Chagas disease is caused by the protozoan *T. cruzi*, transmitted primarily by kissing bugs. Twelve species of kissing bugs are major vectors of *T. cruzi*, but none of these occur in North America. A few species of *Triatoma* from North America, listed above, are minor vectors. These nocturnal insects feed on blood and defecate near the bite site; the parasite enters through broken skin or mucous membranes when the victim scratches. Although endemic in Latin America, locally acquired cases have been confirmed in the southern United States, with *T. cruzi*-infected vectors found as far north as Tennessee and Kentucky. In the United States, most human infections are still considered imported.

The disease progresses through acute and chronic phases. The acute phase is often asymptomatic or presents with mild fever and swelling at the infection site (chagoma). In the chronic phase, which may occur decades later, some individuals develop cardiomyopathy, arrhythmias, heart failure, or megacolon/megaesophagus. Diagnosis requires serological or molecular testing.

Symptoms

- Swelling at bite site (chagoma or Romaña's sign if near eye)
- Fever, fatigue, body aches
- Cardiac complications: arrhythmias, heart failure, cardiomegaly
- Gastrointestinal complications: constipation, esophageal dysmotility
- Often asymptomatic for years before chronic effects emerge

Although currently rare in the United States, Chagas disease is of growing occupational relevance due to shifting vector ranges, increased wildlife contact, and canine involvement. Field personnel in high-risk zones should be trained to recognize kissing bugs and understand the delayed, insidious nature of this disease.

Body Lice

Entomological Parasite and Vector: Order Psocodea: Family Pediculidae: *Pediculus humanus corporis* (human body louse) (Figure 6.19)

Exposure and Severity Ratings (Figure 6.19)

- **Exposure Level: 1**
  - Rare (1) in most ecological fieldwork
  - Only in humanitarian/disaster settings are exposures higher

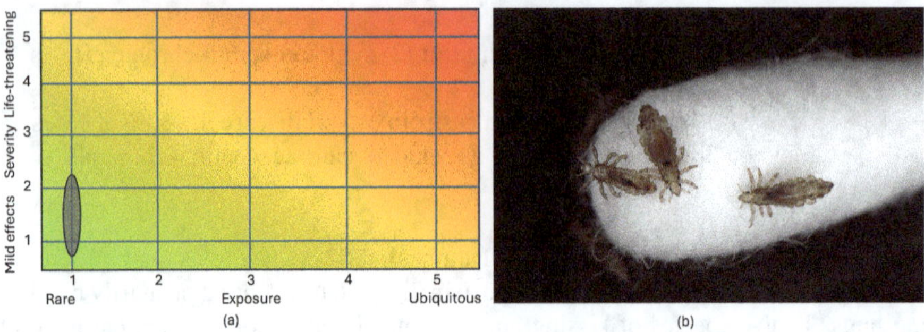

FIGURE 6.19 Body lice. (a) Exposure×severity matrix; (b) Body louse, *Pediculus humanus corporis*.

- **Severity Level: 1–2**
  - Bites and resulting rash can be minimal (1) to mild (2)
  - Disease transmission of epidemic typhus and trench fever is analyzed separately

References: Akhoundi et al. (2020), Amanzougaghene et al. (2020), Fu et al. (2022)

Body lice are blood-feeding ectoparasites that live in clothing and bedding, migrating to the skin only to feed. They differ from head lice by their behavior (residing primarily in clothing) and by their historical role as vectors of serious pathogens including:

- Epidemic typhus (*Rickettsia prowazekii*)
- Relapsing fever (*Borrelia recurrentis*)
- Trench fever (*Bartonella quintana*)

Although uncommon in modern industrialized settings, body lice remain a public health concern in situations of poor hygiene, crowded living conditions, disaster relief camps, and occasionally among homeless populations or refugee camps. It should be noted that louse-borne relapsing fever has not been reported in North America for nearly a century; it is still present in isolated pockets in Africa (e.g., Ethiopia).

In environmental or humanitarian fieldwork, researchers, health workers, and volunteers may encounter infested individuals or living quarters. Prompt recognition and containment are essential.

Symptoms

- Itching, often severe, typically on the trunk and shoulders
- Red bite marks, especially under tight-fitting clothing
- Linear excoriations or thickened skin (lichenification) from chronic infestation
- Nits or live lice in clothing seams, especially in underwear or shirt collars
- Possible secondary bacterial infection due to scratching

Unlike head lice, nits are rarely found on hair; inspection of clothing is key.

Occupational Exposure

Highest risk occurs in:

- Disaster response, conflict zones, or refugee camps
- Field medicine, humanitarian work, or urban outreach to unhoused populations
- Inspection of donated clothing, secondhand gear, or infested shelters
- Shared bedding or sleeping bags in long-duration field stations without laundering
- Wildlife studies involving human-adapted ectoparasites (e.g., primate sanctuaries)

Body lice do not infest animals, but they can spread quickly among humans in unhygienic conditions.

Prevention

- Maintain regular laundering of clothing and bedding with hot water and high heat drying
- Provide individual gear, avoid sharing towels, bedding, or undergarments
- In high-risk areas, wear disposable protective clothing when handling infested individuals or materials
- Use permethrin-treated clothing or repellents in endemic regions or outbreak zones
- Use permethrin-treated clothing in high-risk environments
- Dispose of or isolate infested materials in sealed bags pending decontamination
- Conduct lice surveillance in crowded shelters or camps
- Avoid direct contact with flying squirrels or their nests
- In known endemic areas, prophylactic doxycycline may be used under medical guidance

What To Do If Affected

- Remove and wash clothing and bedding at $\geq$130°F (54°C)
- Apply topical pediculicides (e.g., permethrin or malathion) to the body in affected individuals
- Use oral ivermectin in severe or resistant cases (under medical supervision)
- Treat secondary infections with appropriate antibiotics
- If suspected typhus or relapsing fever, initiate antibiotic therapy immediately and report to public health authorities

Field teams should report exposures and follow up with occupational health guidance.

LOUSE-BORNE DISEASES

Epidemic Typhus

Pathogen: Order Rickettsiales, Family Rickettsiaceae: *Rickettsia prowazekii*
    Entomological Vector: Order Psocodea: Family Pediculidae: *Pediculus humanus corporis* **(human body louse)**

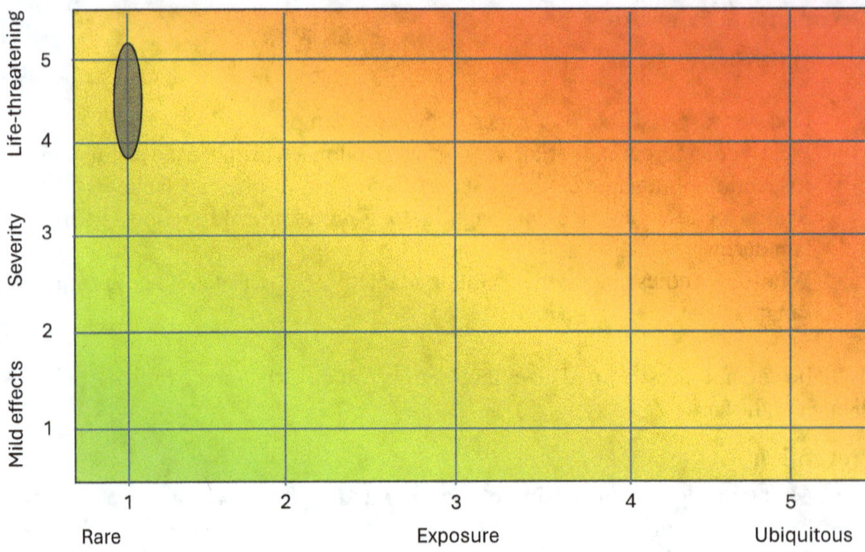

FIGURE 6.20　Epidemic typhus. Exposure × severity matrix.

Exposure and Severity Ratings (Figure 6.20)

- **Exposure Level: 1**
  - Rare (1) in the United States; possibly localized risk in settings with poor hygiene or heavy crowding
- **Severity Level: 4–5**
  - Severe (4) symptoms almost always requiring medical treatment
  - Life-threatening (5) if untreated (20%–60% mortality rate)
  - Historically caused high mortality in wartime and refugee settings

Reference: Badiaga and Brouqui (2012)

Epidemic typhus is a severe, louse-borne rickettsial disease caused by *R. prowazekii*, primarily transmitted through the feces of the body louse (*Pediculus humanus humanus*). It is not transmitted by the head louse. The pathogen enters the human body through scratching of the bite site, mucosal contact, or inhalation of dried louse feces.

Though now rare in the United States, *R. prowazekii* is endemic in some regions of Africa and Central and South America. It persists in North America in a sporadic, zoonotic form called Brill-Zinsser disease; the flying squirrel (*Glaucomys volans*) has been identified as a potential reservoir host in the southeastern United States.

Historically, typhus outbreaks have been linked to warfare, refugee crises, and famine, where lice infestations flourish in unsanitary environments. While rare in modern settings in the United States, ecologists and environmental professionals could feasibly encounter epidemic typhus in settings with poor hygiene or crowding or in international work.

Symptoms

Symptoms appear 7–14 days after exposure and include:

- High fever, often above 40°C (104°F)
- Severe headache
- Muscle aches and chills
- Widespread rash, often starting on the trunk and spreading outward
- Delirium, stupor, or coma in severe cases
- Low blood pressure, vascular collapse, or death in untreated individuals

Mortality rates for untreated epidemic typhus can reach 20%–60%, especially in older or malnourished patients. With prompt antibiotic treatment, the mortality rate drops to near zero. Therefore, if workers are exposed to lice in the extreme circumstances listed above, they should monitor for symptoms for at least 2 weeks and seek medical attention immediately if symptoms develop. Diagnosis is confirmed by serology or PCR, and treatment of choice is predominantly doxycycline. Public health officials must be notified; however, this will be done by medical professionals.

TRENCH FEVER

Pathogen: Order Hyphomicrobiales, Family Bartonellaceae: *Bartonella quintana* **Entomological Vector: Order Psocodea: Family Pediculidae: *Pediculus humanus corporis* (human body louse)**
   Exposure and Severity Ratings (Figure 6.21)

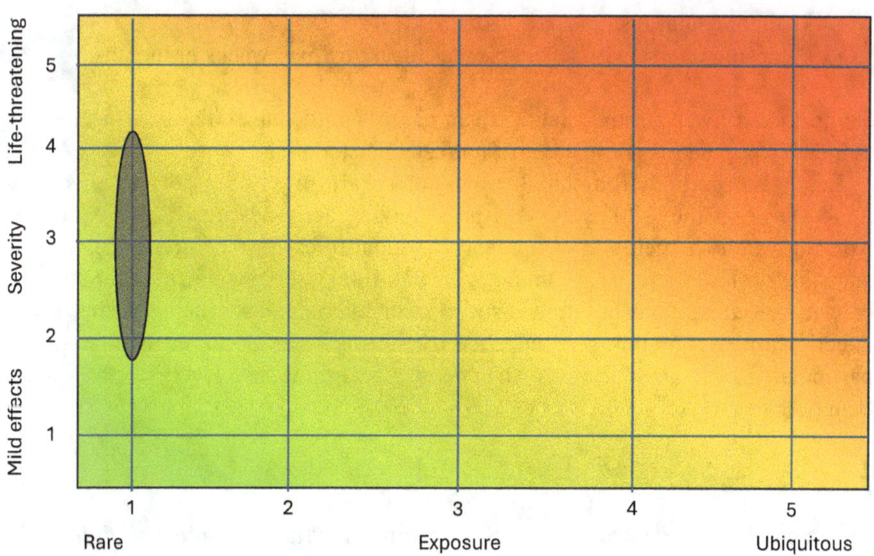

FIGURE 6.21 Trench fever. Exposure × severity matrix.

- **Exposure Level: 1**
  - Rare (1) in the modern United States
  - Documented in certain urban centers (e.g., Seattle, San Francisco, Denver) among homeless populations; a recent study in Denver reported 15% seroprevalence of *B. quintana* in the homeless population
- **Severity Level: 2–4**
  - Often self-limiting and mild (2) but chronic exposure may cause severe (4) harm through prolonged debility or relapse

References: Ohl and Spach (2000), Badiaga and Brouqui (2012)

Trench fever is a bacterial infection caused by *B. quintana* and transmitted by the body louse, *Pediculus humanus corporis*. It was first described during World War I, when it affected large numbers of soldiers in the trenches, hence the name.

Transmission occurs through inoculation of infected louse feces into abrasions or mucous membranes; this happens because of scratching, not through the bite itself. The disease is currently rare in the United States but persists in urban areas with poor sanitation, particularly among people experiencing homelessness. *B. quintana* can survive within macrophages, leading to chronic or relapsing infection, and has been associated with bacillary angiomatosis and endocarditis in immunocompromised hosts.

Symptoms

Symptoms generally appear 5–20 days after exposure and may include:

- Recurrent fevers up to 40°C (104°F), typically lasting 4–5 days
- Severe body and leg pain (especially in the shins and back)
- Headache, malaise, and dizziness
- Maculopapular rash in some cases
- Relapsing course with fever episodes recurring over weeks or months

While trench fever is rarely fatal, it can cause significant disability, especially in vulnerable populations or in cases of untreated bacteremia.

Ecologists and environmental professionals are highly unlikely to encounter trench fever in the wild; however, the following activities may allow exposure: working around homeless encampments or rodent-infested structures in health care or ecology-related activities, humanitarian or military personnel in disaster-stricken or war-torn areas, and building inspection or maintenance when entering abandoned or infested buildings. Body lice infestations may occur in urban settings, particularly during cold seasons when people wear unwashed layers of clothing for long periods.

FLEAS

Entomological Parasites: Order Siphonaptera: notably *Ctenocephalides felis* (cat flea), *Xenopsylla cheopis* (Oriental rat flea), and *Oropsylla* spp. (Figure 6.22)
  Exposure and Severity Ratings (Figure 6.22)

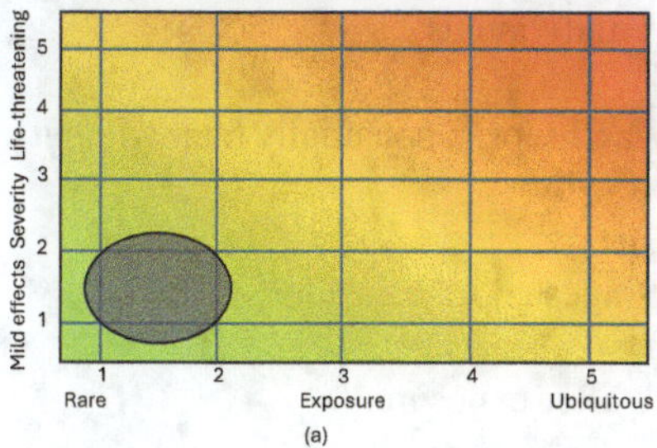

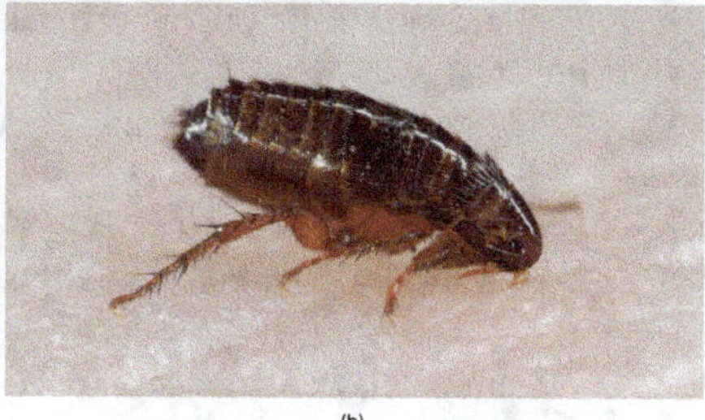

FIGURE 6.22 Fleas. (a) Exposure × severity matrix; (b) Human flea, Pulex irritans.

- **Exposure Level: 2**
  - Uncommon (2) localized risk, especially in areas with infested hosts or abandoned buildings; sometimes in animal nests/burrows
- **Severity Level: 1–2**
  - Typical bites: minimal (1) to mild (2) nuisance irritation
  - Zoonotic diseases (discussed below) spread by fleas have much higher severity

Reference: Akhoundi et al. (2020)

Fleas are small, wingless, blood-feeding insects that parasitize mammals and birds. Their laterally flattened bodies and powerful hind legs allow them to move swiftly through fur and to jump long distances to reach hosts. Flea bites can be a persistent nuisance and a source of allergic dermatitis, particularly in sensitive individuals.

Importantly, fleas are vectors of several serious zoonotic diseases, including:

- Plague (*Yersinia pestis*) – transmitted by *Oropsylla* and *Xenopsylla* spp.
- Murine typhus (*Rickettsia typhi*) – associated with *X. cheopis*
- Cat scratch disease (*Bartonella henselae*) – fleas serve as a reservoir
- Fleas also serve as intermediate hosts for tapeworms (e.g., *Dipylidium caninum*)

Most modern flea exposures in the United States and Canada involve the cat flea (*Ctenocephalides felis*), which can infest a wide range of hosts. Any mammals that have regular nesting or burrowing areas can have fleas. This includes rodents (like squirrels, chipmunks, mice, voles, rats, etc.), rodent-like creatures (like rabbits or pikas), terrestrial carnivores, and others. Some may even have multiple species of fleas, including ones not listed above. These fleas may transfer onto a human opportunistically and are most commonly associated with transfer of pathogens.

Symptoms

Flea bites often appear in clusters, particularly on the ankles, legs, and waistline, and may include:

- Itchy red papules, often with a central puncture point
- Secondary skin infections due to scratching

- Flea allergy dermatitis in hypersensitive individuals
- If infected:
  - Plague: fever, swollen lymph nodes, and sepsis; potentially fatal without treatment
  - Murine typhus: fever, headache, rash
  - Tapeworms: intestinal symptoms if ingested (rare in adults)

Disease symptoms may emerge days to weeks after exposure.

Occupational Exposure

Ecologists and environmental professionals may encounter fleas during:

- Handling wild or domestic animals, especially rodents, opossums, and feral cats
- Entering crawlspaces, attics, or abandoned buildings
- Inspecting wildlife dens, nests, or carcasses
- Conducting pest control, wildlife relocation, or ecological surveys
- Working in endemic plague zones (e.g., Four Corners region)

Fleas may remain dormant in environments for months and be reactivated by vibrations or heat.

Prevention

To minimize risk:

- Wear long pants tucked into socks or boots
- Treat clothing and field gear with permethrin
- Use insect repellents (e.g., DEET) on socks and pant legs
- Avoid contact with wildlife or stray animals, especially in known flea-infested areas
- Use flea control measures for field dogs or other animals accompanying workers
- In plague-endemic areas:
  - Avoid handling rodents directly
  - Use gloves and personal protective equipment (PPE) for animal carcass handling
  - Be alert to sick or dead rodents, which may indicate outbreak

Thorough site inspection and personal hygiene after fieldwork are essential.

What To Do If Affected

- Wash affected skin with soap and water
- Apply antihistamines or anti-itch creams to relieve irritation
- Monitor for signs of systemic illness (fever, rash, swollen glands)

- Seek medical evaluation if symptoms develop; early antibiotic treatment is effective for plague and typhus
- Report suspected exposures in plague-endemic areas to health authorities

Prompt intervention can prevent serious complications from flea-borne diseases.

FLEA-BORNE DISEASES

PLAGUE

Pathogen: Order Enterobacterales, Family Yersiniaceae: *Yersinia pestis*
Entomological Vectors: Order Siphonaptera: *Xenopsylla cheopis* (Oriental rat flea) and other rodent-associated species
Exposure and Severity Ratings (Figure 6.23)

- **Exposure Level: 2**
  - Uncommon (2) and localized to specific fieldwork, primarily around rodent nesting sites, in the western United States
- **Severity Level: 4–5**
  - Severe (4) – Requires urgent medical care and public health notification
  - Potentially life-threatening (5) if untreated

References: Inglesby et al. (2000), Eisen and Gage (2012), Kugeler et al. (2015)
Plague is a bacterial zoonosis caused by *Y. pestis*, a pathogen historically responsible for pandemics such as the Black Death. In modern times, it remains enzootic in

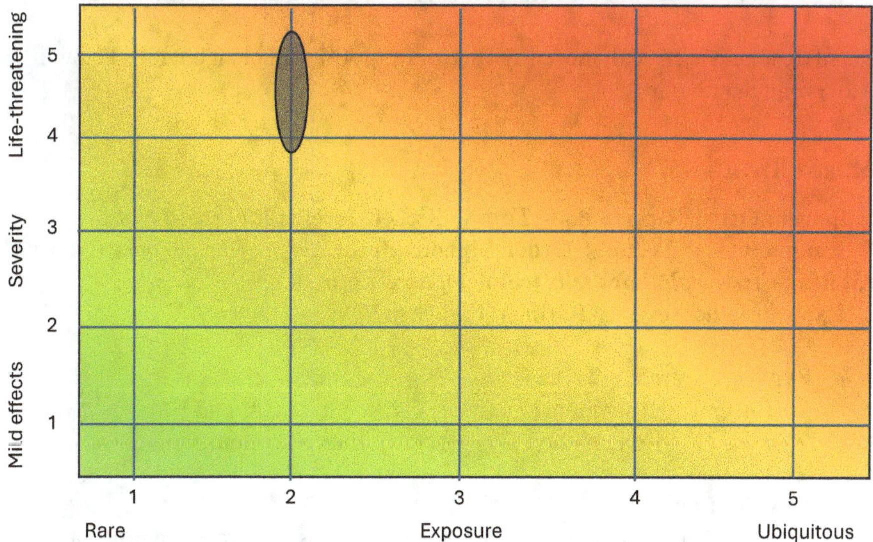

FIGURE 6.23 Plague. Exposure × severity matrix.

wild rodent populations, particularly in the western United States. Humans typically become infected through the bite of infected fleas, most often when working in prairie, desert, or mountainous regions with ground squirrels, prairie dogs, woodrats, or other wild rodents.

Three clinical forms exist:

- Bubonic plague (most common): swollen, painful lymph nodes ("buboes")
- Septicemic plague: bloodstream infection; may occur without buboes
- Pneumonic plague: respiratory form; can be transmitted person-to-person via respiratory droplets

Ecological professionals, biologists, pest control workers, and park staff may be exposed during trapping, handling, or necropsy of wild mammals or their fleas. Outbreaks in rodent populations can trigger epizootics that spill over into humans.

Symptoms

Symptoms typically begin 2–6 days after exposure, depending on form:

- Bubonic plague:
  - Sudden fever, chills, headache, and painful swollen lymph nodes near flea bite site
- Septicemic plague:
  - Fever, weakness, abdominal pain, bleeding, and skin necrosis ("blackening")
- Pneumonic plague:
  - Rapid-onset cough, chest pain, bloody sputum, and respiratory failure

Rapid treatment is critical; mortality approaches 100% without it but falls below 10% with prompt antibiotics.

MURINE TYPHUS

Pathogen: Order Rickettsiales, Family Rickettsiaceae: *Rickettsia typhi*
   Entomological Vectors: Order Siphonaptera: *Xenopsylla cheopis* **(Oriental rat flea),** *Ctenocephalides felis* **(cat flea), rarely others**
   Exposure and Severity Ratings (Figure 6.24)

- **Exposure Level: 1–2**
  - Endemic but sporadic in parts of TX, southern CA, and HI
  - Rare (1) to uncommon (2); generally limited to feral animal nesting locations
- **Severity Level: 2–4**
  - Usually mild (2) and self-limiting but can cause severe (4) significant illness requiring medical care and hospitalization in ~20%–30% of cases

References: Eisen and Gage (2012), Tsioutis et al. (2017)

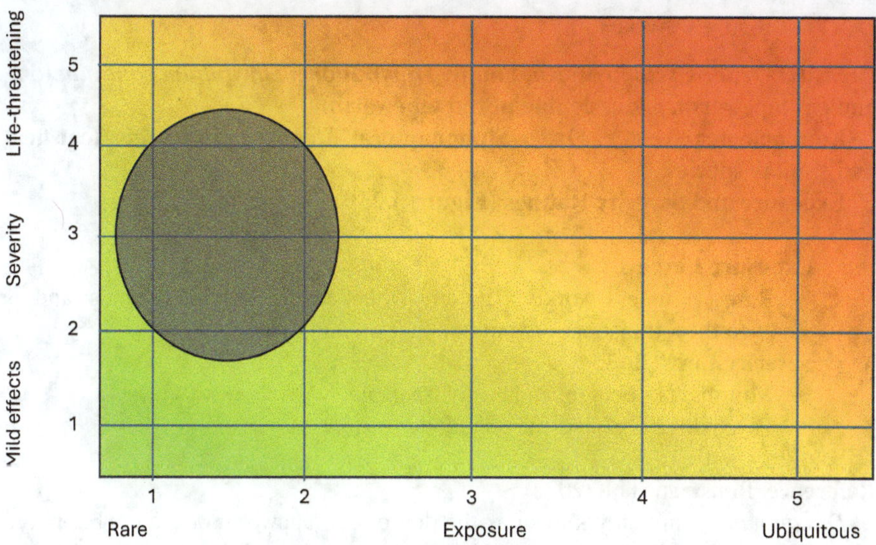

FIGURE 6.24 Murine typhus. Exposure × severity matrix.

Murine typhus, also known as endemic typhus, is a flea-borne disease caused by *R. typhi*, a rickettsial bacterium maintained in rodent-flea cycles. Historically associated with rats and their fleas, the disease has shifted in many urban and suburban U.S. settings to involve opossums and cat fleas. Transmission occurs when infected flea feces contaminate skin abrasions, mucous membranes, or bite sites.

The disease is endemic in parts of the Gulf Coast, Texas (especially south and central regions), southern California, and Hawaii, and often appears in clusters during warmer months when flea populations surge. Most cases are mild to moderate, but serious illness may occur, particularly in the elderly or immunocompromised. Because symptoms mimic viral infections or other febrile illnesses, murine typhus is likely underreported, and diagnosis often depends on clinical suspicion and serologic testing.

Symptoms

Symptoms typically begin 6–14 days after exposure and may include:

- Sudden onset of fever, chills, and headache
- Rash (typically on trunk, spreading to limbs in ~50% of cases)
- Muscle aches, nausea, and vomiting
- Cough or abdominal pain in some patients
- Severe cases: hepatitis, pneumonitis, or meningoencephalitis (rare)

Murine typhus should be considered in occupational settings where flea and rodent exposure is possible, especially in endemic areas. Field personnel and safety officers should treat it as a moderate-severity hazard that is readily preventable with flea control and awareness, yet still capable of significant morbidity if overlooked.

Dog and Cat Tapeworm

Parasite: Order Cyclophyllidea, Family Dipylidiidae: *Dipylidium caninum* (dog and cat tapeworm, a.k.a. double-pored tapeworm)

Entomological Vector: Order Siphonaptera: *Ctenocephalides felis* (cat flea) and similar species

Exposure and Severity Ratings (Figure 6.25)

- **Exposure Level: 1**
  - Rare (1), unless working directly with fleas or infested animals; and even then, transmission requires ingestion of fleas
- **Severity Level: 1–3**
  - Minimal (1), benign, and easily treatable
  - Psychological effects may be moderate (3)

Reference: Rousseau et al. (2022)

D. caninum, commonly known as the dog or cat tapeworm or the double-pored tapeworm, is a flea-transmitted cestode that infects canines, felines, and occasionally humans – typically young children. The tapeworm matures in the small intestine of its definitive host (usually a dog or cat), releasing egg packets that are passed with feces. Flea larvae ingest these eggs, and the infective cysticercoid stage develops within the flea.

When a dog, cat, or human ingests an infected flea, the tapeworm matures in the gut. Humans are accidental hosts, and zoonotic transmission requires direct ingestion of fleas (which, not surprisingly, is rare among adult humans!). Mere contact with feces cannot transmit *D. caninum*. While human infections are generally mild or asymptomatic, they are common in domestic and feral animals.

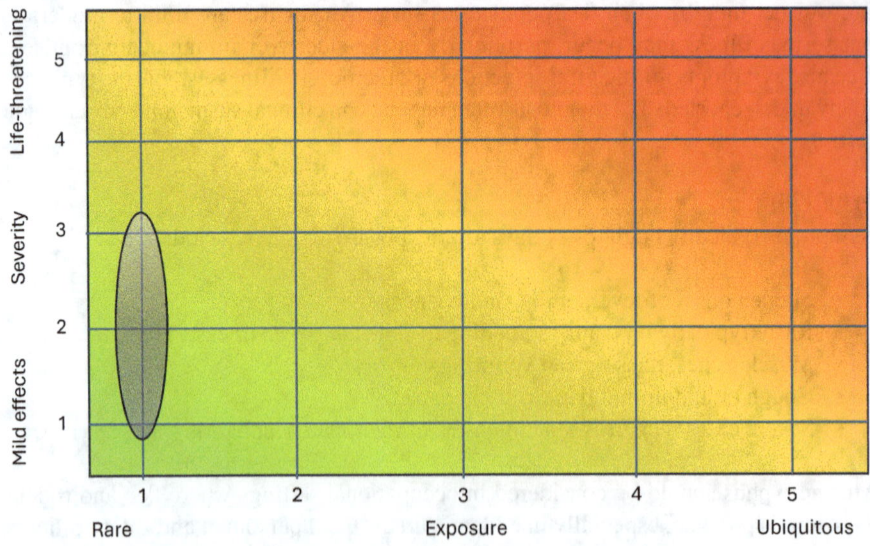

FIGURE 6.25 Dog and cat tapeworm. Exposure × severity matrix.

Symptoms

- Most human infections occur in young children, due to close contact with pets or accidental ingestion of fleas
- Symptoms (if present) may include:
  - Mild abdominal discomfort or digestive upset
  - Irritability, appetite changes, or pruritus ani (itching near the anus)
  - Passing of motile proglottids (rice-like segments) in stool or on perianal region
- No systemic or life-threatening symptoms occur

The infection is benign but psychologically distressing for families or those unfamiliar with parasitology. No long-term health effects result from infection, especially if treated with antihelminthics, but reinfection is possible without follow-up flea control.

Mosquitoes

Entomological Parasites: Order Diptera, Family Culicidae: notably *Aedes*, *Anopheles*, *Culex*, *Ochlerotatus*, and *Psorophora* spp. Many species historically in the genus *Aedes* have been moved to *Ochlerotatus* (Figure 6.26)
Exposure and Severity Ratings (Figure 6.26)

- **Exposure Level: 5**
  - Ubiquitous (5) in warm seasons and environments with any standing water
- **Severity Level: 2–3**
  - Bites may be innocuous (1) or mildly (2) irritating but usually not medically serious; swarms may render greater irritation
  - Hypersensitivity possible, potentially resulting in moderate (3) harm
  - Mosquitoes can be vectors of numerous diseases, addressed separately, that have much higher severity

References: Darsie and Ward (2005), Akhoundi et al. (2020), Duval et al. (2023)

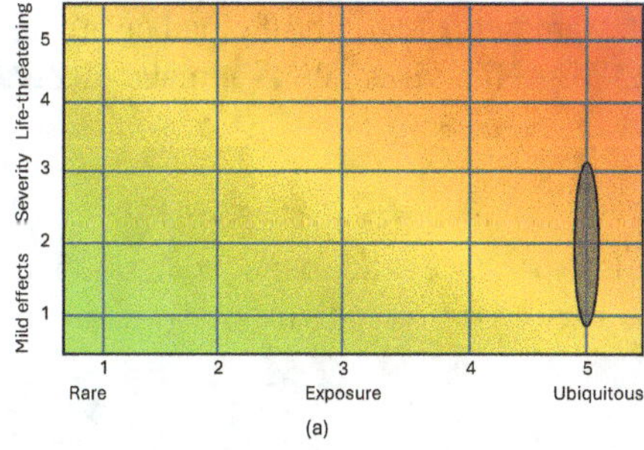

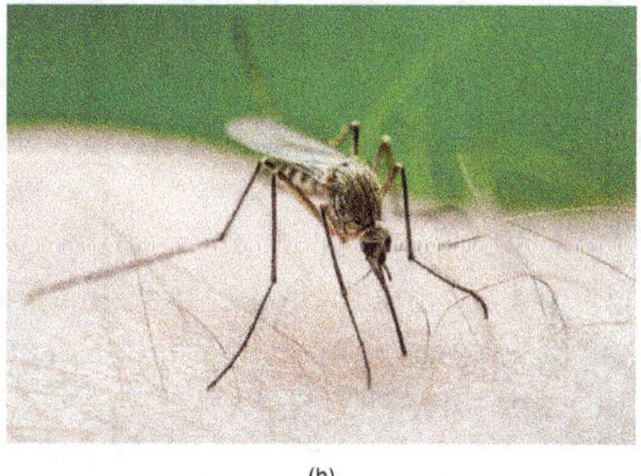

FIGURE 6.26 Mosquitoes. (a) Exposure×severity matrix; (b) Mosquito, *Culex* sp.

Mosquitoes are among the most pervasive and consequential arthropods encountered by environmental professionals across North America. Their importance lies not only in the irritation they cause through biting, but also in their role as vectors for several serious diseases. For professionals working outdoors – and that can be in environments as diverse as wetlands, forests, grasslands, urban greenspaces, or even arid environments – mosquito exposure is often unavoidable and must be proactively managed to minimize both nuisance and health risks.

Understanding mosquito ecology is essential to anticipating where and when risks are highest. Mosquitoes rely on standing water for the development of their aquatic larval and pupal stages, but this water need not be permanent. Traditional breeding habitats include marshes, ditches, swamps, and ponds, but many problematic mosquito species have adapted to much more transient or artificial environments. Some, like *Culex* species, thrive in stagnant water such as that found in clogged gutters, catch basins, and livestock troughs. Others, particularly *Aedes* species, are known as container breeders and readily develop in manmade objects where water can collect and remain undisturbed for a few days, like discarded tires, buckets, birdbaths, tarps, or even upside-down bottle caps.

Floodwater mosquitoes (most notably *Aedes vexans* and *Psorophora* species) lay eggs on moist soil or vegetation in areas prone to episodic flooding, such as river margins, temporary pools, or irrigated fields. These eggs can remain viable for months (up to 3 years in moist conditions!) until heavy rainfall or flooding triggers hatching and leads to sudden and massive adult emergences. These mosquitoes often bite aggressively and travel significant distances from their breeding sites, meaning even well-drained areas can experience outbreaks when regional flooding occurs.

Because mosquito presence is tightly linked to habitat features and weather patterns, professionals must learn to anticipate when mosquito activity will surge. Dusk and dawn tend to be peak periods for many species, though container-breeding *Aedes* mosquitoes are usually active during the day. Activities involving shaded areas, stagnant water, or post-rain fieldwork should be flagged as high risk. While repellents and protective clothing are key, understanding the ecological drivers of mosquito outbreaks allows for more strategic planning of tasks and avoidance measures.

Ultimately, managing mosquito exposure in occupational settings requires not just reactionary control, but proactive ecological awareness. Habitat modification, breeding site identification, and task scheduling based on mosquito ecology can greatly reduce unnecessary risk.

Here, the local effects of mosquito bites are addressed, not the pathogens they may carry. Pathogen-specific entries (e.g., West Nile virus (WNV), malaria, Zika) are treated separately, below.

Symptoms

If a bite is non-pathogenic, most individuals experience mild to moderate skin reactions following a mosquito bite. Reactions vary based on individual sensitivity and prior exposure.

- Itchy, red, raised welts (wheals) appearing shortly after the bite
- Swelling and inflammation, especially in areas of repeated exposure
- Small blisters or more extensive lesions in hypersensitive individuals

- Scratching may lead to:
  - Skin abrasions
  - Secondary bacterial infection (e.g., impetigo)
- Rare: localized or generalized allergic reactions (papular urticaria or anaphylaxis)

Symptoms are usually self-limited but may cause significant discomfort and distraction, especially when bites are numerous.

Occupational Exposure

Risk to ecologists, environmental professionals, and outdoor workers increases when:

- Working at dawn or dusk, when many mosquito species are most active
- Operating in or near wetlands, forests, swamps, riparian areas around streams, or floodplains
- Conducting work during warm, humid months or after heavy rains
  - Especially in the aftermath of hurricanes during late summer and early fall
- Entering shaded or vegetated areas near standing or stagnant water
- Performing biological surveys, vegetation work, or restoration projects in mosquito-prone habitats
- Performing construction, maintenance, or habitat management in swampy or low-lying areas with poor drainage
- Engaging in wildlife handling or bird banding

Mosquitoes are drawn to carbon dioxide, body heat, and sweat, making motionless individuals (e.g., surveyors, observers) particularly vulnerable. Risk is particularly elevated in regions with documented mosquito activity and recent bird mortality.

Prevention

To avoid mosquito bites and related discomfort:

- Wear long sleeves and pants, preferably treated with permethrin
- Avoid perfumes or scented products that may attract mosquitoes
- Apply EPA-approved repellents (e.g., DEET, picaridin, IR3535, or oil of lemon eucalyptus) to exposed skin
- Use head nets and gloves in high-risk areas
- Use permethrin-treated clothing or gear when working in heavily infested areas
- Eliminate nearby standing water when possible (buckets, containers, puddles), especially near work staging or remote sleeping areas
- Use portable fans or smoke sources in temporary field stations or camps
- Monitor conditions in proposed field activities for potential mosquito-borne diseases
- Encourage institutional vector control in public or work areas (e.g., larvicide treatment)

Individual protective measures are highly effective, especially when layered together.

What To Do If Affected

- Wash affected areas with soap and water
- Apply topical antihistamines or hydrocortisone cream for itching
- Use cool compresses to reduce swelling
- Avoid scratching to prevent secondary infection
- Monitor for signs of bacterial infection (pus, spreading redness, warmth)
- Seek medical advice if symptoms worsen or become systemic

While mosquito bites rarely cause serious health effects on their own, persistent exposure can lead to considerable discomfort, loss of focus, or reluctance to engage in essential outdoor work – making bite prevention an important occupational safety measure.

Because of the possibility of pathogenic disease, it is prudent to self-monitor for symptoms for several weeks; a reasonable length of time to monitor and symptoms to watch for are included for each of the following entries. Most of these diseases are viral, so typical diagnosis (or confirmation of suspected diagnosis) is usually by PCR of viral DNA and separation/identification by electrophoresis (this typically works best within the first few days) or serological testing for immunoglobulin M (IgM; this typically works best after about a week, since it is an immunological product of the patient in response to a viral infection). Malaria is protozoan and is diagnosed with microscopic examination of blood smears; dirofilariasis is often unnoticed except incidentally through imaging (X-ray, computed tomography, etc.) for unrelated concerns.

Mosquito-Borne Diseases

These entries for 13 mosquito-borne diseases in North America are listed in order of highest risk to lowest risk considering both exposure risk and potential severity (Table 6.2).

TABLE 6.2

Ranking of 13 Mosquito-Borne Diseases in North America, Considering Both Exposure Risk and Severity

Rank	Disease	Reason for Ranking
1	West Nile Virus (WNV)	Widespread in continental United States; about 1% develop neuroinvasive disease, which can be fatal
2	Eastern Equine Encephalitis (EEE)	Rare but extremely dangerous (30%–50% fatality); most cases in eastern wetlands
3	St. Louis Encephalitis (SLE)	Occasionally re-emerges; older adults especially at risk for severe neurological forms
4	Dengue	Increasing in southern Florida, Puerto Rico, and border areas; severe hemorrhagic forms possible
5	La Crosse Encephalitis	Most common pediatric arbovirus in Appalachia and Midwest; can cause severe brain inflammation in children

(Continued)

TABLE 6.2 (*Continued*)
Ranking of 13 Mosquito-Borne Diseases in North America, Considering Both Exposure Risk and Severity

Rank	Disease	Reason for Ranking
6	Chikungunya Virus	Less severe than dengue but widespread in Caribbean and southern United States; chronic joint pain possible
7	Zika Virus	Declining but still possible in Florida, southern Texas, and Caribbean; fetal birth defects are the major concern
8	Malaria	Rare autochthonous transmission in the United States, but widespread concern for travelers; serious but treatable
9	Western Equine Encephalitis (WEE)	Historically significant but now rarely reported; still potentially dangerous
10	Jamestown Canyon Virus	Emerging in northern states; symptoms often mild, but neuroinvasive forms possible
11	Cache Valley Virus	Rare and primarily an animal pathogen; occasionally causes human infection
12	Dirofilariasis	Rare in humans; usually a concern for pets. In people, it causes a benign nodule rarely noticed unless incidentally through imaging

For each disease, it is best to consult a physician for proper medical diagnosis and treatment and not rely solely on the information provided here. Some diseases require immediate medical care upon notice of symptoms.

West Nile Virus

Pathogens: Order Amarillovirales, Family Flaviviridae: West Nile virus
Entomological Vectors: Order Diptera, Family Culicidae: *Culex pipiens* (northern house mosquito), *Cx. quinquefasciatus* (southern house mosquito), *Cx. tarsalis* (western encephalitis mosquito)
Exposure and Severity Ratings (Figure 6.27)

- **Exposure Level: 2–3**
  - Present in all 48 contiguous states (absent from Alaska, Hawaii, and Guam)
  - Especially common in the Midwest, south, and western United States during late summer and early fall
  - Exposure is uncommon (2) to moderate (3); around 1,000–3,000 cases reported/year
- **Severity Level: 1–5**
  - Most infections (~80%) are asymptomatic/minimal (1) or mild (2)
  - Severe (4) neuroinvasive disease occurs in ~1% of infections, nearly always requires hospitalization, and can be life-threatening (5) with a 6%–11% fatality rate/year

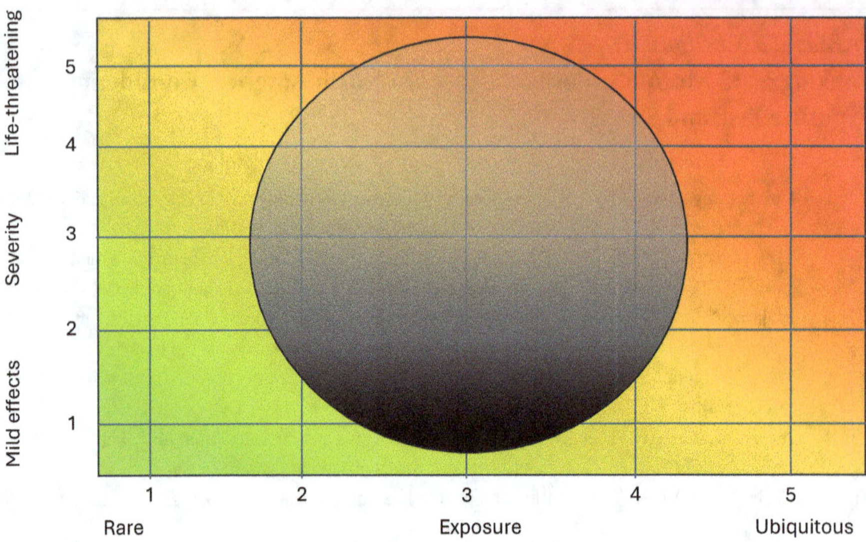

FIGURE 6.27   West Nile virus. Exposure × severity matrix.

References: Petersen (2019), Werner et al. (2019)

WNV is the most common mosquito-borne disease in North America. The virus is transmitted primarily by *Culex* mosquitoes and cycles naturally between mosquitoes and birds. Corvids (ravens, crows, magpies) are susceptible to WNV and may die in large numbers, signaling the presence of WNV in the environment. Humans and other mammals, especially horses, are considered dead-end hosts. Since its introduction to North America in 1999, WNV has spread throughout the United States and is now a seasonal public health concern.

Most human infections are asymptomatic (~80%) or result in a mild febrile illness called West Nile fever, characterized by fever, headache, fatigue, and body aches. However, approximately 1 in 150 infected individuals (particularly elderly or immunocompromised) develop neuroinvasive disease, which includes meningitis, encephalitis, or acute flaccid paralysis. These cases can require intensive medical care and may lead to long-term neurological sequelae or death.

Symptoms

West Nile fever (mild form):

- Fever, chills, body aches, and fatigue
- Headache, sometimes with eye pain
- Skin rash or swollen lymph nodes

Neuroinvasive disease (severe form):

- Stiff neck, confusion, tremors, seizures
- Muscle weakness or paralysis

- Coma or death in severe cases
- Long-term fatigue and neurologic impairment in survivors

This disease is nationally reportable in the United States. Reporting is handled by medical and public health professionals; environmental personnel and their organizations are *not* responsible for direct case reporting. However, ecologists and environmental professionals can even participate in surveillance for WNV: where applicable, report dead birds, especially corvids like ravens, crows, and magpies, to local health departments for monitoring. Support local mosquito control efforts, especially during outbreaks.

Remember that most exposures will not result in illness, and, for mild forms of WNV, supportive care is usually sufficient. Seek medical attention if experiencing signs of neuroinvasive disease. There is no antiviral treatment for WNV; care is supportive only.

EASTERN EQUINE ENCEPHALITIS

Pathogen: Order Martellivirales, Family Togaviridae: *Alphavirus* **Eastern Equine Encephalitis Virus**

Entomological Vectors: Order Diptera, Family Culicidae: *Culiseta melanura* **(black-tailed mosquito),** *Aedes, Coquillettidia,* **and** *Culex* **spp.**

Exposure and Severity Ratings (Figure 6.28)

- **Exposure Level: 2–3**
    - Uncommon (2) and limited to specific wetland ecosystems
    - May be moderately (3) common in the East
    - ~11 cases reported by CDC annually

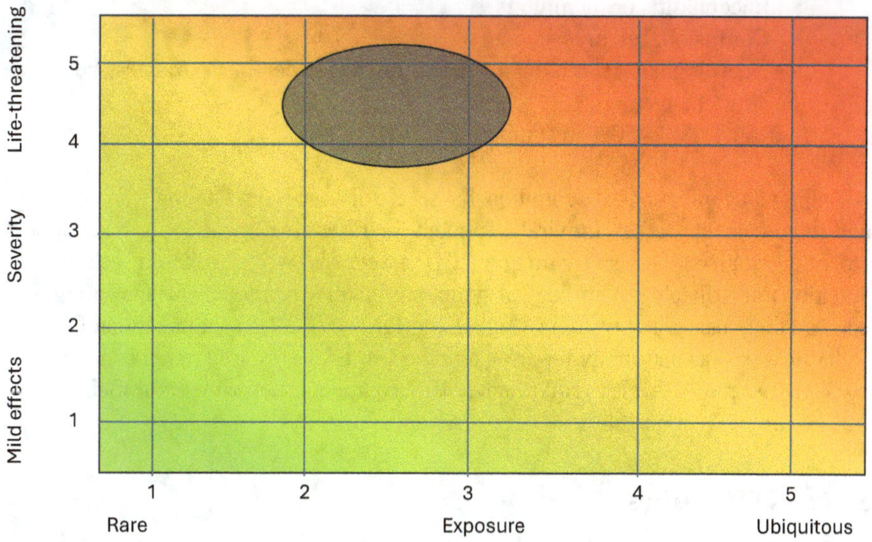

FIGURE 6.28   Eastern equine encephalitis. Exposure × severity matrix.

- **Severity Level: 4**
  - Severe (4): ~50% of cases become neuroinvasive and require hospitalization
  - Can be life-threatening (5): 30%–75% of neuroinvasive cases are fatal; survivors generally suffer long-term neurological damage
  - High mortality and long-term sequelae make Eastern Equine Encephalitis (EEE) one of the most dangerous arboviruses in North America

References: Lindsey et al. (2018), Armstrong and Andreadis (2022)

Eastern Equine Encephalitis virus (EEEV) is one of the most virulent mosquito-borne viruses in North America. It circulates primarily between *Culiseta melanura* mosquitoes and wild passerine birds (perching birds and songbirds) in freshwater swamp ecosystems. Humans and horses are dead-end hosts, infected by bridge vectors such as *Aedes sollicitans*, *Coquillettidia perturbans*, and others that feed on both birds and mammals.

Although human cases are rare, EEEV causes severe neuroinvasive disease in ~30%–50% of symptomatic individuals and has a high case fatality rate (up to 33%). Survivors may experience long-term neurological damage.

EEE is endemic in the eastern United States, especially in the Atlantic and Gulf Coast states, Great Lakes region, and swampy hardwood forest habitats. Professionals working in mosquito-rich wetlands during mid- to late summer are at highest risk.

Symptoms

- Incubation period: 4–10 days after mosquito bite
- Initial symptoms:
  - Sudden onset of fever, chills, malaise
  - Headache and muscle aches
- Severe disease (neuroinvasive form):
  - Encephalitis or meningitis
  - Confusion, seizures, coma
  - Neurological deficits in survivors: cognitive decline, paralysis, behavioral changes
- Mortality: 30%–50% in symptomatic human cases

Asymptomatic infections are common, but severe disease is devastating when it occurs, and there currently is no antiviral treatment for EEE. Treatment is entirely supportive, often requiring intensive care unit (ICU)-level care. Workers should seek medical attention immediately if neurological symptoms begin to occur. Physicians will usually confirm diagnosis with serological screening (IgM) or PCR on cerebrospinal fluid.

This disease is nationally reportable in the United States. Reporting is handled by medical and public health professionals; environmental personnel and their organizations are *not* responsible for direct case reporting.

St. Louis Encephalitis

Pathogen: Order Amarillovirales, Family Flaviviridae: *Orthoflavivirus* St. Louis encephalitis virus

Entomological Vectors: Order Diptera, Family Culicidae: *Culex pipiens* (northern house mosquito), *Cx. quinquefasciatus* (southern house mosquito), *Cx. tarsalis* (western encephalitis mosquito)

Exposure and Severity Ratings (Figure 6.29)

- **Exposure Level: 2**
  - Uncommon (2) but widespread in southern, western, and midwestern United States, including both rural and urban settings
  - 21 cases reported in 2023; average ~14 cases/year (2003–2022)
- **Severity Level: 1–5**
  - Many people experience no to minimal (1) symptoms, while some experience mild (2) febrile illness
  - Severe (4) neuroinvasive disease can occur especially in older adults
  - Can be life-threatening (5): mortality ~10% in neuroinvasive cases

References: Diaz et al. (2018)

St. Louis Encephalitis virus (SLEV) is a flavivirus transmitted primarily by *Culex* mosquitoes. It is endemic to the continental United States, particularly the Midwest, south, and west, and ranges through the Americas, including Mexico, Central America, and northern South America. SLEV circulates in bird-mosquito cycles, with humans as incidental dead-end hosts.

SLEV is closely related to WNV and presents with similar symptoms and ecology. Outbreaks are sporadic but can be severe, particularly in older adults or individuals with compromised immune systems. In contrast to EEE and Western Equine Encephalitis (WEE), urban and suburban settings can also pose a risk due to the adaptability of *Culex* vectors.

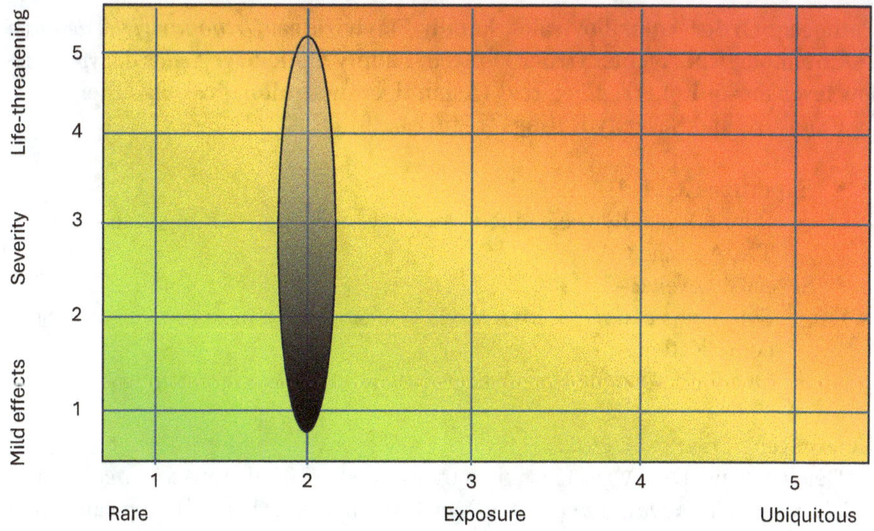

FIGURE 6.29   St. Louis encephalitis. Exposure × severity matrix.

SLEV is an important occupational health concern for field professionals, especially during summer and early fall when *Culex* populations peak.

Symptoms

- Incubation period: 5–15 days post-mosquito bite
- Mild illness (most common):
  - Fever
  - Headache
  - Nausea and fatigue
- Severe cases:
  - Encephalitis or meningitis
  - Neck stiffness, stupor, disorientation
  - Tremors, seizures, and coma (especially in patients >50 years)
- Mortality rate: ~5%–15% in neuroinvasive cases
- Long-term neurological effects may occur, including memory loss and movement disorders

Differentiation from WNV, EEE, or WEE is important for diagnosis and surveillance. Unlike WNV, SLEV rarely causes rash, which may help in differential diagnosis, although it is usually confirmed via serological testing for IgM or PCR. Supportive care is the only recourse as no specific antiviral is currently available, and hospitalization may be required for severe neurologic symptoms.

This disease is nationally reportable in the United States. Reporting is handled by medical and public health professionals; environmental personnel and their organizations are *not* responsible for direct case reporting.

Dengue

**Pathogen: Order Amarillovirales, Family Flaviviridae: *Orthoflavivirus denguei*
    Entomological Agents: Order Diptera, Family Culicidae: *Aedes aegypti* (yellow fever mosquito), *Ae. albopictus* (Asian tiger mosquito), possibly others
    Exposure and Severity Ratings (Figure 6.30)**

- **Exposure Level: 1**
  - Rare (1): locally transmitted cases have recently been reported in FL, TX, AZ, and CA
- **Severity Level: 2–5**
  - Symptoms can range from mild (2) to severe (4); most recover without complications
  - One form, Dengue Hemorrhagic Fever, can be life-threatening (5)

Reference: Werner et al. (2019)

Dengue virus (DENV) is a flavivirus transmitted primarily by *Aedes aegypti* and, to a lesser extent, *Aedes albopictus*. It is endemic in tropical and subtropical regions worldwide and has increasingly been reported in locally transmitted outbreaks in the southern United States, particularly in Florida and Texas, with sporadic cases

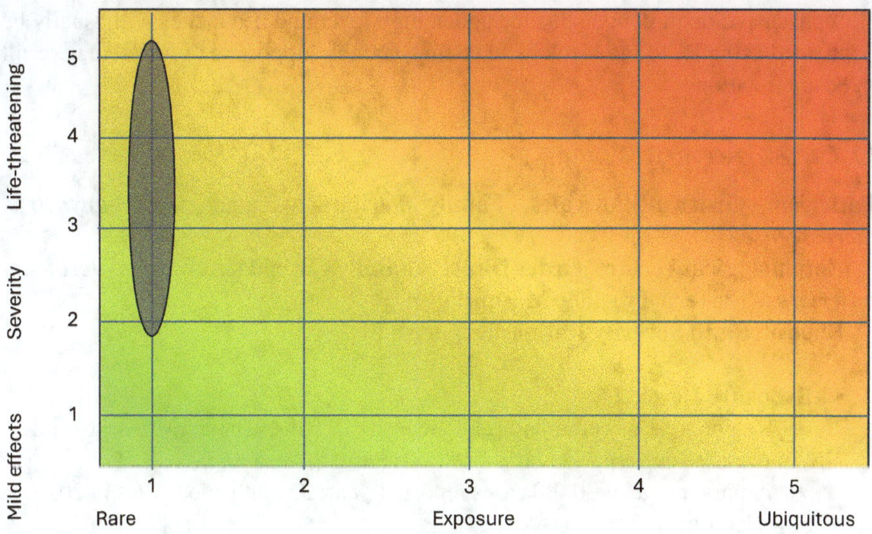

FIGURE 6.30 Dengue. Exposure × severity matrix.

in Arizona and California. In recent years, Florida has reported multiple autochthonous cases annually, especially in urban centers like Miami-Dade County. These outbreaks typically occur in warm months when mosquito populations are at their peak.

Dengue has four serotypes (DENV-1 to DENV-4), and infection with one serotype provides lifelong immunity to that type but increases the risk of severe disease if a person is later infected with a different serotype. Most infections are asymptomatic or mild, but some progress to Dengue Fever, a flu-like illness with high fever, joint and muscle pain (sometimes called "breakbone fever"), rash, and fatigue. Severe forms include Dengue Hemorrhagic Fever and Dengue Shock Syndrome, which require hospitalization and supportive care. There is no antiviral treatment for dengue; clinical management is supportive.

Symptoms

- Incubation time is 4–7 days, but may take as long as 2 weeks
- Sudden high fever (up to 40°C/104°F)
- Severe headache, retro-orbital pain
- Muscle and joint pain ("breakbone fever")
- Rash (appears 3–5 days after fever onset)
- Nausea, vomiting, and fatigue
- In severe cases: bleeding, low platelet count, plasma leakage, and circulatory collapse

Dengue is rare in the continental United States, and most cases are travel-related, but across Mexico, Central America, the Bahamas, and the Caribbean, dengue is endemic, with some countries reporting frequent outbreaks. Monitor for symptoms for up to 2 weeks, and if a fever spikes suddenly, seek immediate medical treatment.

Clinical suspicion of dengue due to sudden high fever and headaches will usually be confirmed using PCR and serological testing. Care is supportive only and may result in hospitalization.

La Crosse Encephalitis

Pathogen: Order Elliovirales, Family Peribunyaviridae: *Orthobunyavirus lacrosseense*

Entomological Vectors: Order Diptera, Family Culicidae: *Aedes/Ochlerotatus triseriatus* **(Eastern Treehole Mosquito)**

Exposure and Severity Ratings (Figure 6.31)

- **Exposure Level: 2**
  - Regionally uncommon (2): focused in the Upper Midwest and Appalachians, particularly in wooded areas
  - Annual range of 30–90 cases reported/year; 35 confirmed cases in 2023
- **Severity Level: 3**
  - Most adults experience moderate (3) illness with good recovery; however, there is ~97% hospitalization rate
  - Long-term neurological sequelae rare

References: Vahey et al. (2021), Goldman and Hamer (2024)

La Crosse Encephalitis is a mosquito-borne viral disease caused by La Crosse virus (LACV), a member of the California serogroup of bunyaviruses. It is transmitted primarily by the Eastern Treehole Mosquito (*Aedes triseriatus*), a species that breeds in natural containers like tree holes, as well as artificial containers like tires, buckets, or birdbaths in forested areas.

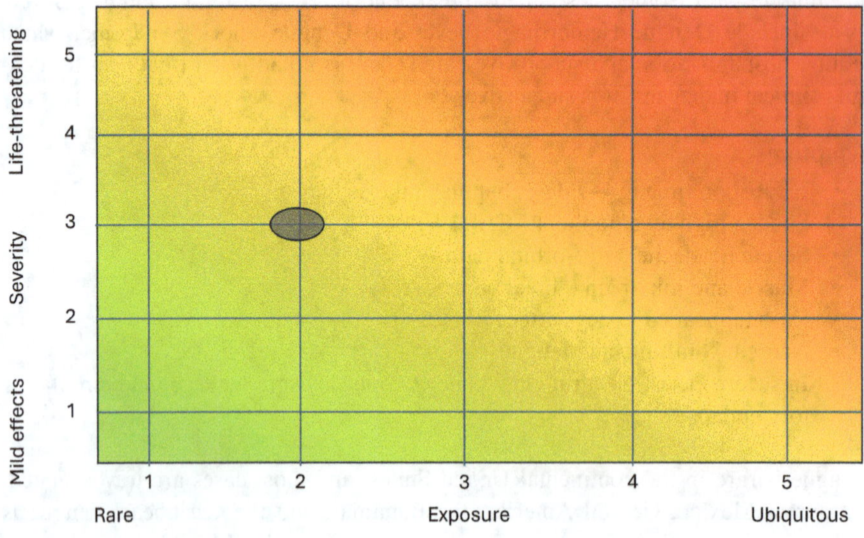

FIGURE 6.31 La Crosse encephalitis. Exposure × severity matrix.

LACV is endemic to the eastern and upper midwestern United States, particularly West Virginia, Ohio, Tennessee, North Carolina, Wisconsin, and surrounding states. While most infections are mild or asymptomatic, the virus can cause serious neuro-invasive disease, especially in children under 16.

Symptoms

- Incubation period: 5–15 days after mosquito bite
- Initial symptoms:
  - Fever
  - Headache
  - Nausea or vomiting
  - Lethargy or drowsiness
- In severe cases (especially in children):
  - Seizures
  - Encephalitis (brain inflammation)
  - Coma or neurological deficits
- Most recover fully, but 1% of cases may result in long-term cognitive or behavioral effects

Adults usually experience mild illness, but children appear to be more likely to develop serious complications. After mosquito exposure in endemic regions at likely times, monitor for symptoms for up to 3 weeks; seek medical evaluation for fever, headache, and especially neurologic signs. Diagnosis is usually made via serological testing for IgM or PCR analysis of cerebrospinal fluid. Treatment is supportive only, and hospitalization may be required in severe cases.

Since there is no vaccine, prevention depends entirely on mosquito avoidance. Medical professionals will report confirmed or suspected cases to local health departments.

CHIKUNGUNYA VIRUS

Pathogen: Order Martellivirales, Family Togaviridae: *Alphavirus chikungunya*
Entomological Vectors: Order Diptera, Family Culicidae: *Aedes aegypti* (yellow fever mosquito), *Ae. albopictus* (Asian tiger mosquito)
Exposure and Severity Ratings (Figure 6.32)

- **Exposure Level: 1**
  - Rare (1) in the southern United States, with only two locally acquired cases documented as of end of 2025
- **Severity Level: 4**
  - Illness can be severely (4) debilitating; however, fatalities are rare

References: Pastula et al. (2016), Werner et al. (2019)
Chikungunya virus is an arthropod-borne alphavirus transmitted by *Ae. aegypti* and *Ae. albopictus* mosquitoes, two introduced species now commonly found in the southern and southeastern United States. The virus is endemic in parts of Africa,

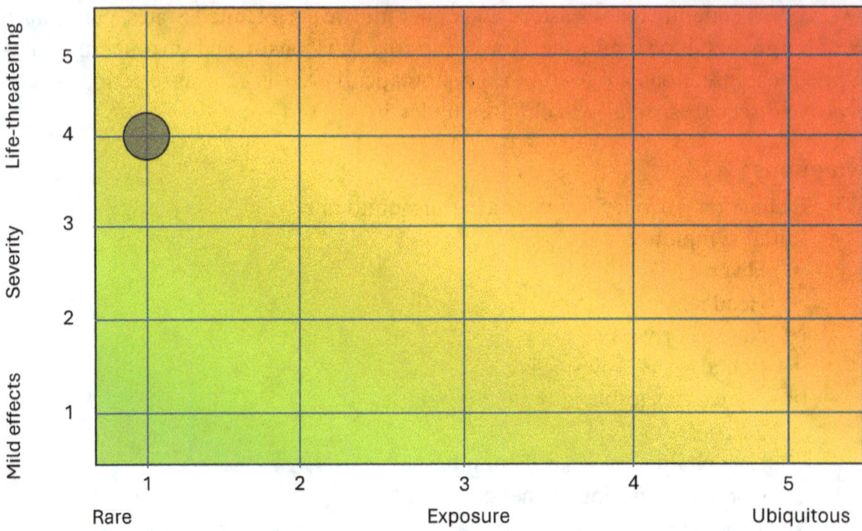

FIGURE 6.32 Chikungunya. Exposure × severity matrix.

Asia, and the Caribbean, and most cases in North America could be linked to a person who had immigrated from or recently traveled to one of those areas. Autochthonous (locally transmitted) cases were first confirmed in the United States in Florida in 2014, with a second confirmed local case in Texas in 2015. These incidents demonstrate that short-term transmission cycles can occur under favorable ecological conditions, especially where *Aedes* mosquitoes are active.

Chikungunya presents with acute febrile illness, typically accompanied by severe joint pain, rash, headache, and fatigue. While most individuals recover within a week, joint symptoms can persist for weeks to months, particularly in older adults. The virus does not usually cause life-threatening complications, but the debilitating arthralgia may limit fieldwork capacity or result in extended recovery periods. The US Food and Drug Administration recently (2023) approved the Ixchiq™ vaccine for people 18 years or older and who at risk for exposure to chikungunya virus.

Symptoms

- Incubation period is typically 3-7 days, but may range up to 12 days
- Sudden high fever (often >39°C/102°F)
- Severe joint pain (often symmetric, involving hands, wrists, ankles, or feet)
- Headache, rash, muscle aches, and fatigue
- In some cases, prolonged joint stiffness or arthritis-like symptoms lasting weeks to months

Although local transmission is rare, outbreaks or isolated cases may occur in the southern United States, especially during periods of increased mosquito activity, such as in the aftermath of hurricanes, or following the introduction of imported cases. Monitor for symptoms for up to 2 weeks, and if a fever spikes suddenly, seek immediate medical treatment. Clinical suspicion of chikungunya due to sudden high fever will usually be confirmed using serological testing for IgM or PCR analysis. Care is supportive only and may result in hospitalization.

This disease is nationally reportable in the United States. Reporting is handled by medical and public health professionals; environmental personnel and their organizations are *not* responsible for direct case reporting.

ZIKA VIRUS

Pathogen: Order Amarillovirales, Family: Flaviviridae: *Orthoflavivirus zikaense*

Entomological Vectors: Order Diptera, Family Culicidae: *Aedes aegypti* (yellow fever mosquito), *Ae. albopictus* (Asian tiger mosquito)

Exposure and Severity Ratings (Figure 6.33)

- **Exposure Level: 1–2**
  - Rare (1) in the United States; only known from the southern tips of FL and TX, where it is uncommon (2)
  - Exposure much higher in American tropics, e.g., Puerto Rico
- **Severity Level: 1–4**
  - Typical adult illness is minimal (1) to mild (2)
  - Pregnancy-related fetal outcomes and possible neurological outcomes are severe (4)

References: Pastula et al. (2016), Werner et al. (2019)

Zika virus (ZIKV) is a mosquito-transmitted flavivirus originally identified in Uganda in 1947, but which rose to global prominence after causing a major outbreak in

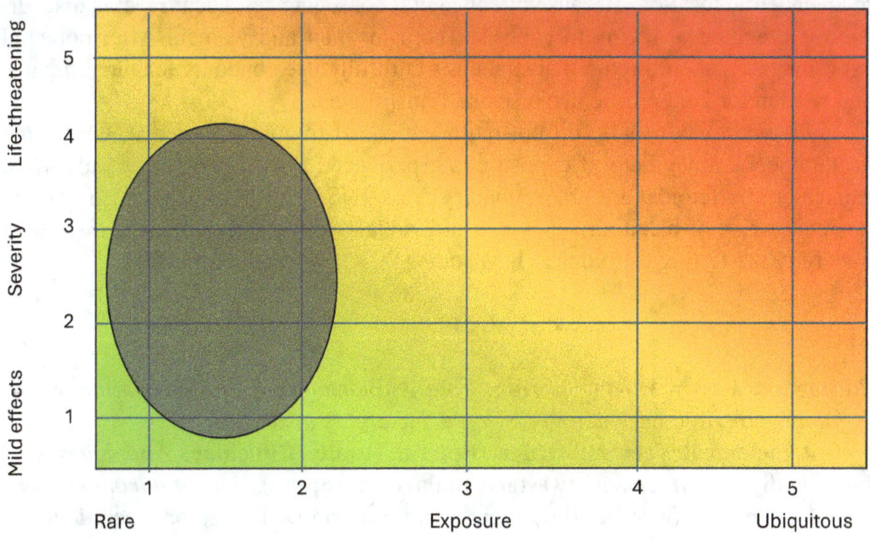

FIGURE 6.33   Zika. Exposure × severity graph.

tropical America (2015–2017) that greatly impacted the 2016 Olympic Games in Rio de Janeiro, Brazil. It is primarily spread by *Ae. aegypti* and *Ae. albopictus*, the same mosquitoes that transmit dengue, chikungunya, and yellow fever. ZIKV is unique among mosquito-borne viruses in that it can also be transmitted sexually and perinatally.

While Zika infection in adults is usually mild or asymptomatic, infection during pregnancy can lead to congenital Zika syndrome, including microcephaly and other severe birth defects. There have also been rare reports of Guillain-Barré syndrome following infection.

Symptoms

- Incubation period: 3–14 days post-mosquito bite
- Most infections are asymptomatic (~80%)
- When symptoms occur:
  - Low-grade fever
  - Rash
  - Joint pain (especially in hands and feet)
  - Conjunctivitis (red eyes)
  - Headache, muscle pain
  - Typically lasts several days to a week
- Complications (rare but serious):
  - Guillain-Barré syndrome (autoimmune paralysis)
  - Congenital Zika syndrome in infants born to infected mothers (microcephaly, brain abnormalities, eye defects)

ZIKV remains rare in the United States, but its prevalence throughout the Caribbean, Mexico, and Central America is uncertain. Most North American ecologists and environmental professionals will not encounter this disease unless they travel abroad to an endemic location. Because of congenital consequences, such travel is discouraged if pregnant or trying to conceive, both for men and women. After potential exposure, men should remain abstinent or faithfully use condoms for three months and women for 2 months to avoid sexual transmission.

Mild symptoms usually do not require medical treatment, but rest, fluids, and acetaminophen may help. If exposure is experienced abroad, workers should avoid aspirin or nonsteroidal anti-inflammatory drugs (NSAIDs) until dengue is ruled out (to reduce risk of bleeding). Pregnant individuals with suspected exposure should undergo Zika testing (serological IgM and/or PCR) and fetal monitoring.

MALARIA

Pathogens: Order Haemosporida, Family Plasmodiidae: *Plasmodium vivax,* *P. falciparum,* **and occasionally** *P. malariae and P. ovale*

Entomological Vectors: Order Diptera, Family Culicidae: *Anopheles* **spp. historically** *An. freeborni* **(western malaria mosquito),** *An.* **quadrimaculatus,** *An.* **punctipennis (woodland malaria mosquito); potential vectors include other** *Anopheles* **spp. present in North America**

Exposure and Severity Ratings (Figure 6.34)

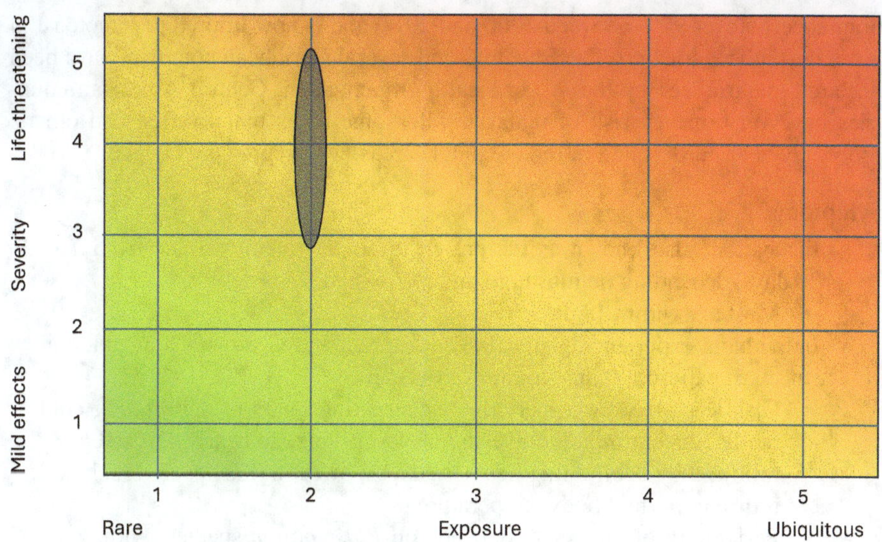

FIGURE 6.34 Malaria. Exposure × severity matrix.

- **Exposure Level: 2**
  - Historically endemic across much of the United States into the mid-20th century; eliminated by the 1950s
  - Currently, uncommon (2): around 2,000–2,500 cases/year, nearly all imported; however, nine locally acquired cases were reported in 2023 (FL, TX, MD)
- **Severity Level: 3–5**
  - Moderate (3) to severe (4) harm, generally; some species cause malaria that can relapse decades later
  - *Plasmodium falciparum* causes severe malaria and is the most life-threatening (5)

References: Griffith et al. (2007), Daily et al. (2022)

Malaria is a mosquito-borne protozoan infection transmitted by female *Anopheles* mosquitoes. Indigenous malaria was historically common across tropical and temperate zones of the United States and into southern Canada near Toronto. Widespread eradication efforts, such as drainage, insecticide use, housing improvements, and screens, in the mid-20th century, have, for the most part, eradicated this disease from North America.

Today, most North American malaria cases are imported, linked to travel. The CDC reports ~2,000–2,500 cases annually (2007–2022) with a mean of seven deaths per year. However, sporadic local transmissions do still occur: in 2023, Florida saw four *Plasmodium vivax* cases, Texas one, and Maryland one, marking the first autochthonous cases since 2003. Historically endemic species like the western malaria mosquito (*Anopheles freeborni*), the woodland malaria mosquito (*An. punctipennis*), and *An. quadrimaculatus* remain capable vectors. In Mexico, malaria cases have dropped dramatically (over 90% between 2000 and 2014) and is now limited to remote rural areas in southern Mexico. The Bahamas and several Caribbean countries have been declared malaria-free by the World Health Organization. Central American countries have very uneven risk of malaria, with some areas malaria-free and others, especially near borders and in remote jungle areas, with raging prevalence.

Symptoms

- Incubation, also known as the pre-erythrocytic stage, can last from 7 to 30 days, depending on mosquito and *Plasmodium* species
  - Most are within 18 days
- Individuals experiencing first infection or infection after a long interval since last exposure (naïve immune systems)
  - Classic paroxysms – periods of alternating bouts of debilitating cold (chills, uncontrollable shivering) as fevers spike to nearly 41°C (106°F), followed by debilitating heat (headache, sweating) as fevers break and return to normal body temperature
  - Periodicity of paroxysm depends on *Plasmodium* species, with some recurring every 2 days and others every 3 days, eventually blurring as variety is introduced into the *Plasmodium* life cycle
  - Paroxysms can continue for up to 2 weeks without treatment or until the body gains sufficient immunological control
- Individuals with repeated or recent infections (experienced immune systems providing limited immunity)
  - Uncomplicated malaria: fever, chills, sweats, headaches, malaise, muscle aches
  - Severe malaria (*falciparum* or delayed treatment): anemia, breathing difficulties, seizures, renal failure – may be fatal without prompt treatment
- Relapsing malaria (*vivax, ovale*): recurrence due to dormant liver forms weeks to months post-infection

Preventing malaria involves a combination of personal protective measures (standard mosquito PPE) and, when warranted, the use of antimalarial prophylaxis. Travelers or field workers operating in malaria-endemic regions should consult healthcare professionals, such as a state health department, to determine if chemoprophylaxis is advisable. There are several common preventive medications, each with distinct dosing schedules and side effects. Even in regions where malaria risk is low or seasonal, local vector activity (especially *Anopheles* mosquitoes) should be monitored, and general mosquito avoidance remains prudent.

Monitor for about a month after potential exposure. If a person develops fever, chills, malaise, or flu-like symptoms within several weeks (or even months) after potential exposure in a malaria-endemic area, immediate medical evaluation is recommended. Malaria diagnosis is typically confirmed by microscopic examination of blood smears, rapid diagnostic tests, or PCR. Waiting until symptoms become severe can delay lifesaving treatment, particularly in *P. falciparum* infections. Treatment depends on the species and severity of infection but often includes artemisinin-based combination therapies or, for relapsing types like *P. vivax* and *P. ovale*, additional medications such as primaquine to eliminate dormant liver stages. Medical care is essential for proper species identification and drug selection, as resistance patterns and individual contraindications vary. Prompt diagnosis and treatment significantly reduce the risk of complications and further transmission.

WESTERN EQUINE ENCEPHALITIS

Pathogen: Order Martellivirales, Family Togaviridae: *Alphavirus*

Entomological Vectors: Order Diptera, Family Culicidae: *Culex tarsalis* (western encephalitis mosquito), *Culex pipiens* (northern house mosquito), *Aedes taeniorhynchus* (black salt marsh mosquito), and possibly other *Aedes/ Ochlerotatus* spp.

Exposure and Severity Ratings (Figure 6.35)

- **Exposure Level: 1–2**
  - Rare (1) to uncommon (2) with declining incidence
  - Vector and reservoir presence remains in western regions
- **Severity Level: 2–4**
  - Usually mild (2) illness
  - Severe (4) neuroinvasive disease occurs especially in children
  - Mortality and long-term effects are lower than EEE, but not negligible

WEE virus is a mosquito-borne alphavirus endemic to western North America, particularly in the Great Plains, desert Southwest, and intermountain regions. The virus cycles primarily between *Culex tarsalis* mosquitoes and wild birds, especially

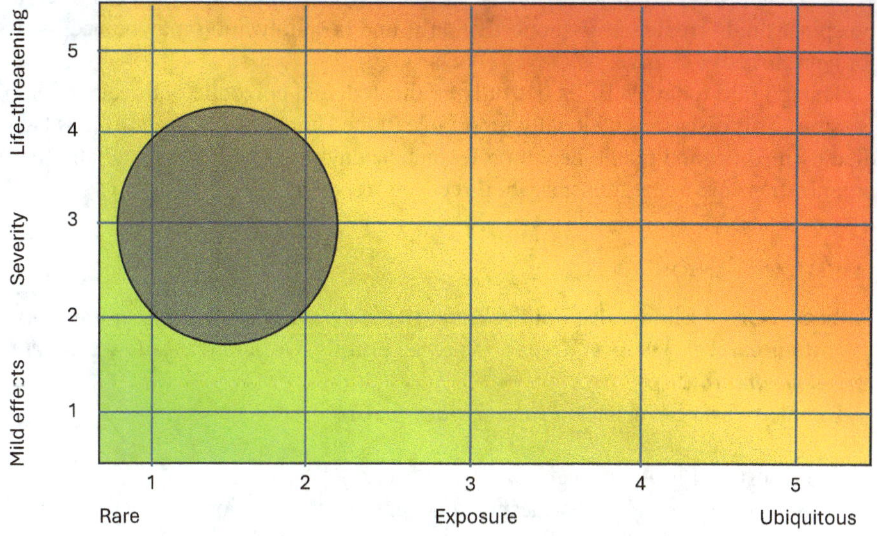

FIGURE 6.35 Western equine encephalitis. Exposure × severity matrix.

passerines (songbirds). Humans and horses are dead-end hosts which means that, while it makes them sick, the virus cannot reproduce or be passed along from these hosts.

Although human cases have become rare in recent decades, WEE was historically an important cause of viral encephalitis, especially in infants and children. Like its eastern counterpart, it can cause severe neurological disease, but mortality and long-term complications are generally lower than for EEE. Due to its vector ecology, WEE presents a potential occupational hazard for those working in wetlands, irrigated farmland, rangelands, and riparian corridors, particularly during mid to late summer.

Symptoms

- Incubation period: 5–10 days after mosquito bite
- Mild cases:
  - Fever
  - Headache
  - Malaise
- Severe cases (neuroinvasive disease, more common in children):
  - Stiff neck
  - Disorientation or confusion
  - Seizures or coma
- Fatality rate: ~3% in humans, with higher risk in the very young or elderly
- Some survivors may have motor deficits or learning disabilities, especially children

WEE often co-circulates with SLEV and WNV, which share similar vectors and habitats. A vaccine exists for horses, so many veterinarians, farmers, ranchers, and horse breeders vaccinate their horses, but no human vaccine yet exists.

Monitor for symptoms for up to 2 weeks and seek medical attention if symptoms occur. Diagnosis is confirmed using serological IgM tests or PCR analysis of cerebrospinal fluid. Treatment is supportive only, and hospitalization may be necessary for neuroinvasive disease.

Though rare today, WEE is not fully eradicated, and epizootic outbreaks remain possible. This disease is nationally reportable in the United States. Reporting is handled by medical and public health professionals; environmental personnel and their organizations are *not* responsible for direct case reporting.

Jamestown Canyon Virus

Pathogen: Order Elliovirales, Family Bunyaviridae: *Orthobunyavirus jamestownense*
Entomological Vectors: Order Diptera, Family Culicidae: *Aedes, Culiseta,* and *Coquillettidia* **spp.**
Exposure and Severity Ratings (Figure 6.36)

- **Exposure Level: 2**
  - Uncommon (2) but widespread geographic distribution
  - Common vectors and reservoirs increase potential risk
  - Twenty-seven reported cases in 2023

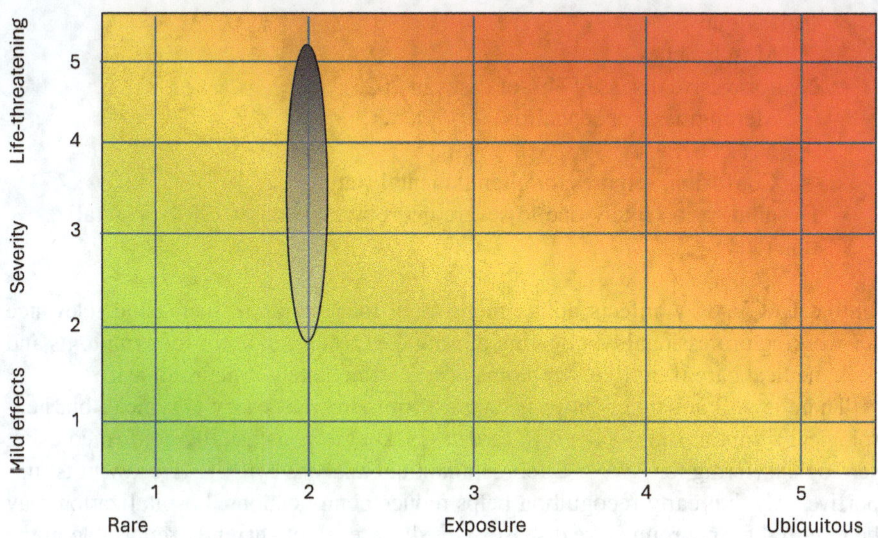

FIGURE 6.36   Jamestown Canyon virus. Exposure × severity matrix.

- **Severity Level: 2–5**
  - Historically, most cases were mild (2)
  - Moderate (3) to severe (4) neuroinvasive disease is becoming more common: CDC reports ~23 neuroinvasive cases/year
  - May be life-threatening (5): ~11% mortality

References: Pastula et al. (2016); Villeneuve et al. (2025)

Jamestown Canyon virus (JCV) is an emerging mosquito-borne *Orthobunyavirus* in the California serogroup, first isolated in Jamestown Canyon, Colorado. It circulates primarily between mosquitoes and wild ungulates, such as white-tailed deer, elk, or moose, throughout much of North America, including the Midwest, northeast, and parts of the south and west. It has recently been detected in *Aedes* mosquitoes in the tundra and other biomes of northern North America.

While most human infections are mild or asymptomatic, JCV has been increasingly recognized as a cause of viral meningitis and encephalitis, particularly in adults, in contrast to LACV, which more often affects children. It is now considered endemic throughout the United States, with cases reported in more than 30 states.

JCV is important to field professionals due to its widespread distribution, multiple mosquito vectors, common wildlife reservoir hosts, and potential severity, especially during spring and summer fieldwork in wooded or wetland regions.

Symptoms

- Incubation period: 3–10 days after bite
- Most cases are mild and self-limiting, but symptoms may include:
  - Fever
  - Headache

- Fatigue
- Muscle aches
- Neuroinvasive disease (74% of cases in 2023):
  - Meningitis or encephalitis
  - Neck stiffness
  - Confusion, seizures, or altered mental status
- Hospitalization likely due to severe neuroinvasive cases (93% hospitalization rate)

Unlike LACV, JCV infects adults more often than children, increasing relevance for working professionals. Following mosquito exposure, monitor for symptoms and seek medical care if flu-like symptoms occur, immediately if neurological.

There is no known person-to-person transmission. Recovery is typical, but neurological symptoms may persist in rare cases. Diagnosis is usually confirmed using serological testing for IgM or cerebrospinal fluid analysis by PCR. Treatment is supportive only, but early recognition helps reduce complications; hospitalization may be required for neuroinvasive disease. This disease is not currently reportable in the United States; however, due to the potential severity, medical and public health professionals often report JCV; environmental personnel and their organizations are *not* responsible for direct case reporting.

CACHE VALLEY VIRUS

Pathogen: Order Elliovirales, Family Bunyaviridae: *Orthobunyavirus cacheense*
Entomological Vectors: Order Diptera, Family Culicidae: primarily *Culiseta inornata* (winter marsh mosquito), but also *Anopheles*, *Aedes*, and other floodwater mosquitoes
Exposure and Severity Ratings (Figure 6.37)

- **Exposure Level: 1–2**
  - Rare (1) to uncommon (2) in rural, wetland, and rangeland habitats across the United States
  - Only seven confirmed human cases in United States to date
- **Severity Level: 4–5**
  - Severe (4) neuroinvasive disease; all cases so far have resulted in encephalitis or meningitis
  - Life-threatening (5): 43% mortality rate

Reference: Hughes et al. (2023)

Cache Valley virus (CVV) is a mosquito-borne *Orthobunyavirus* endemic to North and Central America, especially in the United States and Canada. First isolated in Utah's Cache Valley in 1956, CVV circulates among wild ungulates (especially deer) and domestic livestock, particularly sheep.

While human infections are rare, CVV can cause serious neuroinvasive disease, including meningitis and encephalitis. In animals, especially pregnant ewes, the virus can cross the placenta and cause abortions, congenital malformations,

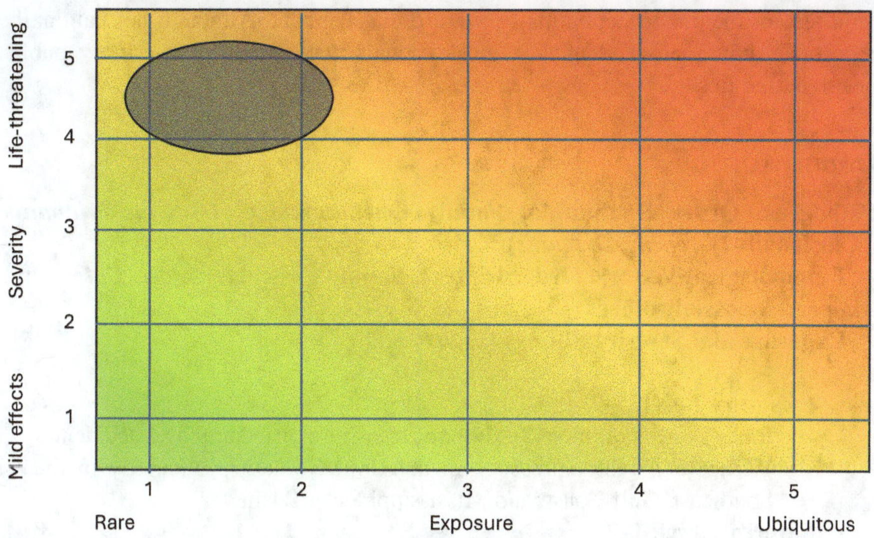

FIGURE 6.37 Cache Valley virus. Exposure × severity matrix.

and stillbirths. CVV is thus of dual importance: as a zoonosis and as a veterinary pathogen.

For field biologists, wildlife professionals, and livestock health workers, CVV presents an occupational risk in wetland, pastureland, or forest edge environments, particularly during mosquito season.

Symptoms

Most human CVV infections are asymptomatic or mild, but in rare cases, severe illness occurs:

- Incubation period: Unknown, likely 3–7 days post-exposure
- Mild symptoms:
  - Fever
  - Fatigue
  - Headache
- Neuroinvasive disease (rare):
  - Meningitis or encephalitis
  - Confusion, stiff neck, seizure, or coma
- Some fatal cases have been reported, but mortality is low and limited to severe presentations

Because CVV is likely underdiagnosed or labeled as unspecified viral encephalitis, its true prevalence may be higher than reported. Monitor for symptoms for up to 2 weeks and seek medical attention if they occur. Diagnosis is made via serological testing for IgM or PCR analysis of cerebrospinal fluid. Treatment is supportive, as no antiviral therapy currently exists, and hospitalization may be required for meningoencephalitis or seizure management. Although not nationally reportable, physicians and medical professionals may report to veterinary public health authorities.

DIROFILARIASIS

Pathogens: Order Rhabditida, Family Onchocercidae: *Dirofilaria immitis* **(occasionally** *D. repens, D. tenuis***)**

Entomological Vectors: Order Diptera, Family Culicidae: *Aedes, Culex,* **and** *Anopheles***, possibly others**

Exposure and Severity Ratings (Figure 6.38)

- **Exposure Level: 1–2**
  - Rare (1) to uncommon (2): zoonotic transmission to humans is accidental
  - Widespread vector presence in the United States, particularly in the Southeast, Gulf Coast, and Mississippi River Basin
- **Severity Level: 1–2**
  - Typically asymptomatic/minimal (1) or results in mild (2) benign, localized lesions

Reference: Simón et al. (2012)

Dog heartworm, caused by the nematode *Dirofilaria immitis*, is a common parasitic infection in domestic and wild canids. Mosquitoes act as vectors, picking up microfilariae from an infected host, allowing it to replicate internally, and then transferring infective larvae to a new host during blood feeding. Worms grow to adulthood and congregate in the pulmonary arteries and the right side of the heart. While the

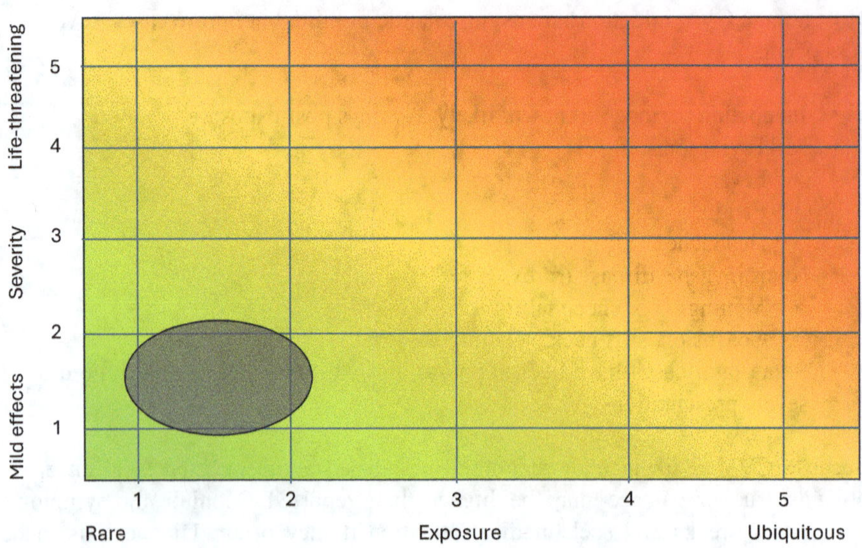

FIGURE 6.38 Dirofilariasis. Exposure × severity matrix.

adult worms continue to release new microfilariae, large numbers can block arteries or fill the chambers of the heart, causing progressive heart failure.

Humans can become accidental hosts, but the parasite cannot complete its life cycle in people. Instead, immature worms may lodge in subcutaneous tissue, lungs, or occasionally the eye; anywhere this happens, they die and form small granulomas. In the United States, pulmonary dirofilariasis is the most common presentation in humans and is usually discovered incidentally on unrelated imaging as a solitary lung nodule – often referred to as a "coin lesion." Subcutaneous or ocular nodules are less frequent and typically associated with other *Dirofilaria* species such as *D. repens* or *D. tenuis*. These infections do not progress to systemic disease and cannot be transmitted between humans.

Symptoms

In human cases, which are rare, symptoms may include:

- Asymptomatic pulmonary nodule (incidental radiographic finding)
- Mild cough or chest discomfort
- Subcutaneous lumps (often painless)
- Ocular irritation if the worm migrates to the eye
- No systemic signs or bloodborne microfilariae in humans

If imaging reveals a suspicious lung lesion, a patient should follow up with a health care provider; biopsy may confirm dead nematode. Subcutaneous or ocular nodules will likely be surgically removed and identified. No antiparasitic treatment is needed; humans are dead-end hosts, and the infection is not transmissible.

SAND FLIES

Entomological Parasites and Vectors: Order Diptera, Family Psychodidae: Subfamily Phlebotominae: *Lutzomyia* spp.
  Exposure and Severity Ratings (Figure 6.39)

- **Exposure Level: 2**
  - Uncommon (2) and localized to extreme southern United States (TX, AZ, FL)
- **Severity Level: 1–2**
  - Sand fly bites result in minimal (1) to mild (2) harm
  - Leishmaniasis (addressed elsewhere), increases severity

Reference: Akhoundi et al. (2020)
  Sand flies are tiny, hairy, moth-like flies known for their nocturnal, silent biting behavior. They thrive in warm, dry climates with organic-rich soils, caves, burrows, or rock outcroppings. Globally, they are most notorious as vectors of leishmaniasis, a disease caused by *Leishmania* parasites. Even in the absence of disease transmission, however, sand fly bites can still cause itchy, painful welts and allergic responses.

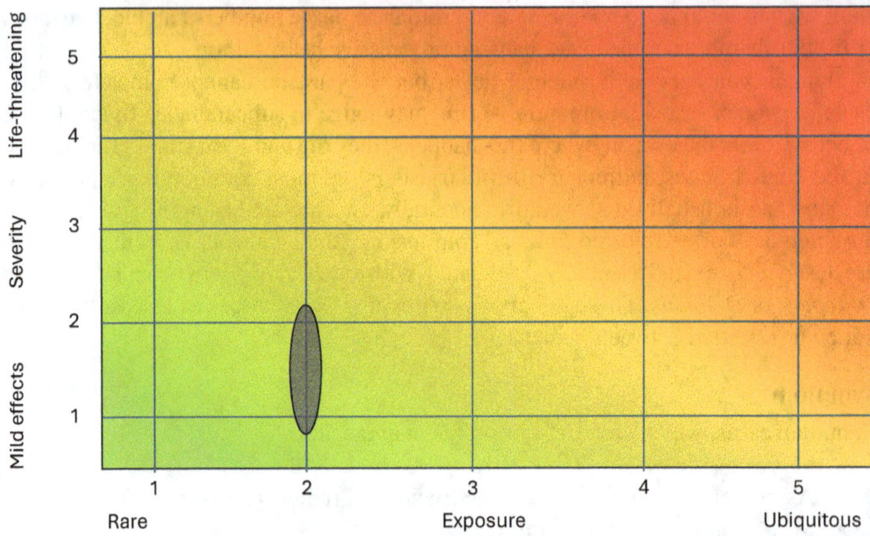

FIGURE 6.39 Sand flies. Exposure × severity matrix.

In the United States, native sand flies (especially *Lutzomyia* spp.) are increasingly recognized as potential vectors of cutaneous leishmaniasis in Texas and the Southwest, particularly where canine reservoirs are present. They are also found in Florida and parts of the Gulf Coast.

Symptoms

Symptoms depend on whether disease is transmitted:

- Non-disease bites:
  - Itchy, painful red bumps or welts
  - Clusters of bites on exposed skin
  - Allergic reactions (swelling, burning, rash)
- Cutaneous leishmaniasis (rare in the United States):
  - Chronic skin sores that may ulcerate
  - Lesions appear weeks to months after bite
  - Typically painless but slow-healing
  - Rare progression to mucocutaneous or visceral forms in certain *Leishmania* species

Leishmaniasis is endemic in Central and South America, the Middle East, and parts of Africa and Asia, but imported and zoonotic cases have been reported in the United States.

Occupational Exposure

Ecologists and environmental professionals are at risk when:

- Working in arid or semi-arid environments with loose soil or rock shelters
- Conducting biological surveys, cave exploration, or burrow inspections

- Performing fieldwork in southern Texas, Arizona, or Florida, or Mexico south through Central America
- Traveling internationally to leishmaniasis-endemic countries

Sand flies are nocturnal, with peak activity from dusk to dawn, and often enter tents, cabins, and poorly sealed structures.

Prevention

Preventing sand fly exposure involves combining barrier methods and chemical repellents:

- Wear long-sleeved shirts, long pants, and closed footwear after dusk
- Use DEET or picaridin-based repellents on skin
- Treat clothing and bed nets with permethrin
- Sleep under fine-mesh netting in endemic or high-risk areas
- Seal tents or structures tightly to prevent entry
- Avoid sitting or sleeping directly on sand or soil

Some sand flies are small enough to pass through standard mosquito netting, so fine mesh is necessary.

What To Do If Affected

- Wash the area with soap and water
- Apply antihistamines or topical steroids to reduce itching
- Monitor for signs of infection or persistent lesions
- If a non-healing sore develops weeks after exposure, especially in endemic regions, seek medical attention and testing for leishmaniasis
- Cutaneous forms are treated with antiparasitic drugs (e.g., miltefosine or amphotericin B), often requiring specialist care

Early diagnosis improves outcomes, especially in mucocutaneous or visceral leishmaniasis cases.

SAND FLY-BORNE DISEASES

Leishmaniasis

Pathogens: Order Kinetoplastida, Family Trypanosomatidae: *Leishmania mexicana, L. infantum*

Entomological Vectors: Order Diptera, Family Psychodidae: *Lutzomyia anthophora* **and** *L. diabolica*

Exposure and Severity Ratings (Figure 6.40)

- **Exposure Level: 1–2**
  - Most cases are introduced
  - Autochthonous cutaneous leishmaniasis rare (1), reported in isolated pockets in TZ, AZ, OK, and a few other southern states

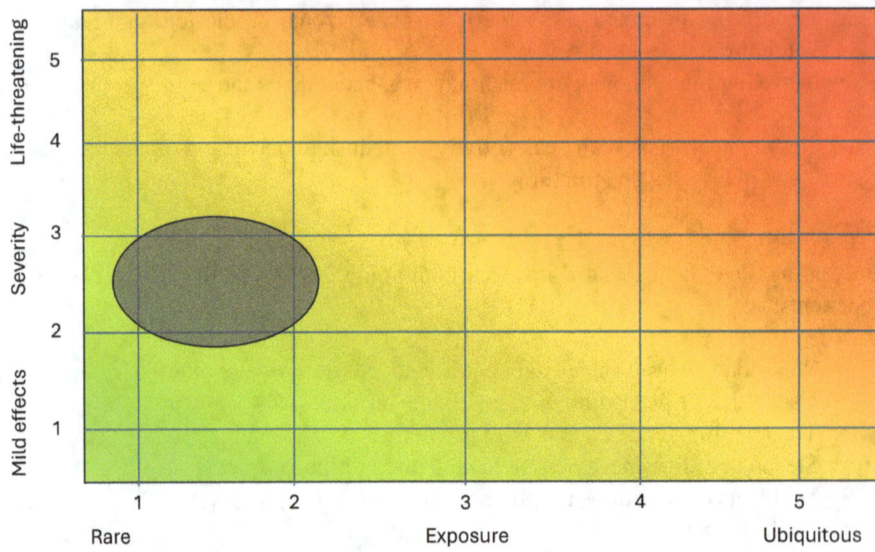

FIGURE 6.40 Leishmaniasis. Exposure × severity matrix.

- **Severity Level: 2–3**
  - Skin ulcers can be chronic but are usually self-limiting; mucocutaneous or visceral forms rare in the United States

References: McIlwee et al. (2018), Beasley et al. (2022)

Leishmaniasis is a parasitic disease caused by *Leishmania* protozoa and transmitted by the bite of infected female sand flies. In the United States, locally acquired cases of cutaneous leishmaniasis, typically caused by *L. mexicana*, have been reported in Texas and occasionally in Arizona and Oklahoma. Reservoir hosts include rodents (e.g., woodrats), and dogs may play a role in parasite maintenance.

Cutaneous leishmaniasis presents as chronic, painless skin ulcers, often at sites of insect bites. While mucocutaneous and visceral forms exist elsewhere (e.g., Latin America, Middle East), they are not endemic in North America. Most U.S. cases resolve spontaneously, though lesions can persist for months and result in disfigurement or secondary infection.

Symptoms

- Painless skin ulcers with raised edges
- Papules or nodules at the bite site that slowly enlarge
- Satellite lesions possible
- Systemic symptoms are rare in the U.S. form
- Scarring and secondary bacterial infection possible

REFERENCES

Acosta-España JD, Herrera-Yela A, Altamirano-Jara B, Bonilla-Aldana K, Rodriguez-Morales AJ. 2025. The epidemiology and clinical manifestations of anaplasmosis in humans: A systematic review of case reports. *J. Infect. Public Hlth.* 18: 102765.

Akhoundi M, Sereno D, Marteau A, Bruel C, Izri A. 2020. Who bites me? A tentative discriminative key to diagnose hematophagous ectoparasites biting using clinical manifestations. *Diagnostics* 10: 308.

Allerdice MEJ, Hecht JA, Lash RR, Karpathy SE, Paddock CD. 2019. *Rickettsia parkeri* and "Candidatus *Rickettsia andeanae*" in *Amblyomma maculatum* (Acari: Ixodidae) collected from the Atlanta metropolitan area, Georgia, United States. *Ticks Tick Borne Dis.* 10: 1066–1069.

Amanzougaghene N, Fenollar F, Raoult D, Mediannikov O. 2020. Where are we with human lice? A review of the current state of knowledge. *Front. Cell. Infect. Microbiol.* 9: 474.

Armstrong PM, Andreadis TG. 2022. Ecology and epidemiology of eastern equine encephalitis virus in the northeastern United States: An historical perspective. *J. Med. Entomol.* 59: 1–13.

Badiaga S, Brouqui P. 2012. Human louse-transmitted infectious diseases. *Clin. Microbiol. Infect.* 18: 332–337.

Beasley EA, Mahachi KG, Petersen CA. 2022. Possibility of *Leishmania* transmission via *Lutzomyia* spp. sand flies within the USA and implications for human and canine autochthonous infection. *Curr. Trop. Med. Rep.* 9: 160–168.

Borchers AT, Keen CL, Huntley AC, Gershwin ME. 2013. Lyme disease: A rigorous review of diagnostic criteria and treatment. *J. Autoimmun.* 57: 82–115.

Brault, AC, Savage HM, Duggal NK, Eisen RJ, Staples JE. 2018. Heartland virus epidemiology, vector association, and disease potential. *Viruses* 10: 498.

Campbell O, Krause PJ. 2020. The emergence of human Powassan virus infection in North America. *Ticks Tick Borne Dis.* 11: 101540.

Castelli E, Caputo V, Morello V, Tomasino RM. 2008. Local reactions to tick bites. *Am. J. Dermatopathol.* 30: 241–248.

Daily JP, Minuti A, Khan N. 2022. Diagnosis, treatment, and prevention of malaria in the US: A review. *JAMA.* 328: 460–471.

Darsie Jr RF, Ward RA. 2005. *Identification and Geographical Distribution of the Mosquitoes of North America, North of Mexico.* University Press of Florida, Gainesville, FL.

Dennis DT, Inglesby TV, Henderson DA, Bartlett JG, Ascher MS, Eitzen E, Fine AD, Friedlander AM, Hauer J, Layton M, Lillibridge SR, McDade JE, Osterholm MT, O'Toole T, Parker G, Perl TM, Russell PK, Tonat K. 2001. Tularemia as a biological weapon: Medical and public health management. *JAMA.* 285: 2763–2773.

Diaz A, Coffey LL, Burkett-Cadena N, Day JF. 2018. Reemergence of St. Louis encephalitis virus in the Americas. *Emerg. Infect. Dis.* 24: 2150–2157.

Duval P, Antonelli P, Aschan-Leygonie C, Moro CV. 2023. Impact of human activities on disease-spreading mosquitoes in urban areas. *J. Urban Health* 100: 591–611.

Edlow JA, McGillicuddy GC. 2008. Tick paralysis. *Infect. Dis. Clinics N.* Am. 22: 397–413.

Eisen RJ, Gage KL. 2012. Transmission of flea-borne zoonotic agents. *Ann. Rev. Entomol.* 57: 61–82.

Eisen RJ, Kugeler KJ, Eisen L, Beard CB, Paddock CD. 2017. Tick-borne zoonoses in the United States: Persistent and emerging threats to human health. *ILAR J.* 58: 319–335.

Foley J, López-Pérez AM, Álvarez-Hernández G, Labruna MB, Angerami RN, Zazueta OE, Bermudez S, Rubino F, Salzer JS, Brophy M, Pinter A, Paddock CD. 2025. A wolf at the door: The ecology, epidemiology, and emergence of community- and urban-level Rocky Mountain spotted fever in the Americas. *Am. J. Vet. Res.* https://doi.org/10.2460/ajvr.24.11.0368

Fu YT, Yao C, Deng YP, Elsheikha HM, Shao R, Zhu X-Q, Liu G-H. 2022. Human pediculosis, a global public health problem. *Infect. Dis. Poverty* 11: 58.

Garcia MN, O'Day S, Fisher-Hoch S, Gorchakov R, Patino R, Feria Arroyo TP, Laing ST, Lopez JE, Ingber A, Jones KM, Murray KO. 2016. One health interactions of chagas disease vectors, canid hosts, and human residents along the Texas-Mexico border. *PLoS Negl. Trop. Dis.* 10: e0005074.

Garcia MN, Woc-Colburn L, Aguilar D, Hotez PJ, Murray KO. 2015. Historical perspectives on the epidemiology of human chagas disease in Texas and recommendations for enhanced understanding of clinical chagas disease in the Southern United States. *PLOS Negl. Trop. Dis.* 9: e0003981.

Goddard J, Varela-Stokes AS. 2009. Role of the lone star tick, *Amblyomma americanum* (L.), in human and animal diseases. *Vet. Parasitol.* 160: 1–12.

Goldman T, Hamer DH. 2024. Current status of La Crosse virus in North America and potential for future spread. *Am. J. Trop. Med. Hyg.* 110: 850–855.

Griffith KS, Lewis LS, Mali S, Parise ME. 2007. Treatment of malaria in the United States: A systematic review. *JAMA.* 297: 2264–2277.

Gygax L, Schudel S, Kositz C, Kuenzli E, Neumayr A. 2025. Human monocytotropic ehrlichiosis: A systematic review and analysis of the literature. *PLoS Nglect. Trop. Dis.* https://doi.org/10.1371/journal.pntd.0012377

Haddad Jr V, Haddad MR, Santos M, Costa Cardosa JL. 2018. Skin manifestations of tick bites in humans. *An. Bras. Dermatol.* 93: 251–255.

Harris EK, Foy BD, Ebel GD. 2023. Colorado tick fever virus: A review of historical literature and research emphasis for a modern era. *J. Med. Entomol.* 60: 1214–1220.

Hassett EM, Thangamani S. 2021. Ecology of Powassan virus in the United States. *Microorganisms* 9: 2317.

Hughes HR, Kenney JL, Calvert AE. 2023. Cache Valley virus: An emerging arbovirus of public and veterinary health importance. *J. Med. Entomol.* 60: 1230–1241.

Inglesby TV, Dennis DT, Henderson DA, Bartlett JG, Ascher MS, Eitzen E, Fine AD, Friedlander AM, Hauer J, Koerner JF, Layton M, McDade J, Osterholm MT, O'Toole T, Parker G, Perl TM, Russell PK, Schoch-Spana M, Tonat K. 2000. Plague as a biological weapon: Medical and public health management. *JAMA.* 283: 2281–2290.

Jakab A, Kahlig P, Kuenzli E, Neumayr A. 2022. Tick borne relapsing fever: A systematic review and analysis of the literature. *PLoS Neglect. Trop. Dis.* 16: e0010212.

Klotz JH, Dorn PL, Logan JL, Stevens L, Pinnas JL, Schmidt JO, Klotz SA. 2010. "Kissing bugs": Potential disease vectors and cause of anaphylaxis. *Clin. Inf. Dis.* 50: 1629–1634.

Klotz SA, Dorn PL, Mosbacher M, Schmidt JO. 2014a. Kissing bugs in the United States: Risk for vector-borne disease in humans. *Environ. Hlth. Insights* 8(s2): 49–59.

Klotz SA, Schmidt JO, Dorn PL, Ivanyi C, Sullivan KR, Stevens L. 2014b. Free-roaming kissing bugs, vectors of chagas disease, feed often on humans in the Southwest. *Am. J. Med.* 127: 421–426.

Kugeler KJ, Staples JE, Hinckley AF, Gage KL, Mead PS. 2015. Epidemiology of human plague in the United States, 1900–2012. *Emerg. Inf. Dis.* 21: 16–22.

Lindsey NP, Staples JE, Fischer M. 2018. Eastern equine encephalitis virus in the United States, 2003–2016. *Am. J. Trop. Med. Hyg.* 98: 1472–1477.

Mantlo EK, Haley NJ. 2023. Heartland virus: An evolving story of an emerging zoonotic and vector-borne disease. *Zoonotic Dis.* 3: 188–202.

McIlwee BE, Weis SE, Hosler GA. 2018. Incidence of endemic human cutaneous leishmaniasis in the United States. *JAMA Dermatol.* 154: 1032–1039.

Mead, PS. 2015. Epidemiology of Lyme disease. *Infect. Dis. Clinics* 29: 187–210.

Moffitt JE, Venarske D, Goddard J, Yates AB, deShazo RD. 2003. Allergic reactions to *Triatoma* bites. *Ann. Allergy Asthma Immunol.* 91: 122–128.

Morshed MG, Drews SJ, Lee M-K, Fernando K, Mann S, Mak S, Simpson Y, Wong Q, Patrick D. 2017. Tick-borne relapsing fever in British Columbia: A ten-year review (2006–2015). *Brit. Columbia Med. J.* 59: 412–417.

Nelson CA, Winberg J, Bostic TD, Davis KM, Fleck-Derderian S. 2024. Systematic review: Clinical features, antimicrobial treatment, and outcomes of human tularemia, 1993–2023. *Clin. Infect. Dis.* 78: S15–S28.

Nicholson WI, Masters E, Wormser GP. 2009. Preliminary serologic investigation of '*Rickettsia amblyommii*' in the aetiology of Southern tick associated rash illness (STARI). *Clin. Microbiol. Infect.* 15: 235–236.

Ohl ME, Spach DH. 2000. *Bartonella quintana* and urban trench fever. *Clin. Inf. Dis.* 31: 131–135.

Ord RL, Lobo CA. 2015. Human babesiosis: Pathogens, prevalence, diagnosis, and treatment. *Curr. Clin. Micro. Rep.* 2: 173–181.

Pastula DM, Smith DE, Beckham JD, Tyler KL. 2016. Four emerging arboviral diseases in North America: Jamestown Canyon, Powassan, chikungunya, and Zika virus diseases. *J. Neurovirol.* 22: 257–260.

Petersen LR. 2019. Epidemiology of West Nile Virus in the United States: Implications for arbovirology and public health. *J. Med. Entomol.* 56: 1456–1462.

Peterson CJ, Mohankumar P, Tarbox JA, Nugent K. 2025. Alpha-gal syndrome: A review for the general internist. *Am. J. Med. Sci.* 369: 313–320.

Radolf JD, Strle K, Lemieux JE, Strle F. 2021. Lyme disease in humans. *Curr. Iss. Mol. Biol.* 42: 333–384.

Richardson M, Khouja C, Sutcliffe K. 2019. Interventions to prevent Lyme disease in humans: A systematic review. *Prevent. Med. Rep.* 13: 16–22.

Roe MK, Huffman ER, Batista YS, Papadeas GC, Kastelitz SR, Restivo AM, Stobart CC. 2023. Comprehensive review of emergence and virology of tickborne Bourbon Virus in the United States. *Emerg. Infect. Sis.* 29: 1–7.

Rousseau J, Castro A, Novo T, Maia C. 2022. *Dipylidium caninum* in the twenty-first century: Epidemiological studies and reported cases in companion animals and humans. *Parasites Vectors* 15: 131.

Schudel S, Gygax L, Kositz C, Kuenzli E, Neumayr A. 2024. Human granulocytotropic anaplasmosis: A systematic review and analysis of the literature. *PLoS Neglect. Trop. Dis.* 18: e0012313.

Simón F, Siles-Lucas M, Morchón R, González-Miguel J, Mellado I, Carretón E, Montoya-Alonso JA. 2012. Human and animal dirofilariasis: The emergence of a zoonotic mosaic. *Clin. Microbiol. Rev.* 25: 507–544.

Talagrand-Reboul E, Boyer PH, Bergström S, Vial L, Boulanger N. 2018. Relapsing fevers: Neglected tick-borne diseases. *Front. Cell. Infect. Microbiol.* 8: 98.

Tian Y, Durden C, Hamer GL. 2024. A scoping review of triatomine control for Chagas disease prevention: Current and developing tools in Latin America and the United States. *J. Med. Entomol.* 61: 1290–1308.

Tsioutis C, Zafeiri M, Avramopoulos A, Prousali E, Miligkos M, Karageorgos SA. 2017. Clinical and laboratory characteristics, epidemiology, and outcomes of murine typhus: A systematic review. *Acta Trop.* 166: 16–24.

Vahey GM, Lindsey NP, Staples JE, Hills SL. 2021. La Crosse virus disease in the United States, 2003–2019. *Am. J. Trop. Med. Hyg.* 105: 807–812.

Villeneuve C-A, Snyman J, Snyman LP, Gouin GG, Jenkins E, Martinez V, Hobman T, Kumar A, Dusfour I, Lecomte N, Leighton PA. 2025. Expanding knowledge of mosquito (Diptera: Culicidae) and California serogroup viruses distributions in the North America arctic. *J. Med. Entomol.* 62: 1590–1598.

Waked R, Krause PJ. 2022. Human babesiosis. *Infect. Dis. Clin.* 36: 655–670.

Werner SL, Banda BK, Burnsides CL, Stuber AJ. 2019. Zoonosis: Update on existing and emerging vector-borne illnesses in the USA. *Curr. Emerg. Hosp. Med. Rep.* 7: 91–106.

Yendell SJ, Fischer M, Staples JE. 2015. Colorado tick fever in the United States, 2002–2012. *Vector-Borne Zoonotic Dis.* 15: 311–316.

Yeni DK, Büyük F, Ashraf A, Salah ud Din Shah M. 2021. Tularemia: A re-emerging tick-borne infectious disease. *Folia Microbiol.* 66: 1–14.

7 Physical Irritants and Allergens

ARACHNIDS

HOUSE DUST MITES

Entomological Agent: Order Sarcoptiformes, Family Pyroglyphidae: *Dermatophagoides farinae* **(American house dust mite) (Figure 7.1)**
  Exposure and Severity Ratings (Figure 7.1)

- **Exposure Level: 5**
  - Pest is ubiquitous (5) indoors; nearly impossible to avoid in certain climates
- **Severity Level: 1**
  - Symptoms are allergic, not infectious; most individuals experience minimal (1) harm

Reference: Miller (2019)

House dust mites are microscopic arachnids that feed on organic material in household dust, particularly shed human and animal skin cells. Though harmless to most people, their shed body parts and fecal pellets are potent allergens and a major trigger for asthma, allergic rhinitis, and eczema.

Dermatophagoides farinae is especially prevalent east of the Mississippi River and along the Pacific Coast, where humidity levels support its reproduction. Though not parasitic or biting arthropods, these mites are still medically significant due to their contribution to chronic allergic conditions.

Symptoms

Exposure to house dust mites may lead to:

- Allergic rhinitis (sneezing, nasal congestion, runny nose)
- Asthma exacerbation (coughing, wheezing, shortness of breath)
- Itchy, red eyes
- Eczema flare-ups or skin irritation
- Scratching-induced secondary infections
- Rarely, severe allergic responses in hypersensitive individuals

Symptoms are generally chronic or recurrent, especially in settings with long-term indoor exposure.

DOI: 10.1201/9781003745709-9

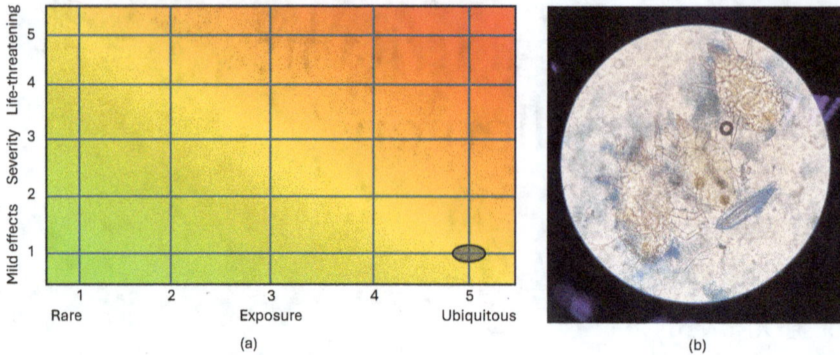

FIGURE 7.1 House dust mites. (a) Exposure × severity matrix; (b) house dust mite, *Dermatophagoides farina*.

Occupational Exposure

Ecology and environmental professionals may be exposed during:

- Lodging in hotels, dormitories, or bunkhouses, especially in humid regions
- Structure inspections of buildings, crawlspaces, or attics
- Monitoring in dust-laden indoor environments, including older homes or closed spaces
- Handling archived materials, fabrics, or carpets in poorly ventilated facilities

Exposure risk increases with extended time in dusty environments, especially without proper cleaning or filtration.

Prevention

To reduce risk:

- Enclose mattresses and pillows in dust-mite-proof covers during extended stays
- Wash bedding, towels, and clothing regularly in hot water (≥130°F)
- Avoid disturbing accumulated dust in old buildings or storage areas
- Use High-Efficiency Particulate Air (HEPA) filters or respirators when working in visibly dusty indoor environments
- Maintain clean, dry, and well-ventilated field accommodations when possible
- Choose lodging that uses hard flooring and washable bedding when available

Controlling environmental conditions (humidity, dust) is essential to limiting exposure.

What To Do If Affected

- Use over-the-counter antihistamines or decongestants to control mild allergy symptoms
- For asthma or eczema, follow prescribed maintenance medications

- Seek medical attention if symptoms are severe, persistent, or interfere with fieldwork
- Long-term exposure may require environmental allergen reduction strategies

Dust mite exposure is not dangerous for most individuals, but it can significantly impact productivity and comfort for allergic persons.

WHIP SCORPIONS/VINEGAROONS

Entomological Agents: Order Uropygi, Family Thelyphonidae: *Mastigoproctus giganteus*, plus about three additional species in southern Mexico (Figure 7.2)
    Exposure and Severity Ratings (Figure 7.2)

- **Exposure Level: 1**
    - Rare (1) but memorable when encountered
    - Limited to dry, rocky environments from southern CA east to central TX, western OK, south into Mexico
- **Severity Level: 1–2**
    - Most exposures result in minimal (1) harm unless sprayed with acetic acid, which may cause mild (2) irritation in the skin or eyes
    - May induce a moderate (2) psychological effect due to their large size

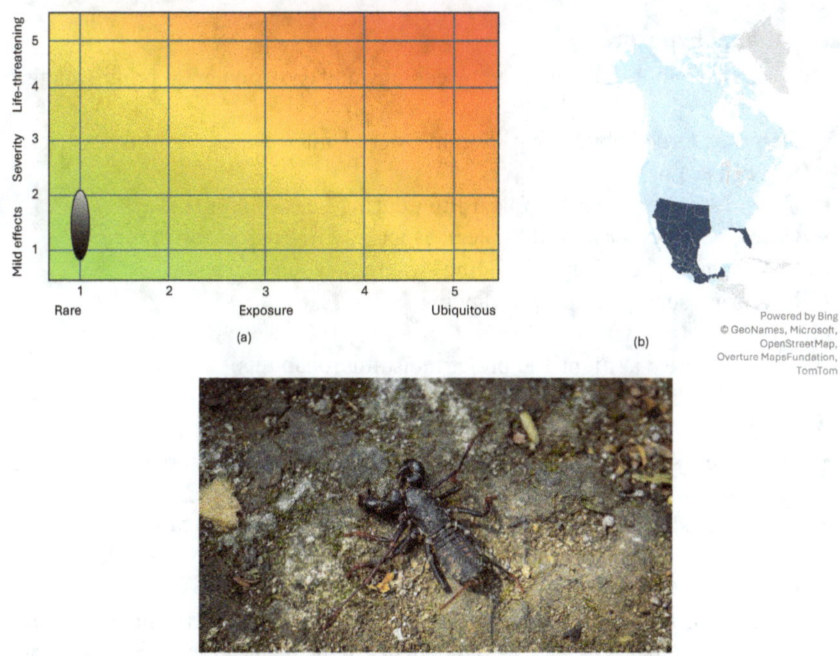

FIGURE 7.2 Whip scorpions. (a) Exposure × severity matrix; (b) geographic distribution; (c) giant vinegaroon, *Mastigoproctus giganteus*.

References: Smolinske et al. (2022), Castro-Pereira et al. (2025)

Whip scorpions, also called vinegaroons, are large (up to 85 mm/3.3 in.), nocturnal arachnids with a striking appearance: a flattened body, long pedipalps, and a thin whiplike tail that gives them their name. Whip scorpions are common in arid, sub-tropical, and tropical habitats, often hiding under rocks, logs, or leaf litter during the day and emerging at night to beneficially hunt small insects, spiders, scorpions, and sometimes mice. Despite their intimidating look, they are nearly harmless to humans – non-venomous, non-stinging, and generally non-aggressive.

Their primary defense is the ability to spray a concentrated solution of acetic acid (vinegar) and other chemicals from glands near the tail. This mist or spray is effective at repelling predators and can cause mild skin and mucous membrane irritation in humans.

Symptoms

- Skin exposure to spray:
  - Mild burning, tingling, or irritation
  - Temporary redness or discomfort
- Eye or mucous membrane exposure:
  - Stinging, tearing, or conjunctival redness if spray enters eyes or nose
  - Rare, short-lived discomfort; no permanent damage
- No bites or venom injection – they do not possess fangs or stingers

The most common "symptom" is startled overreaction due to their appearance.

Occupational Exposure

Whip scorpions may be encountered by ecology and environmental professionals in:

- Desert or scrub habitats (e.g., Southwestern United States, Central America, Southeast Asia)
- Under logs, stones, bark, or leaf litter during fieldwork or surveys
- Caves, burrows, or humid shelters, especially in tropical forest regions
- Field camps, sheds, or outbuildings where they may seek shelter
- Nocturnal surveys or pitfall trapping

They are most active at night and prefer moist microhabitats.

Prevention

- Wear gloves when handling logs, rocks, or ground cover in desert or tropical areas
- Do not handle whip scorpions directly, especially near the tail
- Avoid placing hands or face near disturbed individuals, as they may spray defensively
- Educate personnel that these creatures are harmless and beneficial predators
- Instruct field teams to relocate rather than kill them when found in work areas
- Keep camping and storage areas dry and elevated in high-density regions

Whip scorpions are non-aggressive and will retreat if given the chance.

What To Do If Affected

- If skin is affected:
  - Rinse with cool water and soap
  - Apply topical hydrocortisone or antihistamines if irritation persists
- If eyes are exposed:
  - Rinse with clean water or saline for at least 10–15 minutes
  - Seek medical attention if pain, blurred vision, or redness persists
- No treatment is needed for brief contact unless discomfort continues

Reassure affected individuals: the chemical is unpleasant but not harmful.

MYRIAPODA

MILLIPEDES

Entomological Agents: Class Diplopoda: particularly *Narceus*, *Orthoporus*, *Apheloria*, and related genera (Figure 7.3)
    Exposure and Severity Ratings (Figure 7.3)

- **Exposure Level: 2–3**
  - Uncommon (2) to moderately (3) common in moist, shaded, or litter-rich habitats
- **Severity Level: 1–3**
  - Chemical defenses may result in minimal (1) to mild (2) skin irritation/staining or moderate (3) irritation in eye exposures

References: Girardin and Steveson (2002), Júnior et al. (2025)

Millipedes are slow-moving, cylindrical arthropods with two pairs of legs per body segment, commonly found in leaf litter, soil, and decaying vegetation. Unlike centipedes, millipedes are not venomous and do not bite. Instead, when threatened, they may curl into a coil and secrete defensive chemicals, including benzoquinones, phenols, and cyanogenic compounds, depending on the species.

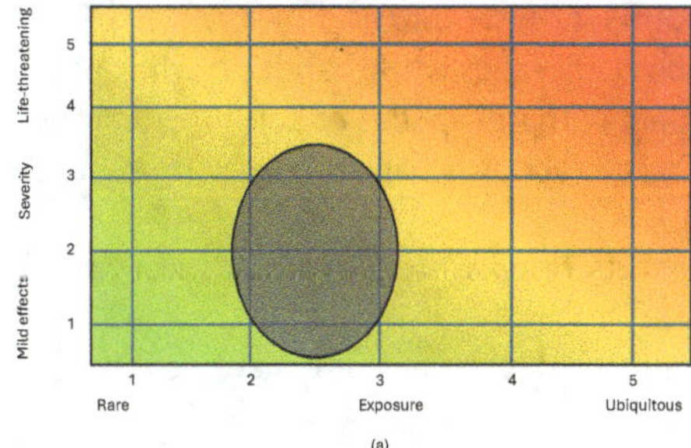

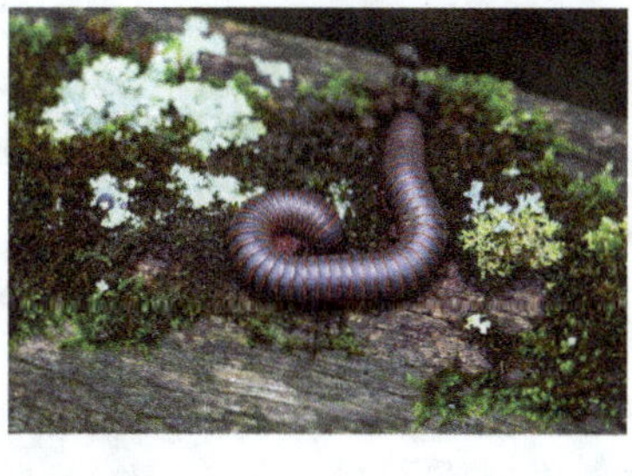

FIGURE 7.3 Millipedes. (a) Exposure × severity matrix; (b) American millipede, *Narceus americanus*.

These secretions can irritate thin skin areas and some may cause eye irritation, particularly in large tropical or Appalachian species. Some species may also produce foul odors or cause temporary staining of skin or clothing. Millipedes pose no serious medical risk, but their chemical defenses can interfere with fieldwork, handling, or laboratory use.

Millipedes are most active in moist environments and are especially common during rainy seasons or after soil disturbance.

Symptoms

- Skin exposure:
  - Redness, itching, or temporary staining (brownish/yellow discoloration)
  - Some secretions can cause chemical dermatitis or blistering in sensitive individuals, often in paired dots where legs touched skin surfaces
- Eye exposure:
  - Conjunctivitis, pain, tearing, or blurred vision if secretions are rubbed into the eye
- Mucous membranes:
  - Irritation of lips, nose, or mouth if contact occurs

Symptoms typically resolve within hours to a few days. There is no envenomation or systemic toxicity from contact with North American millipedes.

Occupational Exposure

Millipedes may be encountered by ecology and environmental professionals in:

- Soil sampling, leaf litter surveys, and restoration ecology
- Under logs, stones, mulch, or bark, especially in damp conditions
- Tents, labs, or cabins, especially during heavy rains or in high humidity
- Biodiversity assessments, where millipedes are collected by hand
- Agricultural or forestry work involving mulch, compost, or debris piles

They may inadvertently be handled or crushed, releasing defensive secretions.

Prevention

- Wear gloves when handling soil, debris, or litter fauna
- Avoid touching face, eyes, or mucous membranes while handling arthropods
- Wash hands immediately after contact with millipedes or soil invertebrates
- Educate workers on chemical defense reactions, particularly staining and eye risk
- Do not encourage handling for curiosity or classroom demonstration without caution
- Instruct workers to avoid smashing millipedes – squashing increases chemical exposure

Millipedes are ecologically beneficial decomposers and should not be killed unnecessarily.

What To Do If Affected

- For skin exposure:
  - Rinse with soap and cool water
  - Apply topical hydrocortisone or antihistamines if irritation persists
- For eye exposure:
  - Flush with clean water or sterile saline for 15 minutes
  - Seek medical evaluation if pain, redness, or blurred vision persists
- Staining will fade over time; do not use abrasives or solvents on skin

In rare cases of persistent dermatitis or blistering, medical attention may be warranted.

INSECTS

COCKROACHES

Entomological Agents: Order Blattodea, Families Blattidae: *Blatta orientalis* **(Oriental cockroach),** *Eurycotis floridana* **(Florida woods cockroach),** *Periplaneta americana* **(American cockroach),** *P. fuliginosa* **(smoky-brown cockroach), and other species; Family Ectobiidae:** *Blattella germanica* **(German cockroach),** *Supella longipalpa* **(brown-banded cockroach), and other genera (Figure 7.4)**

Exposure and Severity Ratings (Figure 7.4)

- **Exposure Level: 2–3**
  - Cockroaches of health and safety concern are widespread, with uncommon (2) to moderate (3) exposure throughout the built environment
  - Difficult to eliminate in some settings
- **Severity Level: 1–3**
  - Many exposures produce minimal (1) harm
  - Some mild (2) allergy or contact dermatitis can lead to moderate (3) asthma, especially with chronic exposure to heavy infestations

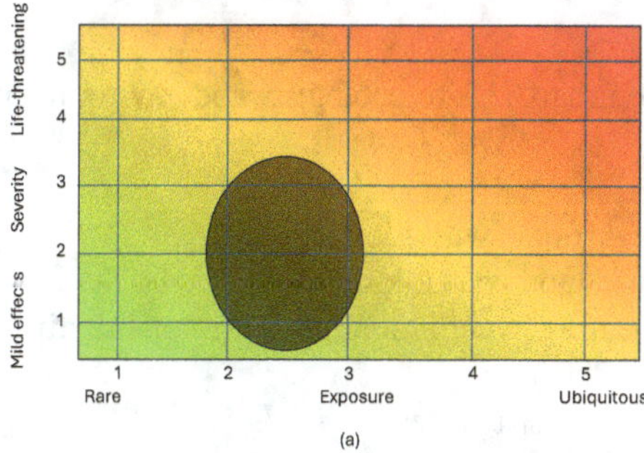

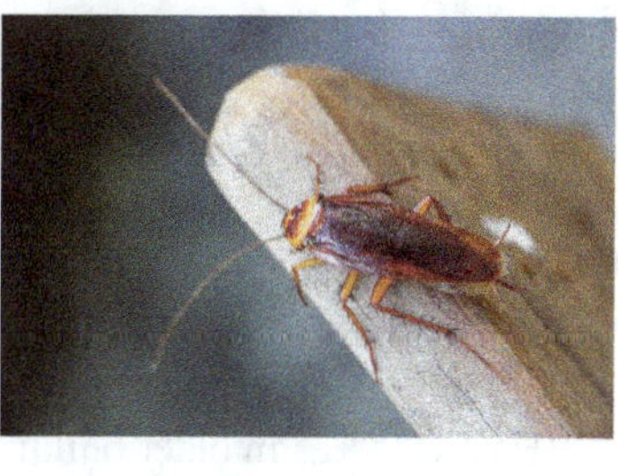

FIGURE 7.4 Cockroaches. (a) Exposure × severity matrix; (b) American cockroach, *Periplaneta americana*.

References: Arlina (2002), Do et al. (2015), Weihmann et al. (2015)

Cockroaches are ubiquitous scavengers found in human structures, animal facilities, and warm outdoor environments. Although they tend not to bite and cannot sting, they pose significant public and occupational health risks due to their role in triggering allergies and asthma and their capacity to mechanically transmit pathogens.

There are ~4,600 species of cockroaches globally, of which ~80 species are reported from North America. Most prefer outdoor habitats and shun human presence. Only a handful of species are of particular concern in occupational settings, including:

- German cockroach (*Blattella germanica*)
- American cockroach (*Periplaneta americana*)
- Smoky-brown cockroach (*Periplaneta fuliginosa*)
- Oriental cockroach (*Blatta orientalis*)
- Brown-banded cockroach (*Supella longipalpa*)

The Florida woods cockroach (*Eurycotis floridana*) has the ability to emit a foul-smelling noxious secretion, spraying it up to a distance of 1 m (3.3 ft). Primarily hexenal, hexenol, and hexenoic acid, the spray is not particularly medically harmful, although it can irritate eyes and mucous membranes.

Cockroach frass (droppings), exuviae (shed exoskeletons), and body secretions are highly allergenic. Infestations can also contaminate instruments, lab spaces, and stored goods, creating both sanitation and regulatory issues.

Symptoms

- Allergic rhinitis (sneezing, runny nose, congestion)
- Wheezing, coughing, and asthma attacks, particularly in sensitized individuals
- Skin rashes or eye irritation from airborne allergens
- Nausea or vomiting in cases of severe contamination (odor or visual presence)
- Risk of secondary bacterial infections from contaminated surfaces
- Minor irritation if Florida woods roach spray enters the eye

Cockroach allergens are persistent in indoor dust and can be hard to eliminate without thorough sanitation.

Occupational Exposure

Since most of the major pest species are urban, risk to ecologists and environmental professionals is highest in:

- Laboratories, classrooms, and breakrooms with food residues
- Animal facilities with bedding, feed, and warm, humid conditions
- Storage rooms, basements, or heating, ventilation, and air-conditioning (HVAC) areas in older buildings
- Urban field sites, sewers, or abandoned structures
- Food service areas and institutional kitchens
- Florida woods roaches can be encountered in leaf litter, bushes and shrubs, and palmettos

Cockroaches are nocturnal and often remain hidden, so infestations may go unnoticed until symptoms appear.

Prevention

To prevent infestation and allergen exposure:

- Implement integrated pest management (IPM) strategies
- Keep food sealed and workspaces clean of crumbs, spills, and residues
- Use sticky traps to monitor population presence
- Store paper goods and bedding in sealed containers
- Eliminate moisture and clutter, particularly around appliances or drains
- Seal cracks, baseboards, and access points to limit entry

For Florida woods cockroach exposure, use caution when moving leaf litter and other moist organic debris, wearing gloves, if necessary. Professional pest control may be needed for moderate to severe infestations in installations.

What To Do If Affected

- Clean and ventilate the area; vacuum with HEPA filtration
- Remove or relocate affected personnel, especially those with asthma
- Treat allergy symptoms with antihistamines or inhalers as prescribed
- Report the infestation to facility management or occupational health
- In severe cases, deep-clean the workspace and consider temporary relocation
- Rinse eyes and mucous membranes if secretions are encountered

Prompt intervention helps prevent sensitization and improves workplace safety.

Two-Striped Walkingstick

Entomological Agent: Order Phasmatodea, Family Pseudophasmatidae: *Anisomorpha buprestoides* **(Figure 7.5)**
  Exposure and Severity Ratings (Figure 7.5)

- **Exposure Level: 3**
  - Moderately (3) common in specific habitats in the southeastern United States (eastern Texas through the coastal states to NC, inland to OK, AR, and TN)
- **Severity Level: 1–3**
  - Skin exposure: mild (1) irritation
  - Eye or rare inhalation exposure: moderate (3) harm (potentially serious, temporarily disabling)

Reference: Brutlag et al. (2011)

The two-striped walkingstick is a large, diurnal phasmid native to the southeastern United States, especially common in Florida, Georgia, and coastal plains habitats. Adults are slender, up to 7.5 cm long, with parallel light stripes along a brown

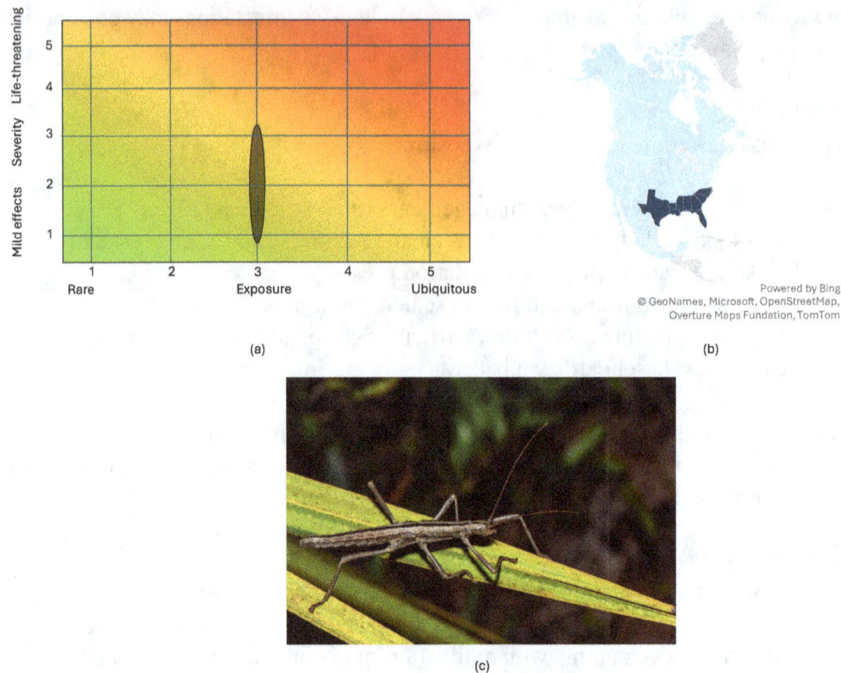

FIGURE 7.5 Two-stripe walkingstick. (a) Exposure × severity matrix; (b) geographic distribution; (c) two-stripe walkingstick, *Anisomorpha buprestoides.*

body. They are often found on shrubs, oaks, or palmettos and are most active in late summer to fall.

This species is notable for its chemical defense: when threatened, it can spray a milky secretion from thoracic glands that contains terpenoid compounds (including anisomorphal and dolichodial). This spray is highly irritating to the eyes and may cause temporary blindness, conjunctivitis, and intense burning. The spray can reach up to 30–40 cm (12–16 in.) and appears to be intentionally aimed toward the eyes of perceived predators, including humans.

While they are non-biting, non-venomous, and beneficial in the ecosystem, improper handling poses a significant eye safety risk.

Symptoms

- Ocular exposure:
  - Immediate stinging or burning sensation, excessive tearing, blurred vision, or temporary blindness
  - Conjunctival inflammation or corneal damage if not flushed quickly
- Skin exposure:
  - Mild burning, redness, or rash, especially on sensitive skin
- Inhalation or mucosal contact (rare):
  - Coughing, sneezing, or throat irritation

Ocular effects may last hours to several days, depending on exposure and treatment.

Occupational Exposure

Exposure risk to ecologists and environmental professionals is most likely in:

- Vegetation surveys in pine-oak scrub, coastal hammocks, or palmetto habitats
- Shrub or foliage disturbance, especially during late summer or fall
- Entomological fieldwork, sweep netting, or collection of herbivorous insects
- Educational or outreach activities, where individuals may handle walking-sticks unaware of the risk
- Backyard or residential landscaping in the southeastern United States

Walkingsticks are slow-moving and often spotted during daylight hours.

Prevention
- Do not handle and examine closely two-striped walkingsticks without eye protection
- Wear safety glasses or sunglasses when surveying vegetation in regions where they are common
- Train personnel to identify the species and understand its defensive capabilities
- Avoid placing face or eyes close to insects resting on foliage
- Do not crush or provoke; spraying is most likely when the insect feels cornered or grabbed
- Educate outreach personnel and students to observe, not handle

Proper identification is critical to avoid unnecessary panic or injury.

What To Do If Affected
- Eyes:
  - Immediately flush with copious water or saline for 15–20 minutes
  - Avoid rubbing the eyes
  - Seek medical evaluation, especially if pain, blurred vision, or redness persists
- Skin:
  - Wash thoroughly with soap and cool water
  - Apply topical hydrocortisone or antihistamines if irritation develops
- Mucous membranes:
  - Rinse with water and monitor for symptoms

Prompt decontamination typically resolves symptoms, but eye exposure requires medical attention.

BOMBARDIER BEETLES, FIERY SEARCHERS, BLISTER BEETLES, AND OTHER NOXIOUS BEETLES

Entomological Agents: Order Coleoptera, Family Carabidae: *Brachinus* spp. (bombardier beetles), *Calosoma scrutator* (fiery searcher), and similar species;

Family Meloidae: *Epicauta, Lytta,* **and** *Meloe* **species (blister beetles); Family Staphylinidae:** *Paederus* **spp. and a few other genera (rove beetles); Family Tenebrionidae:** *Eleodes* **spp. and several other genera (darkling beetles) (Figure 7.6)**

Exposure and Severity Ratings (Figure 7.6)

- **Exposure Level: 1–3**
  - Bombardier beetles rare (1) and localized; most often found under rocks or bark or in dry habitats
  - Other species uncommon (2) to moderate (3) exposure; localized risk during fieldwork in forests, deserts, weedy and agricultural fields, and disturbed habitats
- **Severity Level: 1–4**
  - Can cause mild (2) to moderate (3) harm due to brief but painful burning sensation on skin
  - Blister beetle effects on skin range from minimal (1) to moderately (3) painful skin lesions
  - Eye exposure causes moderate (3) harm and frequently requires medical treatment
  - Severe (4) systemic effects possible if blister beetles ingested (very rare in humans, unfortunately common in horses)
  - If sprayed, workers may experience mild (2) psychological effects
  - All effects tend to resolve over time

References: Haddad et al. (2012), Krinsky (2019), Villada et al. (2021)

Several North American beetles from several different families produce noxious chemical secretions as a defense mechanism. These species do not bite or sting, but may cause skin irritation, eye inflammation, or blistering reactions when disturbed or handled.

Bombardier beetles (Carabidae: *Brachinus* spp.) are a remarkable group of ground beetles that inhabit dry, sandy areas, under rocks, or in debris, often overlooked during field activity. They defend themselves by explosively ejecting boiling hot (>100°C) chemicals from their abdomen. The discharge is typically a mix of hydroquinones, enzymes, and hydrogen peroxide and is expelled with audible popping

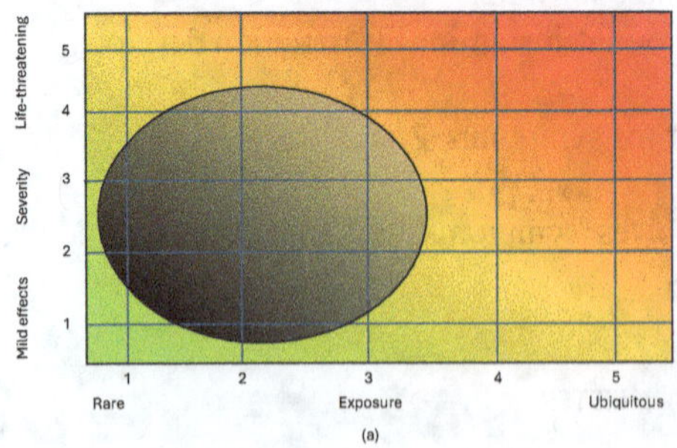

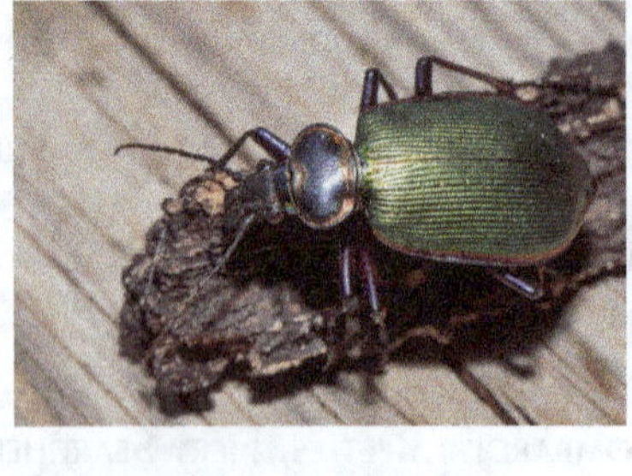

FIGURE 7.6 Noxious beetles. (a) Exposure × severity matrix; (b) fiery searcher, *Calosoma scrutator*.

that can burn or irritate human skin and eyes if contact occurs. The defensive spray is highly targeted but may ricochet off surfaces. Though these beetles are small (~1 cm), the chemical reaction can surprise and alarm field workers, especially if beetles are unknowingly handled.

The fiery searcher, *Calosoma scrutator*, and some other large ground beetles in the family Carabidae can produce a weak spray of pungent compounds such as formic acid and aldehydes from abdominal glands. While generally harmless, direct contact may cause burning or staining of the skin and mucous membranes.

Blister beetles (family Meloidae) are soft-bodied, elongate beetles found in fields, grasslands, and disturbed areas, often on flowers. They do not bite or sting, but when threatened or crushed, they exude a defensive compound called cantharidin, a potent blistering agent that can cause severe skin irritation and, if ingested, toxicity in humans and livestock. Cantharidin itself is odorless and colorless, sometimes making exposure difficult to detect until after symptoms develop, although several species include dark exudates that stain skin. Because of its blistering properties, medical doctors use cantharidin to treat warts and molluscum contagiosum. *Epicauta* species are particularly notorious in North America for contaminating alfalfa hay, leading to fatal poisoning in horses and other animals.

Paederus beetles, small and elongate with a metallic or reddish thorax, are medically significant. When crushed against the skin, they release pederin, a potent vesicant. Contact with this toxin causes a delayed blistering reaction known as Paederus dermatitis, often appearing as linear or streaky lesions.

Eleodes beetles are common in arid and semi-arid regions of the western United States. Sometimes called pinacate beetles, desert stink beetles, or headstand beetles, they perform a distinctive "headstand" before releasing strong-smelling quinones from abdominal glands. These chemicals can stain skin and cause eye or nasal irritation if aerosolized in close quarters.

Symptoms

Symptoms vary by species but may include:

- Burning or tingling sensations on skin lasting minutes (bombardier beetles, fiery searchers) to hours (blister beetles)
- Discoloration, redness, or localized rash at contact site
- Blister formation (vesicles or bullae) within 12–24 hours, especially if blister beetles or *Paederus* are crushed against the skin
- Eye irritation, conjunctivitis, or mucous membrane irritation if contact occurs near face or if transferred by touch
- Mild respiratory irritation (rare, with *Eleodes*)
- If ingested (e.g., contaminated food or water):
  - Oral and gastrointestinal ulceration
  - Abdominal pain, bloody urine, or kidney failure (in severe cases)

Blister reactions are localized but can be severe, especially on thin skin or if ingested. With the exception of internal exposure leading to systemic pathology, lesions are typically self-limited but may persist for several days to over a week.

Occupational Exposure

Risk to ecologists and environmental professionals increases when:

- Conducting fieldwork in woodlands, desert scrub, or disturbed soils
- Working at night or turning over logs, stones, or debris (ground beetle hiding sites)
- Handling insects or sweep netting in areas with high beetle density, such as weedy fields
- Sleeping outdoors or in unscreened buildings where *Paederus* may be drawn to light
- Low-light field conditions where beetles may be mishandled
- Conducting vegetation surveys or agricultural fieldwork, especially among flowering plants or in hayfields
- Working in pastures, roadsides, or recently burned areas where beetles aggregate
- Collecting insects for educational, research, or ecological surveys
- Feeding livestock with hay baled from infested fields

Unintentional crushing of beetles against the skin is the most common route of exposure.

Prevention

To minimize risk of exposure to noxious beetles:

- Wear long sleeves, pants, and gloves during field activities
- Avoid bare-handed collection of unknown beetles; use forceps or collection vials
- Do not crush beetles against the skin; gently flick or brush them away
- Use yellow or sodium vapor lights at night to avoid attracting *Paederus*
- Train field personnel to recognize color patterns
  - Bombardier beetles are <1cm long, have a dark body, reddish head or legs
  - Blister beetles range from 1 to 3cm, are typically narrow and soft-bodied, with a pronounced neck
  - Fiery searchers are 2–3cm in length, with iridescent red/green/gold coloration
- In agricultural settings:
  - Monitor hay crops for beetle infestations before harvesting
  - Avoid crimping hay if beetles are present to prevent crushing and toxin spread

Awareness of beetle behavior and appearance reduces accidental contact.

What To Do If Affected
- Immediately wash affected skin with soap and water
- Do not scrub or rub exposed area – this can spread vesicants
- Avoid touching face, eyes, or other sensitive areas

- Apply cool compresses and, if needed, topical corticosteroids for inflammation
- For extensive blistering, ocular exposure, or ingestion, seek medical care promptly
- Irrigating the eyes with sterile saline or water is essential if contact occurs
- Do not pop blisters; apply cool compresses and topical corticosteroids if needed

Prompt decontamination and symptomatic treatment are effective in most cases.

MEALWORMS AND OTHER GRAIN BEETLES, CARPET BEETLES, AND OTHER DERMESTIDS

Entomological Agents: Order Coleoptera, Family Tenebrionidae: *Tenebrio molitor* **(mealworm),** *Tribolium castaneum* **(red flour beetle),** *T. confusum* **(confused flour beetle),** *Zophobas morio* **(superworm); Family Curculionidae:** *Sitophilus granarius* **(grain weevil); Family Dermestidae:** *Dermestes lardarius* **(larder beetle) and others,** *Attagenus, Anthrenus,* **and related genera (Figure 7.7)**

Exposure and Severity Ratings (Figure 7.7)

- **Exposure Level: 1–4**
  - Rare (1) to uncommon (2) in natural settings
  - Moderate (3) to frequent (4) in enclosed locations with dried biological materials, such as closets (furs, wools), dried grain or meat products, and museums
  - Dermestids may be frequent (4) on old, dried carrion
  - Frequent (4) in animal care, teaching, and, unfortunately, museum environments; preventable with good lab colony hygiene
- **Severity Level: 1–2**
  - Most exposures result in minimal (1) harm
  - Allergic reactions (dermatitis, respiratory irritation) may be mild (2) depending on chronic exposure and sensitization; asthma may also be triggered

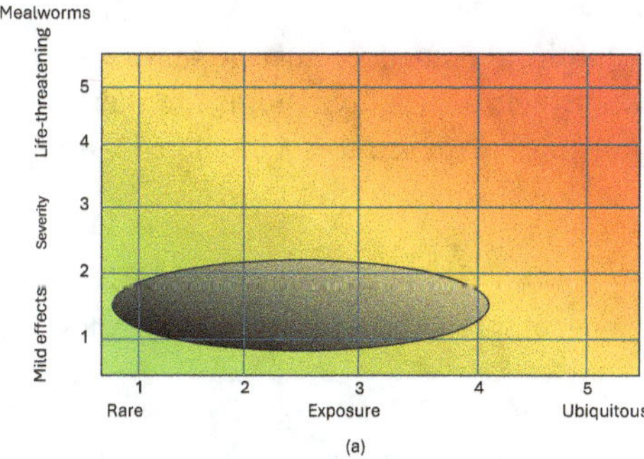

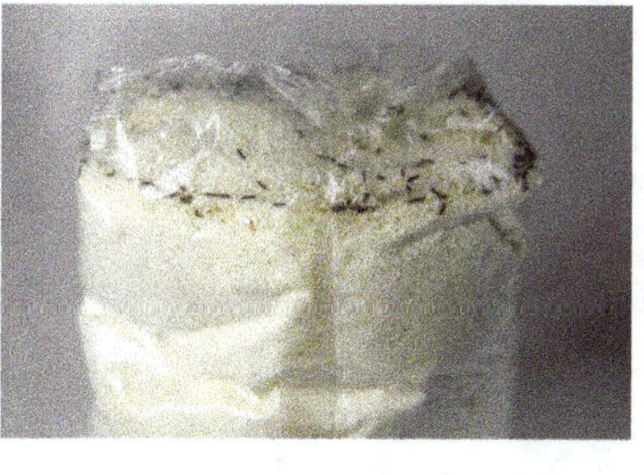

FIGURE 7.7   Mealworms, grain beetles, and dermestid beetles. (a) Exposure × severity matrix; (b) confused flour beetle, *Tribolium confusum.*

References: Arlina (2002), Lunn (1966), Ruzzier et al. (2020)

Mealworms (*Tenebrio molitor*) and superworms (*Zophobas morio*) are widely used in research, pet food, animal feed, and education. These beetles and the *Tribolium* spp. are rarely encountered outdoors; instead, they thrive in stored grain products and animal bedding, and infestations may arise in entomology labs, animal rooms, or feed storage. They can easily penetrate paper-wrapped grain products, such as flour or meal. While these beetles and their larvae are not harmful by bite or sting, they can cause allergic sensitization through prolonged contact or inhalation of shed exoskeleton fragments, frass (feces), and body hairs. Repeated exposure can lead to respiratory symptoms, contact dermatitis, and in sensitized individuals, occupational asthma; allergy attributed to the grain weevil, *Sitophilus granarius*, is called "millworker's asthma."

Dermestid beetles, commonly known as carpet beetles, hide beetles, or larder beetles, are scavengers that feed on dried animal material, including skin, feathers, fur, dead insects, and preserved specimens. While they are extremely useful in museum settings for cleaning bones and skeletons and can be used as forensic indicators, they can also become occupational pests in entomology labs, taxidermy shops, natural history collections, and animal housing facilities.

The larvae of most dermestids and a few other grain beetles are covered in bristly, detachable hairs, called "hastisetae," which are responsible for most health-related concerns. Contact with these hastisetae can cause dermatitis or allergic respiratory reactions, especially with chronic exposure in enclosed spaces. Larvae and adults of both groups are hearty scavengers, able to survive in a range of conditions, and their presence may go unnoticed until allergenic symptoms appear.

Symptoms

- Sneezing, nasal congestion, watery eyes, especially during cleaning
- Asthma-like symptoms (coughing, wheezing, shortness of breath)
- Itchy rash or contact dermatitis, typically on arms or hands
- Irritated eyes and throat, particularly in enclosed, dusty spaces, due to airborne larval hairs
- Symptoms may intensify over time with continued exposure
- Dermatitis that may be mistaken for bed bug bites or flea bites
- Rarely, secondary skin infection from scratching

Symptoms are not caused by bites, but by physical contact or allergic sensitization to the insects, detached hastisetae, exuviae, or their debris. Symptoms are more common in workers with frequent handling or those exposed to accumulated frass and shed skins.

Occupational Exposure

Mealworms are commonly encountered by ecologists and environmental professionals in:

- Animal care facilities, especially those that house reptiles, birds, or amphibians
- Entomology and biology teaching labs using live insects for instruction
- Research colonies maintaining beetles as feeder insects

- Feed mills or storage facilities where contamination of grain or feed occurs
- Breeding operations for pet stores or zoos

Carpet beetles and other dermestids are encountered by ecologists and environmental professionals in:

- Outdoor settings, where carrion has entered a dried remains stage of decomposition
- Entomology labs that store insect collections or rearing colonies
- Natural history museums using dermestid colonies for skeleton cleaning
- Taxidermy and forensic science settings
- Rodent or insect colonies, where dried food, bedding, or corpses attract dermestids
- Stored product facilities (e.g., animal feed, grain, leather goods)

Beetles may also escape from improperly sealed containers and infest surrounding environments. Contamination can also occur via infested specimens, boxes, or insulation brought into workspaces.

Prevention

To minimize exposure:

- Use sealed containers for food products
- Avoid open storage of dried animal materials
- Clean animal cages and containers frequently, disposing of frass and old bedding
- Install ventilation systems with HEPA filtration in colony rooms
- Wear gloves, long sleeves, and dust masks or respirators when handling infested materials or large numbers of beetles
- Wash hands and exposed skin after handling beetles or larvae
- Monitor and contain dermestid colonies with sealed enclosures and strict hygiene protocols
- Freeze or heat-treat newly acquired specimens to prevent introduction of larvae

Routine sanitation and stringent colony management and housekeeping protocols reduce both allergen buildup and infestation risk. Many natural history museums use small amounts of naphthalene or paradichlorobenzene ("moth balls") to deter these pests in collections; use of these products should be monitored carefully as they are considered by the U.S. Environmental Protection Agency (EPA) to be possibly carcinogenic.

What To Do If Affected

- Remove yourself from exposure and wash skin thoroughly
- Remove and clean infested clothing or gear, and vacuum workspaces thoroughly
- Treat mild dermatitis with topical corticosteroids or antihistamines

- For respiratory symptoms, use bronchodilators or corticosteroid inhalers as prescribed by medical authorities
- Seek occupational health evaluation if symptoms are recurrent or severe
- Consider transferring duties or modifying workspace if sensitization develops
- Infested food should be disposed of properly; infested natural history specimens can be heat treated to >75°C for 30 minutes or frozen for at least 96 hours (twice, about a week apart) to decontaminate

Long-term sensitization may necessitate relocation of dermestid colonies (if this is the source) or the worker from the exposure source.

URTICATING CATERPILLARS

Entomological Agents: Order Lepidoptera, Family Limacodidae: *Acharia stimulea* (saddleback caterpillar) and others; Family Megalopygidae: *Megalopyge*; Family Saturniidae (subfamily Hemileucinae): *Automeris*, *Hylesia*; some members of the Families Lasiocampidae, Notodontidae, and Nymphalidae (Figure 7.8)

Exposure and Severity Ratings (Figure 7.8)

- **Exposure Level: 1–2**
  - Rare (1) in most contexts; uncommon (2) in certain natural areas
  - Localized but notable in wooded or tropical areas, especially during larval season
- **Severity Level: 2–3**
  - Typically mild (2) irritation; can be moderate (3) if continuous/chronic exposure or exposed on or near mucous membranes
  - The most serious species do not occur in North America

References: Diaz (2005), Hossler (2010), Battisti et al. (2011), Haddad et al. (2012)

While most caterpillars are medically harmless, some species possess defensive hairs, spines, or venom glands that can cause dermatitis, burning pain, or systemic symptoms. These urticating caterpillars pose particular concern to field biologists, agricultural workers, forestry crews, and others working in vegetated or wooded areas.

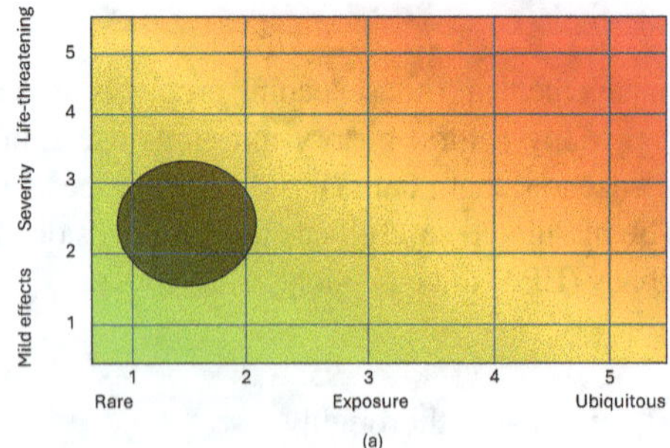

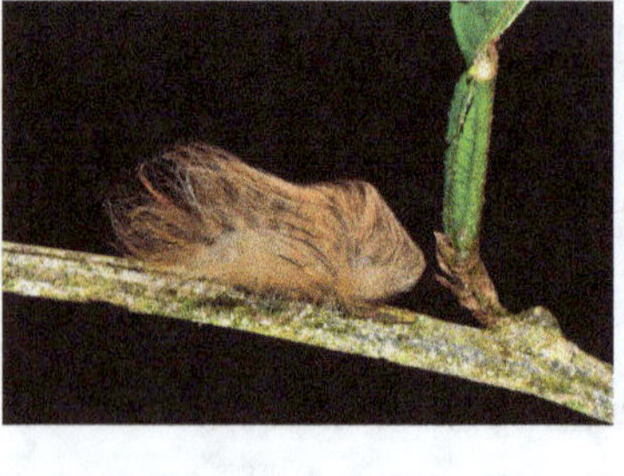

FIGURE 7.8 Urticating caterpillars. (a) Exposure×severity matrix; (b) flannel moth, *Megalopyge opercularis*.

In North America, only about a dozen of the 14,000 or so species of butterflies and moths have urticating hairs. The severity of symptoms depends on species, region, and degree of exposure. Some caterpillars (e.g., *Megalopyge opercularis*, the "asp" or "puss caterpillar") can cause intense localized pain, while others (e.g., *Lonomia* spp. in South America) are capable of inducing systemic coagulopathy and internal bleeding – a medical emergency.

In a few species, urticating hairs can also become airborne, leading to eye and respiratory irritation without direct contact.

Symptoms

Depending on the species and exposure, symptoms may include:

- Burning or stinging pain, often described as intense or radiating
- Redness, swelling, hives, or blistering at the contact site
- Numbness, nausea, headache, or lymph node tenderness
- Eye irritation or conjunctivitis from airborne hairs
- In rare cases (e.g., *Lonomia*), bleeding disorders, shock, or death

Most of the 11 North American species of caterpillars that have urticating hairs cause painful but self-limiting dermal reactions.

Occupational Exposure

High-risk situations for ecologists and environmental professionals include:

- Forestry and brush-clearing in warm months
- Tree pruning or vegetation sampling in deciduous forests
- Wildlife trapping and handling, especially where caterpillars may hide under leaves or bark
- Working near oak, elm, or citrus trees, which support many urticating species
- Accidentally brushing against foliage, logs, or equipment with resting larvae

Exposure is most likely during spring through fall, when larvae are active.

Prevention

To minimize exposure:

- Wear long sleeves, pants, and gloves when working around dense foliage
- Avoid handling caterpillars or brushing against tree trunks and leaves
- Train field crews to identify high-risk species, especially *Acharia*, *Megalopyge*, *Automeris*, and *Hylesia*
- Use safety goggles or face shields when operating under canopies in infested areas
- Avoid drying clothing or sleeping gear outdoors in outbreak zones

When caterpillars are encountered in quantity, postpone work or cordon off infested trees.

What To Do If Affected

- Do not rub or scratch the affected area
- Remove spines with adhesive tape, applied and peeled repeatedly
- Wash area with soap and water
- Apply cold compresses, oral antihistamines, or topical steroids
- For systemic symptoms (e.g., nausea, dizziness, abnormal bleeding), seek medical attention immediately
- If hairs contact eyes or mucous membranes, flush thoroughly and consult a health care provider

Most cases resolve within a few days, but some reactions may intensify over time if hairs remain embedded in clothing.

ADULT BUTTERFLIES AND MOTHS, CADDISFLIES

Entomological Agents: Orders Lepidoptera and Trichoptera (Figure 7.9)
   Exposure and Severity Ratings (Figure 7.9)

- **Exposure Level: 2–4**
  - May be uncommon (2) in most natural settings, flowering fields during the day and lights at night may increase exposure to frequent (4) for butterflies and moths
  - Localized, but high-density emergence of caddisflies from large water bodies may occur in season
- **Severity Level: 1–2**
  - A typical exposure is minimal (1) or less
  - If moth densities are high (such as around lights at night), abraded scales or hairs may be mildly (2) irritating

References: Henson (1966), Arlina (2002), Hossler (2010), Haddad et al. (2012), Dublon and Sumpter (2014)

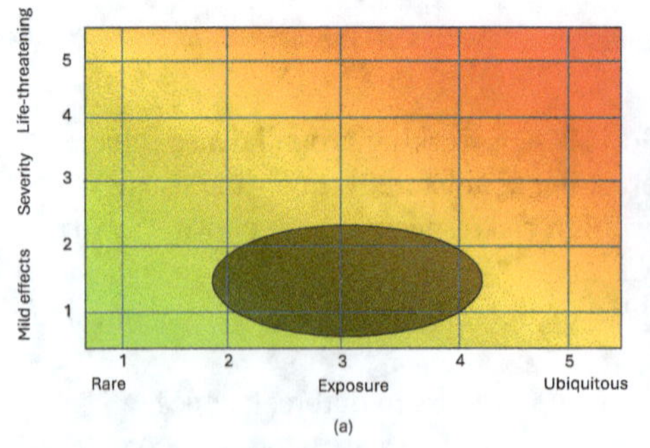

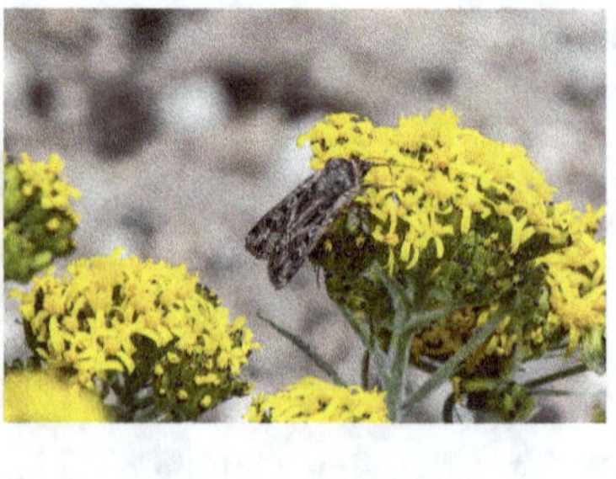

FIGURE 7.9 Adult butterflies and moths, caddisflies. (a) Exposure×severity matrix; (b) army cutworm moth, *Euxoa auxiliaris*.

While some caterpillars are typically of primary concern for causing dermatological reactions, adult moths (and a few butterflies) can also pose health hazards. In particular, the loose scales and defensive secretions of certain species can trigger allergic responses, respiratory irritation, and contact dermatitis. In some cases, scales from adult moths may become airborne and settle on exposed skin, eyes, or mucous membranes, resulting in irritation even without direct handling.

The physical irritation caused by adult Lepidoptera is much less severe than that caused by larvae with urticating hairs, but it can still disrupt work in forested environments. Populations of moths may aggregate in large numbers around lights, on structures, or near field camps. During outbreaks, airborne hairs or scales can infiltrate clothing, bedding, or ventilation systems, affecting both indoor and outdoor personnel.

Caddisflies are aquatic insects that appear very similar to moths, characterized by hairy wings, long antennae, and aquatic larvae that build protective cases. As larvae, they are indicators of clean freshwater ecosystems and play a key role in nutrient cycling.

However, adult caddisflies may emerge synchronously and in large numbers, particularly near large lakes and rivers, causing significant nuisance and operational hazards. Though they do not bite or sting, their presence can overwhelm lighting systems, obstruct visibility, and trigger allergies in sensitive individuals. Caddisfly emergences are often nighttime events, with swarms drawn to artificial light sources. In some regions, especially around hydroelectric dams, bridges, and riparian corridors, the volume of insects can be substantial. Operational hazards due to caddisflies are discussed in Chapter 9.

Symptoms

Symptoms vary by species and exposure type, but may include:

- Itching, rash, or red blotches on exposed skin
- Eye irritation, tearing, or conjunctivitis
- Sneezing, nasal congestion, or respiratory discomfort
- Dermatitis from contact with clothing contaminated with moth scales or hairs

While these symptoms are usually mild and self-limiting, individuals with preexisting allergies or asthma may experience more pronounced reactions.

Occupational Exposure

Exposure to adult Lepidoptera and Trichoptera is more likely under the following conditions:

- Nighttime field operations near lights and/or riparian zones during emergence periods
- Construction or road activity at night where illumination is provided by high-output halide or mercury vapor lights, especially near aquatic habitats
- Work in forests or orchards where adult moth species are active

- Night operations in wetland or streamside environments
- Handling equipment, tents, or laundry that has been left outdoors in infested areas
- Entering poorly sealed buildings or structures with moth infestations

Outbreaks may be seasonal or cyclical, depending on climate and species.

Prevention

To reduce risk of exposure:

- Avoid direct contact with adult moths, especially hairy-bodied species
- Use insect netting or fine mesh around sleeping quarters and ventilation in infested areas
- Wear long sleeves and gloves when handling equipment left outdoors
- Avoid bright outdoor lights near sleeping areas, or use yellow "bug-safe" lighting
- Launder and store clothing in sealed containers when not in use
- Educate field teams about the risks of moths during outbreak periods

What To Do If Affected

- Rinse affected skin or eyes gently with clean water
- Use adhesive tape to remove any visible scales or hairs
- Apply topical antihistamines or hydrocortisone creams for rash or itching; oral antihistamines for more generalized symptoms
- Seek medical care if respiratory symptoms worsen, or if eye symptoms do not resolve
- Avoid scratching or rubbing the area

Most reactions subside within 24–72 hours.

REFERENCES

Arlina A. 2002. Arthropod allergens and human health. *Ann. Rev. Entomol.* 47: 395–433.

Battisti A, Holm G, Fagrell B, Larsson S. 2011. Urticating hairs in arthropods: Their nature and medical significance. *Ann. Rev. Entomol.* 56: 203–220.

Brutlag AG, Hovda LR, Della Ripa MA. 2011. Corneal ulceration in a dog following exposure to the defensive spray of a walkingstick insect (*Anisomorpha* spp.). *J. Vet. Emerg. Crit. Care* 21: 382–386.

Castro-Pereira D, Pinto-da-Rocha R, Prendini L. 2025. *Mastigoproctus spinifemoratus*, a new species of giant vinegaroon (Thelyphonida: Thelyphonidae) from Mexico. *Arthropoda* 3: 2.

Diaz JH. 2005. The evolving global epidemiology, syndromic classification, management, and prevention of caterpillar envenoming. *Am. J. Trop. Med. Hyg.* 72: 347–357.

Do DC, Zhao Y, Gao P. 2015. Cockroach allergen exposure and risk of asthma. *Allergy* 71: 463–474.

Dublon IAN, Sumpter DJT. 2014. Flying insect swarms. *Curr. Biol.* 24: R828–R830.

Girardin BW, Steveson S. 2002. Millipedes: Health consequences. *J. Emerg. Nurs.* 28: 107–110.

Haddad V, Costa Cardoso JL, Lupi O, Tyring SK. 2012. Tropical dermatology: Venomous arthropods and human skin: Part I. Insecta. *J. Am. Acad. Dermatol.* 67: 331.e1–331.e14.

Henson EB. 1966. Aquatic insects as inhalant allergens: A review of American Literature. *Ohio J. Sci.* 66: 529–532.

Hossler EW. 2010. Caterpillars and moths: Part I. Dermatologic manifestations of encounters with Lepidoptera. *J. Am. Acad. Dermatol.* 62: 1–10.

Júnior VH, Haddad AMV, Barreiros JB. 2025. Myriapods (Diplopoda and Chilopoda): Medical aspects of envenomations. *J. Braz. Soc. Trop. Med.* 58: e00300–2025.

Krinsky WL 2019. Beetles (Coleoptera). Ch. 9 in: Mullen GR, Durden LA (eds.) *Medical and Veterinary Entomology*. Academic Press, Cambridge, MA.

Lunn JA. 1966. Millworkers' asthma: Allergic responses to the grain weevil (*Sitophilus granarius*). *Brit. J. Industr. Med.* 23: 149–152.

Miller JD. 2019. The role of dust mites in allergy. *Clinic. Rev. Allerg. Immunol.* 57: 312–329.

Ruzzier E, Kadej M, Battisti A. 2020. Occurrence, ecological function and medical importance of dermestid beetle hastisetae. *PeerJ.* 8: e8340.

Smolinske SC, Seifert SA, Warrick BW, Tadfor Y. 2022. Vinegaroon exposures reported to a poison center. *Toxicon* 219: e106928.

Villada JR, Panos MI, Del Cerro I, Granados JM. 2021. Ocular injury caused by the bombardier beetle. *Case Rep. Ophthalmol.* 12: 629–633.

Weihmann T, Reinhardt L, Weißing K, Siebert T, Wipfler B. 2015. Fast and powerful: Biomechanics and bite forces of the mandibles in the American Cockroach *Periplaneta americana*. *PLoS One* 10: e0141226.

Potentially Pathogenic Non-Biting Contact Hazards

INSECTS

Gastrointestinal Diseases Mechanically Spread by Arthropods

Filth flies, particularly house flies (*Musca domestica*) and oriental latrine flies (*Chrysomya megacephala*), are notorious vectors of gastrointestinal pathogens. Although they do not transmit these organisms biologically like mosquitoes or ticks, their role in mechanical transmission makes them a serious public health concern, especially in settings with inadequate sanitation. These flies frequently land on feces, garbage, and decaying organic matter where they pick up bacteria, protozoa, and helminth eggs on their body surfaces, mouthparts, and in their digestive tracts. When they subsequently land on human food, eating utensils, or open wounds, they can deposit these pathogens through regurgitation, defecation, or simply by physical contact.

A wide range of bacterial pathogens have been associated with filth flies, including *Escherichia coli, Salmonella* spp., *Shigella* spp., and *Campylobacter jejuni.* These bacteria can cause anything from mild gastrointestinal discomfort to severe and even life-threatening illnesses, especially in vulnerable populations such as children, the elderly, or the immunocompromised. Outbreaks of bacterial gastroenteritis in urban and rural areas alike have implicated house flies as key contributors to disease spread, particularly where hygiene infrastructure is compromised.

In addition to bacteria, protozoan parasites such as *Entamoeba histolytica, Giardia duodenalis, Cryptosporidium parvum*, and *Cyclospora cayetanensis* can also be mechanically transmitted by flies. These protozoa are typically passed in feces and persist in the environment as hardy cysts or oocysts, which flies can easily carry to human food sources. Ingesting these contaminated materials can lead to significant gastrointestinal distress, including diarrhea, dysentery, and chronic malabsorption syndromes. These parasites are especially problematic in developing regions but can also pose risks in industrialized nations through contaminated produce or poor sanitation.

Filth flies are also known to transmit helminth eggs, especially those of intestinal nematodes and cestodes. Species such as *Ascaris lumbricoides, Trichuris trichiura,* and *Hymenolepis nana* can have their infective stages transferred via flies. These eggs may adhere to the exoskeleton or be ingested and later excreted by the flies. In regions where open defecation is practiced or sewage systems are insufficient, the potential for widespread helminth transmission via flies increases dramatically, contributing to the high burden of intestinal parasitism (Box 8.1).

    DOI: 10.1201/9781003745709-10

BOX 8.1 UNIFIED GASTROINTESTINAL DISEASE PREVENTION STRATEGIES

Regardless of the specific pathogen or parasite, preventive actions are largely the same:

- Water Safety
  - Boil water for at least 1 minute, longer at high elevations
  - Use filters rated ≤1 μm, or chemical treatments with iodine or chlorine dioxide (not always effective for *Cryptosporidium*).
  - Use bottled water when available
  - Avoid ice or raw water in high-risk areas
- Food Hygiene
  - Cook meat and eggs thoroughly (especially poultry and ground beef)
  - Avoid raw produce in high-risk areas unless peeled or washed with safe water
  - Keep food preparation and eating areas clean and covered
  - Cover food and utensils to prevent insect contact
  - Store food in fly-proof sealed containers
- Sanitation and Personal Hygiene
  - Wash hands with soap and water after latrine use and before handling food
  - Use alcohol-based sanitizer when soap is unavailable
  - Clean dishes and utensils with safe water
- Insect Control
  - Screen kitchens, sleeping quarters, and latrines
  - Keep waste enclosed and then disposed away from kitchens, sleeping quarters, and latrines
  - Use fly traps, bait, or insecticides, if needed
- Educate workers on the risk posed by insects landing on feces and food

Mechanical transmission by flies is distinct from vector-borne disease in that the pathogen does not replicate or develop within the insect. Instead, flies serve as passive carriers, picking up and dropping off pathogens as they go about their scavenging. Despite the indirect nature of this transmission, the impact can be substantial, particularly where fly populations are dense and sanitation is poor. For this reason, control of filth flies is a key component of public health strategies aimed at reducing gastrointestinal diseases, particularly in food preparation and waste management contexts.

BACTERIAL GASTROINTESTINAL DISEASES

Pathogens: Order Enterobacterales, Family Enterobacteriaeae: pathogenic *Escherichia coli* (ETEC, EHEC, etc.), *Shigella* spp., *Salmonella* spp.;

Family Yersiniaceae: *Yersinia enterocolitica*; **Order Campylobacterales, Family Campylobacteraceae:** *Campylobacter* **spp.; Order Vibrionales, Family Vibrionaceae:** *Vibrio* **spp.; and others.**

Entomological Vectors: Order Blattodea, Family Blattidae: *Blatta orientalis* **(Oriental cockroach),** *Periplaneta americana* **(American cockroach),** *P. fuliginosa* **(smoky-brown cockroach), and other species; Family Ectobiidae:** *Blattella germanica* **(German cockroach),** *Supella longipalpa* **(brown-banded cockroach), and others; Order Diptera, Family Muscidae:** *Musca domestica* **(house fly) and others; Family Calliphoridae:** *Chrysomya megacephala* **(oriental latrine fly) and others**

Severity and Exposure Ratings (Figure 8.1)

- **Exposure Rating: 3–4**
  - Moderately (3) common in most environments
  - May be frequently (4) encountered wherever unsanitary conditions predominate, including urban landscapes where dogs are kept
- **Severity Rating: 1–4**
  - Minimal (1) for self-limiting diseases
  - Mostly mild (2) to moderate (3), but can be severe (4)
  - See Table 8.1 for more specific details

References: Greenberg (1971, 1973), Graczyk et al. (2001), Junqueira et al. (2017), Nayduch et al. (2023)

A wide range of bacterial pathogens can cause gastrointestinal illness via fecal-oral transmission, particularly in field conditions where water is untreated, sanitation is limited, and flies or cockroaches have access to food or waste. While these bacteria differ in severity, incubation periods, and complications, they share several key features.

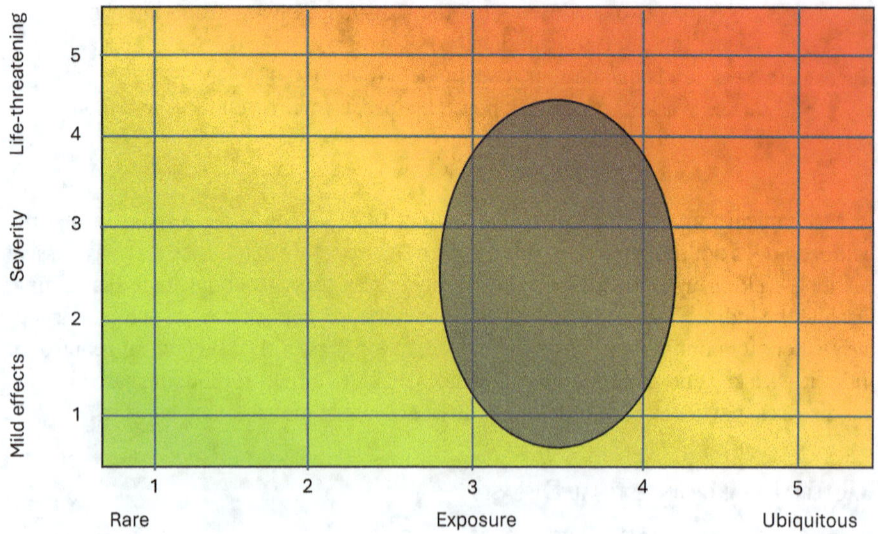

FIGURE 8.1 Bacterial gastrointestinal pathogens. Exposure × severity matrix.

TABLE 8.1

Key Bacterial Gastrointestinal Pathogens, of Which Insects Are a Potential Vector

Pathogen	Incubation	Key Symptoms	Notes	Antibiotics?	Severity (1–5)
Shigella spp.	1–3 days	Bloody diarrhea, fever, tenesmus	Extremely contagious, low infectious dose	Often needed	Mild (2) to Moderate (3)
Salmonella spp.	6–72 hours	Diarrhea, fever, vomiting	Often obtained from raw eggs, poultry, handling amphibians and reptiles	Sometimes (severe only)	Minimal (1) to Moderate (3)
Campylobacter spp.	2–5 days	Watery/bloody diarrhea, cramps	Associated with livestock, poultry	Sometimes	Mild (2) to Moderate (3)
Escherichia coli (ETEC)	1–3 days	Watery diarrhea, cramps	Traveler's diarrhea	Rarely	Minimal (1) to Mild (2)
Escherichia coli (EHEC)	3–4 days	Bloody diarrhea, fever uncommon	Can cause hemolytic uretic syndrome	No, contraindicated	Moderate (3) to Severe (4)
Vibrio spp.	12–72 hours	Watery diarrhea ("rice-water stool")	Risk with shellfish, warm seawater	Yes	Mild (2) to Moderate (3)
Yersinia enterocolitica	4–7 days	Fever, abdominal pain, diarrhea	Mimics appendicitis	Sometimes	Moderate (3) to Severe (4)
Listeria monocytogenes	1–4 weeks	Fever, muscle aches, gastrointestinal symptoms	Mostly affects pregnant women and immunocompromised	Yes	Moderate (3) to Severe (4)

Symptoms

- Transmitted via ingestion of fecal-contaminated material
- Mechanically spread by flies and cockroaches that walk on feces, then on food, tools, or hands
- Cause diarrhea, vomiting, abdominal pain, sometimes fever or blood in stool
- Present major risks in developing nations, post-disaster zones, or backcountry settings

Field professionals must consider not only food and water safety, but also insect exclusion and waste management to prevent outbreaks.

PROTOZOAN GASTROINTESTINAL PATHOGENS

Pathogens: Order Diplomonadida, Family Hexamitidae: *Giardia duodenalis*; **Order Eucoccidiorida, Family Cryptosporidiidae:** *Cryptosporidium* **spp.; Family Eimeriidae:** *Cyclospora cayetanensis*; **Phylum Amoebozoa, Family Entamoebidae:** *Entamoeba histolytica*; **Order Vestibuliferida, Family Balantidiidae:** *Balantidium coli*; **and others**

Entomological Vectors: Order Blattodea, Family Blattidae: *Blatta orientalis* **(Oriental cockroach),** *Periplaneta americana* **(American cockroach),** *P. fuliginosa* **(smoky-brown cockroach), and other species; Family Ectobiidae:** *Blattella germanica* **(German cockroach),** *Supella longipalpa* **(brown-banded cockroach), and others; Order Diptera, Family Muscidae:** *Musca domestica* **(house fly) and others; Family Calliphoridae:** *Chrysomya megacephala* **(oriental latrine fly); and others**

Severity and Exposure Ratings (Figure 8.2)

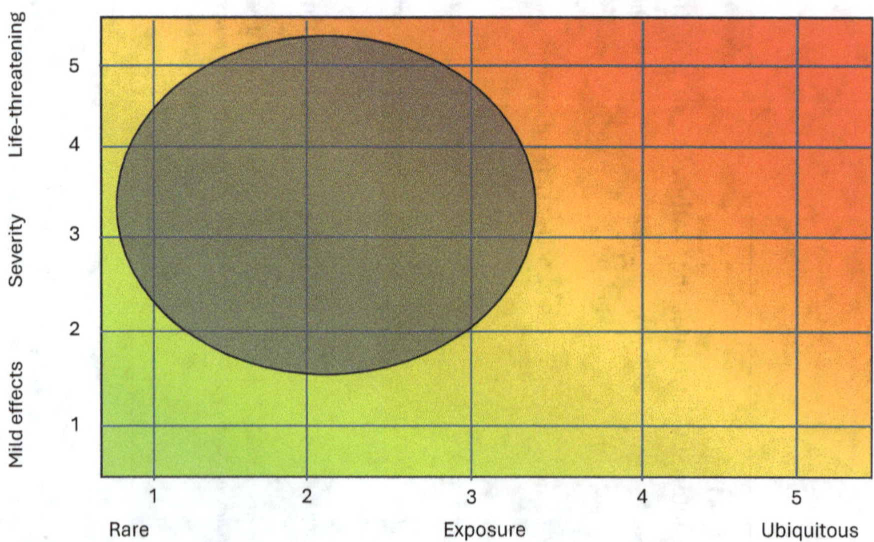

FIGURE 8.2 Protozoan gastrointestinal pathogens. Exposure × severity matrix.

- **Exposure Level: 1–3**
  - Rare (1) in most natural settings with good hygiene and treated water
  - Uncommon (2) to moderately (3) common in warm, fly-prone, unsanitary settings
- **Severity Level: 2–5**
  - Most immunocompetent individuals experience mild (2) symptoms
  - Untreated disease may become severe (4), and may even be life-threatening (5) in compromised individuals
  - See Table 8.2 for more specific details

References: Greenberg (1971, 1973), Graczyk et al. (2001, 2005), Nayduch et al. (2023)

Protozoan parasites from a variety of phyla are responsible for a wide range of gastrointestinal illnesses that can affect ecological and environmental professionals in the field. Most are spread by ingesting hardy cysts or oocysts (immature life stages of the protozoa) found in contaminated water, soil, or food. The most common transmission routes in North America involve contaminated produce where contaminated fecal material that was used as fertilizer was allowed to contact produce. Entomological agents can similarly spread these diseases, albeit far more rarely than they do bacterial diseases; however, some cases have been documented or suspected.

TABLE 8.2

Key Protozoan Gastrointestinal Pathogens, of Which Insects Are a Potential Vector

Pathogen	Incubation	Key Symptoms	Transmission Notes	Treatment	Severity (1–5)
Giardia duodenalis	1–2 weeks	Gas, greasy stools, cramps, fatigue	Common in surface water, fly contact possible	Usually metronidazole or tinidazole	Mild (2) to Moderate (3)
Cryptosporidium spp.	2–10 days	Watery diarrhea, cramps, fever	Resistant to chlorine, fly/cockroach contact likely	Usually nitazoxanide (only effective in immunocompetent)	Moderate (3) to Severe (4)
Entamoeba histolytica	2–4 weeks	Bloody diarrhea, fever, liver and intestinal abscesses	House fly transmission documented	Usually metronidazole + paromomycin	Moderate (3) to Severe (4)
Cyclospora cayetanensis	~1 week	Watery diarrhea, relapses, bloating	Fresh produce; flies may carry oocysts	Usually TMP-SMX (Bactrim)	Mild (2) to Severe (4)
Balantidium coli	Days to weeks	Bloody diarrhea, nausea, weight loss	Pig feces, contaminated water, possible fly route	Usually tetracycline or metronidazole	Moderate (3) to Severe (4)

GASTROINTESTINAL HELMINTHS

Pathogens: Phylum Nematoda, Order Rhabditida, Family Ascarididae: *Ascaris lumbricoides*; **Order Trichocephalida, Family Trichuridae:** *Trichuris trichiura*; **Phylum Platyhelminthes, Order Cyclophyllidea, Family Hymenolepididae:** *Hymenolepis nana*; **Family Dipylidiidae:** *Dipylidium caninum*; **and others**

Entomological Vectors: Order Blattodea, Family Blattidae: *Blatta orientalis* (Oriental cockroach), *Periplaneta americana* (American cockroach), *P. fuliginosa* (smoky-brown cockroach), and other species; Family Ectobiidae: *Blattella germanica* (German cockroach), *Supella longipalpa* (brown-banded cockroach), and others; Order Diptera, Family Muscidae: *Musca domestica* (house fly) and others; Family Calliphoridae: *Chrysomya megacephala* (oriental latrine fly) and others

Severity and Exposure Ratings (Figure 8.3)

- **Exposure Level: 1–2**
  - Rare (1) in most natural conditions
  - Uncommon (2) even in unsanitary conditions
- **Severity Level: 1–4**
  - Most infections minimal (1) to mild (2) harm
  - Severe (4) only in very heavy infections, highly unlikely in North America
  - See Table 8.3 for more specific details.

References: Greenberg (1971, 1973), Graczyk et al. (2001)

Helminths (parasitic worms) that infect the gastrointestinal tract may be mechanically transmitted by flies, particularly in warm, unsanitary environments. While

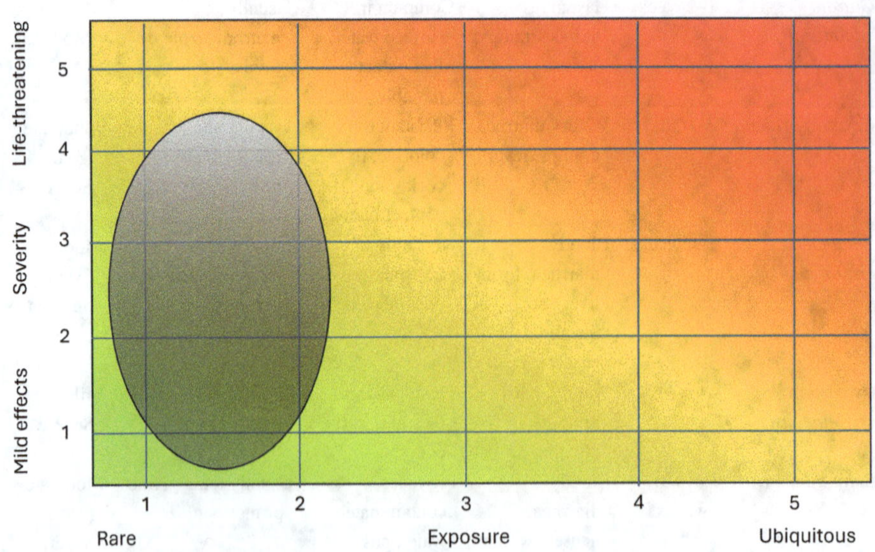

FIGURE 8.3 Gastrointestinal helminths. Exposure × severity matrix.

TABLE 8.3

Key Gastrointestinal Helminths, of Which Insects Are a Potential Vector

Helminth	Transmission Form	Key Symptoms	Treatment	Severity (1–5)
Ascaris lumbricoides (human roundworm)	Eggs	Intestinal discomfort, obstruction in heavy parasite loads	Albendazole, mebendazole	Minimal (1) to Moderate (3)
Trichuris trichiura (whipworm)	Eggs	Diarrhea, anemia, rectal prolapse in severe cases	Albendazole	Mild (2) to Moderate (3)
Hymenolepis nana (dwarf tapeworm)	Eggs	Often asymptomatic; can cause GI symptoms	Praziquantel	Minimal (1) to Mild (2)
Dipylidium caninum (dog and cat tapeworm)	Flea ingestion	Rare symptoms in humans (mostly children)	Praziquantel	Minimal (1) to Mild (2)

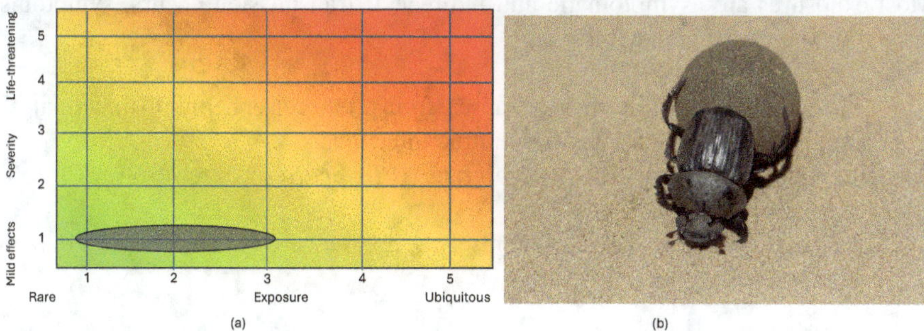

FIGURE 8.4   Dung beetles. (a) Exposure × severity matrix; (b) Dung beetle.

these helminths are not transmitted biologically through insect bites, their eggs or larvae can adhere to flies that contact feces, animal dung, or latrines, and subsequently contaminate human food, water, or surfaces. Bacterial and protozoan parasites are far more likely to be transmitted by flies than helminths.

Dung Beetles

Entomological Agents: Order Coleoptera, Family Scarabaeidae (subfamilies Scarabaeinae and Aphodiinae): *Onthophagus, Canthon, Aphodius,* and related genera (Figure 8.4)

Exposure and Severity Ratings (Figure 8.4)

- **Exposure Level: 1–3**
    - Rare (1) to uncommon (2) in most natural settings
    - Moderate (3) for workers in livestock, wildlife, or conservation settings where dung is abundant

- **Severity Level: 1**
  - Minimal (1) risk of indirect transmission of enteric pathogens or parasites through mechanical contact or contamination

Reference: Krinsky (2019)

Dung beetles play an essential ecological role by burying and decomposing feces, thus improving soil health and reducing pest populations. However, their frequent contact with animal feces raises concern for the potential mechanical transmission of gastrointestinal pathogens or parasites. Unlike biting or stinging insects, dung beetles do not directly infect humans, but they may act as mechanical vectors by carrying viable helminth eggs or protozoan cysts on their exoskeletons, especially in environments where sanitation is poor or where they encounter human or animal feces contaminated with pathogens. Studies have identified various parasitic organisms on or within dung beetles, including *Ascaris, Trichuris, Toxocara, Giardia*, and *Entamoeba* species, though evidence of actual transmission to humans via beetles remains limited.

Symptoms

Most exposures are asymptomatic and indirect. If transmission occurs, symptoms vary with pathogen but may include:

- Abdominal cramps, diarrhea, or nausea (from protozoan or helminth infection)
- Fatigue and eosinophilia in helminthic infections
- Rarely, ocular or visceral larva migrans (if *Toxocara* spp. are involved)

Symptoms arise from the parasites themselves, not the beetles. The beetles are passive carriers of infectious stages.

Occupational Exposure

Occupational exposure to dung beetles is typically incidental; some risk may exist when handling feces-contaminated soil or beetles in field settings, agricultural work, or wildlife management, such as:

- Agricultural and livestock operations (cattle, horses, swine)
- Wildlife reserves, conservation areas, and zoos
- Field ecology studies involving dung or soil sampling
- Public health surveys of enteric parasite distribution
- Composting facilities that incorporate manure or feces

Handling of beetles, dung pats, or contaminated equipment may result in unintentional exposure to infectious stages of enteric parasites.

Prevention

To reduce occupational risks:

- Wear gloves and protective clothing when handling dung or beetles
- Avoid hand-to-mouth contact and wash hands thoroughly after exposure

- Use dedicated tools for feces collection and clean them regularly
- Educate workers on the risks of fecal-oral transmission
- In endemic areas, consider routine deworming of livestock and appropriate use of latrines to reduce environmental contamination

Proper hygiene and awareness are the most effective means of preventing pathogen transmission in environments where dung beetles are abundant.

What To Do If Affected

- If symptoms of enteric illness occur after fieldwork, seek medical evaluation and disclose potential exposure
- Stool testing may be required to identify specific parasitic infections
- Antiparasitic treatments (e.g., albendazole, metronidazole) may be prescribed depending on the diagnosis
- Report suspected occupational transmission to health and safety personnel
- Implement stricter hygiene protocols for future exposures

Although dung beetles themselves are not inherently hazardous, they may act as vehicles for parasite dissemination in occupational contexts. Appropriate precautions and sanitation minimize this risk.

FILTH FLIES

Entomological parasites and vectors: Order Diptera, Families Muscidae (house flies), Calliphoridae (blow flies), Fanniidae (lesser house flies), Sarcophagidae (flesh flies) (Figure 8.5)

Exposure and Severity Ratings (Figure 8.5)

- **Exposure Level: 4–5**
  - Frequent (4) to ubiquitous (5)
  - Most common around stockyards, animal facilities, and in carcass-related work

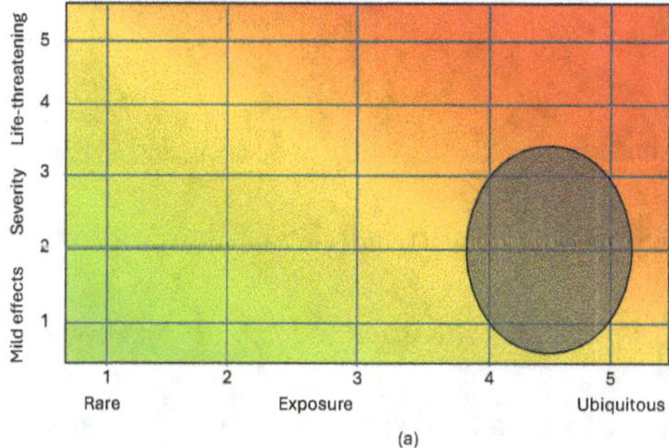

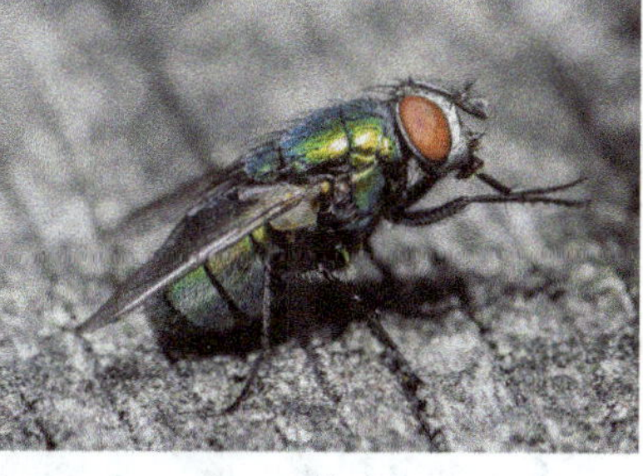

FIGURE 8.5 Filth flies. (a) Exposure × severity matrix; (b) blow fly, *Lucilia* sp.

- In addition to the ubiquity of the gastrointestinal diseases potentially spread by these flies, *Thelazia californiensis* has been documented in California and adjacent areas
- **Severity Level: 1–3**
  - Houseflies and blowflies tend to be a minimal (1) to mild (2) nuisance, but they do not bite
  - Some muscid species can bite with mild (2) pain
  - Moderate (3) effects from wound contamination or myiasis; occupationally rare, but can occur in incapacitated individuals
  - May be vectors of various bacteriological, protozoan, and helminth parasites, treated separately

References: Greenberg (1971, 1973), Graczyk et al. (2001), Nayduch et al. (2023), Omkar (2025)

House flies, horn flies, stable flies (Muscidae), blow flies (Calliphoridae), and flesh flies (Sarcophagidae) are small- to medium-sized, fast-flying flies commonly associated with decomposing organic matter, including animal carcasses, feces, and garbage. While they perform critical ecological functions as decomposers and are important in forensic entomology, they can also pose entomological health risks to humans and animals. Some of these flies (e.g., horn flies, stable flies) can bite; although each bite can be relatively mild, these flies often occur in large numbers and the accumulated bites can be highly annoying. Livestock may also be highly irritated by these flies, resulting in a secondary risk to workers.

Of the flies that do not bite, many are capable of mechanically transmitting pathogens or contaminating wounds and food. Typically, they do this by landing on and ingesting contaminated fecal material and then subsequently landing on food or open wounds, transmitting the pathogen. House flies and lesser house flies can also biologically transmit *Thelazia* eyeworms, a type of worm that affects the eyes.

In rare cases, usually involving incapacitated persons, some species cause myiasis, the infestation of living tissue by fly larvae. Flesh flies may also larviposit (deposit live maggots) directly onto necrotic tissue or mucous membranes.

These species are cosmopolitan and found in urban, rural, and natural environments, often appearing rapidly after defecation, death, or carcass decay begins – and very quickly attracted to human food.

Symptoms

While usually a nuisance, exposure can lead to:

- Irritation and psychological discomfort due to persistent landing or swarming
- Pathogen transmission, including *Salmonella*, *Shigella*, and *E. coli*, via contact with feces or carrion
- Contamination of tools, specimens, or food in field stations and remote labs
- Contamination of open wounds, leading to delayed healing or infection
- Maggot infestations (myiasis) in open sores, surgical wounds, or nasal/oral cavities – more likely in compromised individuals or animals

Occupational Exposure

Ecologists and environmental professionals may encounter these flies and potential gastrointestinal disease pathogens when:

- Spending prolonged time outdoors during fly season in endemic regions
- Cooking, eating, or sleeping outdoors
- Working with animal carcasses, such as roadkill surveys, necropsies, or scavenger studies
- Engaged in waste management, sanitation, or dead animal removal

Ecologists and environmental professionals may encounter *Thelazia* carried by these flies when:

- Working in regions with high densities of face flies or eye-seeking non-biting flies
- Handling livestock, particularly cattle, horses, or dogs
- Conducting wildlife health assessments, including trapping or handling injured animals
- Handling wild mammals, especially rodents, rabbits, and large ungulates

Myiasis by filth flies is rare unless the individual is more-or-less incapacitated, but some other flies may invade living tissues. Primarily restricted to tropical locations outside North America, these flies invade through small wounds (e.g., *Cochliomyia hominivorax*) or through another vector (e.g., mosquitoes and *Dermatobia hominis*) when ecologists and environmental professionals are:

- Working primarily in tropical locations, especially where mosquito-borne transmission of *D. hominis* may occur
- Working around rodent burrows, dens, or abandoned structures
- Collecting or processing biological specimens/necropsies in the field
- Working in rural veterinary or field hospital conditions

Prevention

To reduce exposure risk:

- Use insect repellents and mosquito nets to deter egg-laying vectors
- Wear gloves and eye protection when handling potential host species or their carrion
- Avoid direct contact with wild animal nests, carcasses, or burrows
- Keep wounds clean and covered with breathable dressings
- Maintain strict sanitation protocols in field labs or kitchens
- Store animal remains in sealed containers or bags for transport
- Dispose of carcasses promptly and away from work areas
- Use fly nets or traps in shelters or food prep areas
- Avoid drying clothes outdoors without ironing (eggs may be laid on fabric)

In tropical environments, constant vigilance is required to prevent fly contact.

What To Do If Affected

- For gastrointestinal disease
  - Follow recommendations provided above
- For wound exposure, clean thoroughly with antiseptics and monitor for signs of infection
- Inspect unusual insect bites or persistent lesions after fieldwork abroad
- If myiasis is suspected (i.e., presence of larvae in a wound):
  - Do not attempt forceful removal at home which may leave part of the larvae embedded and worsen the situation
  - Seek prompt medical care, which will involve
    - Physical removal of larvae by occlusion of breathing hole, forcing larva to the surface, and surgical extraction
    - Antibiotic treatment to prevent or treat secondary infection
    - Lesion care, depending on depth and tissue damage
  - For eye or nasal infestation, this constitutes a medical emergency
  - Seek psychiatric help if psychological trauma exists or persists
- Report infestations at field sites to public health or veterinary personnel

FLY-RELATED DISEASE

THELAZIASIS

Parasites: Order Rhabditida, Family Thelaziidae: *Thelazia californiensis* **and** *T. gulosa*

Entomological Agents: Order Diptera, Family Muscidae: *Musca autumnalis* **(lesser house fly)**

Exposure and Severity Ratings (Figure 8.6)

- **Exposure Level: 1–4**
  - Rare (1) in most natural settings
  - Frequent (4) for workers in close proximity to livestock or wildlife, especially in rural or agricultural settings
- **Severity Level: 2–3**
  - Mild (2) to moderate (3) ocular discomfort, usually requiring medical intervention

References: O'Hara and Kennedy (1989), Sobotyk et al. (2021)

Thelaziasis is an ocular parasitic disease caused by nematodes of the genus *Thelazia*, commonly referred to as "eyeworms." The lesser house fly, *Musca autumnalis*, acts as an intermediate host when feeding, which is by "sponging" up liquids since these flies do not actually bite. Adult female worms residing in the eye of an infected host release larvae that are ingested by flies when they feed on ocular secretions at an infected animal. The larvae develop within the fly and migrate to the fly's mouthparts, where they can be deposited into the conjunctival sac of a new host during subsequent feeding.

Eyeworms are normally veterinary parasites primarily affecting domestic animals (especially cattle, horses, and dogs), but human cases of thelaziasis have been

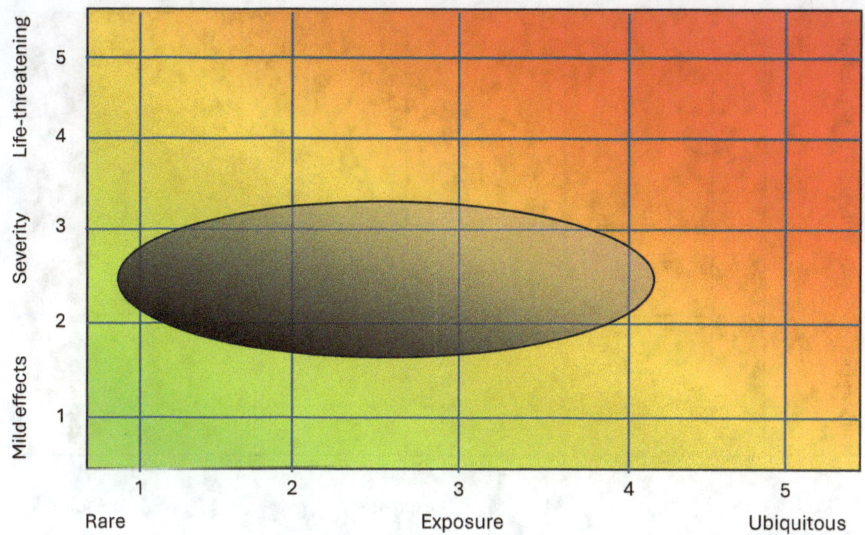

FIGURE 8.6   Thelaziasis. Exposure × severity matrix.

recorded in both North America and Eurasia. The condition is typically benign but can cause conjunctivitis, corneal ulceration, or secondary bacterial infections if left untreated. Occupational exposure is of particular concern for veterinary personnel, livestock handlers, and outdoor field workers in endemic regions.

Symptoms

- Foreign body sensation or irritation in one or both eyes
- Excessive tearing (epiphora)
- Conjunctivitis with redness and swelling
- Visual disturbances or blurry vision
- Presence of motile nematodes in conjunctival sac (diagnostic)
- Secondary bacterial infection or corneal ulceration in severe or neglected cases

Symptoms typically emerge within days to weeks after infection and may persist or worsen if not treated.

MYIASIS

Entomological Parasites: Order Diptera, Family Oestridae: *Cuterebra* spp., *Hypoderma* spp., *Oestrus ovis* (sheep nose bot fly); Family Muscidae: *Musca domestica* (house fly) and others; Family Calliphoridae: *Chrysomya* spp., *Lucilia sericata* (green bottle fly); and a few other fly families (Phoridae, Piophilidae, Stratiomyidae, Syrphidae)

Exposure and Severity Ratings (Figure 8.7)

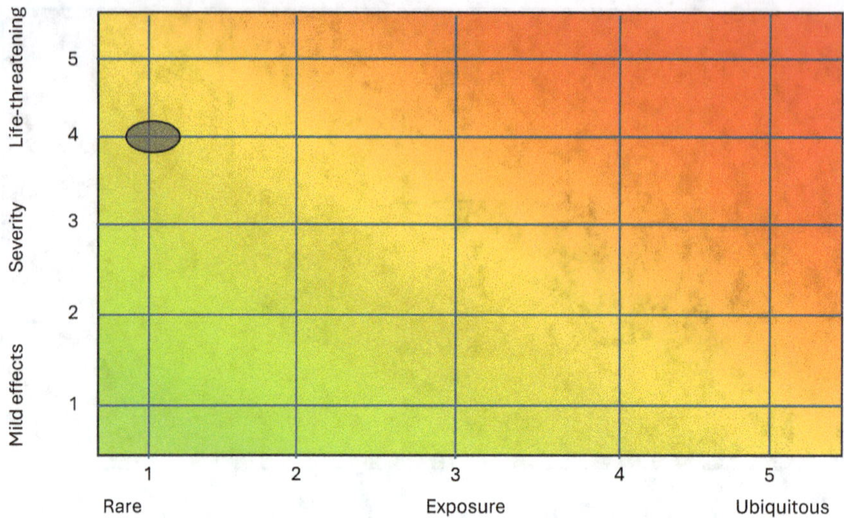

FIGURE 8.7 Myiasis. Exposure × severity matrix.

- **Exposure Level: 1**
  - Rare (1) across North America in humans (more common in wildlife)
- **Severity Level: 4**
  - Severe (4), as it is unpleasant and potentially disfiguring; some cases may require medical or surgical intervention
  - May result in psychological trauma

References: Haddad et al. (2012), Panadero-Fontán (2015), Bernhardt et al. (2019)

Myiasis is the infestation of live human or animal tissue by the larvae (maggots) of certain fly species. While many flies are harmless scavengers, several families exploit vertebrate hosts, either as obligate parasites or opportunistic invaders. Myiasis can range from relatively benign to severely disfiguring or even life-threatening, depending on the location, fly species involved, and health status of the host.

Myiasis is generally classified by its type of parasitism:

- Obligate myiasis involves species that require a live host to complete their larval development. Notable examples include *D. hominis* (the human bot fly) and *C. hominivorax* (New World screwworm), which must develop in living tissue
- Facultative myiasis occurs when species that typically breed in decaying organic matter, such as blowflies and flesh flies, invade necrotic wounds or unclean orifices in debilitated patients
- Accidental myiasis (pseudomyiasis) happens when non-parasitic larvae are ingested or contaminate wounds unintentionally, often through poor hygiene or contaminated food

Myiasis can also be described by its clinical presentation:

- Cutaneous myiasis is the most common form, often appearing as boil-like lesions that contain a single larva, with symptoms including localized pain, itching, and a visible breathing pore
- Furuncular myiasis is a subtype of cutaneous infestation involving deeper tissue invasion and a painful inflammatory response
- Cavitary or internal myiasis can affect the eyes (ophthalmic), nasal sinuses, ears, intestines, or even the urogenital tract. These cases are rarer and more dangerous, often requiring medical or surgical intervention

The usual fly families implicated in human myiasis include Oestridae (bot flies), Calliphoridae (blow flies), Sarcophagidae (flesh flies), Muscidae (house flies and relatives), and less commonly Phoridae, Piophilidae, and others. In North America, most human cases are rare and accidental, though hunters, professionals working in close contact with wildlife, or travelers to tropical regions should be aware of the risks. Prevention includes avoiding exposure to fly-infested environments, using protective clothing and repellents, and inspecting persistent skin lesions following travel or fieldwork.

Myiasis in humans is much more common in tropical areas, involving many more species, including the New World screwworm fly, *C. hominivorax*, which has been eradicated from North America. Although it historically was distributed as far north as the central United States, its northernmost persistent populations appear to be in Panama and the Greater Antilles in the Caribbean. Despite this, occasional reports of populations in southern Mexico periodically arise, while travelers bring infestations into the mainland United States.

Symptoms

Symptoms depend on species and location of larval development:

- Cutaneous myiasis:
    - Swollen, boil-like skin lesions
    - Pain, itching, and sensation of movement within lesion
    - Serosanguinous discharge and visible breathing pore
    - Secondary bacterial infection is possible
- Furuncular and cavitary/internal myiasis (rare):
    - Inflammation and pain in affected tissues, such as eyes, sinuses, genito-urinary openings, anus
    - Pustulant erupting sores
    - Neurological symptoms (in severe cases)
    - Often associated with travel or poor hygiene in tropical settings

Lesions may persist for weeks or months unless larvae are removed.

REFERENCES

Bernhardt V, Finkelmeier F, Verhoff MA, Amendt J. 2019. Myiasis in humans: A global case report evaluation and literature analysis. *Parasitol. Res.* 118: 389–397.

Graczyk TK, Knight R, Gilman RH, Cranfield MR. 2001. The role of non-biting flies in the epidemiology of human infectious diseases. *Microbes. Inf.* 3: 231–235.

Greenberg B. 1971. *Flies and Disease. I. Ecology, Classification, and Biotic Associations.* Princeton University Press, Princeton, NJ.

Greenberg B. 1973. *Flies and Disease. II. Biology and Disease Transmission.* Princeton University Press, Princeton, NJ.

Haddad V, Costa Cardoso JL, Lupi O, Tyring SK. 2012. Tropical dermatology: Venomous arthropods and human skin: Part I. Insecta. *J. Am. Acad. Dermatol.* 67: 331.e1–331.e14.

Junqueira ACM, Ratan A, Acerbi E, Drautz-Moses DI, Premkrishnan BNV, Costea PI, Linz B, Purbojati RW, Paulo DF, Gaultier NE, Subramanian P, Hasan NA, Colwell RR, Bork P, Azeredo-Espin AML, Bryant DA, Schuster SC. 2017. The microbiomes of blowflies and houseflies as bacterial transmission reservoirs. *Sci. Rep.* 7: 16324.

Krinsky WL 2019. Beetles (Coleoptera). Ch. 9 in: Mullen GR, Durden LA (eds.) *Medical and Veterinary Entomology.* Academic Press, Cambridge, MA.

Nayduch D, Neupane S, Pickens V, Purvis T, Olds C. 2023. House flies are underappreciated yet important reservoirs and vectors of microbial threats to animal and human health. *Microorganisms* 11: 583.

O'Hara JE, Kennedy MJ. 1989. Prevalence and intensity of *Thelazia* spp. (Nematoda: Thelazioidea) in a *Musca autumnalis* (Diptera: Muscidae) population from Central Alberta. *J. Parasitol.* 75: 803–806.

Omkar GM. 2025. *Flies: Agricultural and Public Health Perspectives.* CRC Press, Boca Raton, FL.

Panadero-Fontán R, Otranto D. 2015. Arthropods affecting the human eye. *Vet. Parasitol.* 208: 84–93.

Sobotyk C, Foster T, Callahan RT, McLean NJ, Verocai GG. 2021. Zoonotic *Thelazia californiensis* in dogs from New Mexico, USA, and a review of North American cases in animals and humans. *Vet. Parasitol. Region. Stud. Repts.* 24: 100553.

9 Transportation, Equipment, and Operations Hazards

ARACHNIDS

TARANTULAS

Entomological Agents: Order Araneae, Family Theraphosidae: *Aphonopelma*, *Brachypelma*, **and related genera (Figure 5.9)**
  Exposure and Severity Ratings

- **Exposure Level: 2–3**
  - Uncommon (2) to moderately (3) common in southwestern rangelands in CO, NM, OK panhandle, and TX
  - Annual "migrations" occur in late summer and early fall, sometimes large
  - Tarantulas do not occur outside of the western rangelands
- **Severity Level: 1–3**
  - Swarming impact can range from negligible (1) to moderate (3) by causing slippery roads

During late summer and early fall, large numbers of male tarantulas (*Aphonopelma* spp.) become active as they leave their burrows in search of mates. This seasonal behavior, often referred to as a "tarantula migration," is not a true migration in the ecological sense, but rather a mass dispersal of sexually mature males traveling across landscapes, including roadways, to locate sedentary females. These movements tend to peak during dusk and evening hours, coinciding with cooler ground surface temperatures.

The primary risk associated with this behavior is not bites from the tarantulas themselves, which is addressed in Chapter 5, but rather from road safety concerns. Tarantulas crossing highways and dirt roads in large numbers can cause motorists to brake abruptly or swerve to avoid them, leading to vehicular accidents or collisions with other wildlife. In some cases, the squashed bodies of many tarantulas can create traction issues, particularly on narrow or winding rural roads. Additionally, the sight of large spiders in high numbers can provoke panic or distraction, especially for individuals with arachnophobia, adding a psychological component to the physical hazard.

For environmental professionals, field vehicles parked on roadsides during tarantula movement periods may be at risk of attracting curious onlookers or startling

DOI: 10.1201/9781003745709-11

passersby. Workers in these areas should be aware of the timing of tarantula activity and should anticipate potential delays or distractions when working near affected roadways. Safety signage and advance planning may be prudent in heavily affected zones. While tarantulas pose no medical threat unless provoked, and bites are rare and minor, their seasonal movement has genuine implications for logistics, travel planning, and rural field operations.

Symptoms

- Slick roadways due to crushing by vehicles, which may cause administrative closure of roads
- Slips and falls due to slippery road surfaces
- Vehicle accidents, including motorcycle crashes and pileups

Occupational Exposure

- Ecologists and environmental professionals may encounter tarantula migrations when:
  - Driving on paved roads in areas where tarantulas live
  - Walking on or along the sides of roads

Migrating tarantulas usually do not cause a slickness hazard away from roads, but it is still advisable to watch footing in these locations to avoid stepping on individual tarantulas.

Prevention

There are not many options for prevention of tarantula migrations. Best practices would be to monitor areas in which these kinds of migrations occur during time frames (e.g., autumn) in which they are likely.

What To Do If Affected

- Avoid driving on roads which are impacted by tarantula migrations
- Keep abreast of road closures
- If driving is necessary, reduce speed, increase following distance, and make all maneuvers (steering, braking, accelerating) in a slow and gradual manner

INSECTS

SPRINGTAILS

Entomological Agents: Class Collembola, Order Entomobryomorpha, Family Entomobryidae: *Entomobrya* **and other genera; Order Symphypleona, Family Sminthuridae:** *Sminthurus* **and other genera; Order Poduromorpha, Family Neanuridae:** *Anurida maritima* **(seashore springtail); Family Hypogastruridae:** *Hypogastrura* **and other genera; and others (Figure 9.1)**
Exposure and Severity Ratings

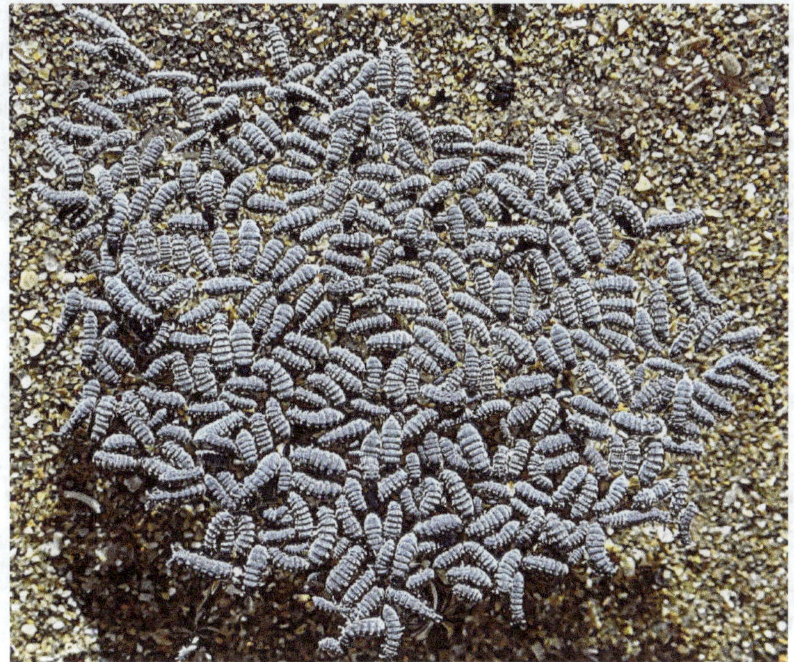

FIGURE 9.1 Collembola. Aggregation of seashore springtails, *Anurida maritima*.

- **Exposure Level: 1–5**
  - Ubiquitous (5) in most field conditions, especially in natural soils
  - Particularly abundant in tundra regions, and may form large aggregations in sea wrack or rocks in tidepools
  - Indoors, normally rare (1), but can be moderately (3) common in moist environments; rarely problematic unless populations surge
- **Severity Level: 0–1**
  - Direct health risk: 0 (none)
  - Minimal (1) nuisance or psychosomatic impact

References: Lim et al. (2009), Cranshaw (2011)

Springtails are tiny, wingless, soil-dwelling arthropods that thrive in moist environments rich in organic matter, such as leaf litter, mulch, potting soil, compost, and drainage areas. They are often considered to be insects because they have six legs but have recently been reclassified as non-insect hexapods. Although completely harmless to humans, they are frequently the subject of misattributed infestations or dermatological complaints and are among the ten most reported nuisance pests in buildings in the United States.

In some work environments, especially in greenhouses, crawlspaces, wet laboratories, or field research in moist habitats, springtails may be found in large numbers.

Natural densities in optimal conditions in natural soils or on rocks in intertidal zones can range from 10,000 to 200,000 individuals/m^2; in greenhouses, densities up to 400,000 individuals/m^2 have been reported. These kinds of densities can increase slickness on walking surfaces, potentially leading to slips and falls. Large collembolan presence can lead to worker discomfort, incorrect diagnosis of parasitosis, or anxiety about hygiene or contamination. There is no evidence that springtails bite, sting, or transmit pathogens, though some species may trigger psychological distress due to their sudden appearance.

Symptoms

- No direct medical symptoms caused by springtails
- Rare, unproven claims of bites or crawling sensations, often attributed to delusional parasitosis
- Anxiety, distraction, or disruption of routine due to unexpected swarming

Springtails are attracted to high humidity, and their presence indoors often indicates a moisture problem rather than a medical issue.

Occupational Exposure

Springtails are encountered in:

- Greenhouses and nurseries, particularly in potting media
- Moist basements, crawlspaces, and Heating, Ventilation, and Air Conditioning (HVAC) systems
- Soil sampling, wetland ecology, or riparian zone work
- Wrack and intertidal zones along lakes and seashores
- Zoological or veterinary facilities with moist bedding or feed
- Entomological fieldwork, especially involving collection of material for Berlese funnels or leaf litter sorting

Prevention

If they are indoors, collembolans control is part of maintaining sanitary work environments:

- Reduce moisture and humidity in workspaces with dehumidifiers or improved drainage
- Avoid overwatering plants in enclosed areas
- Use well-draining substrates in greenhouses and lab colonies
- Seal cracks in floors, walls, or equipment that allow soil organisms indoors
- Educate workers about non-biting arthropods to reduce anxiety and misdiagnosis
- Avoid treating for "bites" unless other evidence supports parasitic infestation

Springtail infestations are not a cause for pesticide application and usually resolve with improved sanitation.

What To Do If Affected

- For anxiety or skin irritation, assess for underlying mold, allergens, or chemical exposure
- Reassure affected workers that springtails are harmless and non-parasitic
- Remove individuals from overly humid or mold-prone environments
- Clean and ventilate affected areas to reduce microarthropod populations
- Consult occupational health or entomology staff to confirm identification and advise next steps

If individuals persist in reporting "bites" without evidence, consider referral to medical or psychological support.

MAYFLIES AND CADDISFLIES

Entomological Agents: Order Ephemeroptera, although most of the risk involves a small number of species in the Family Ephemeridae: *Hexagenia limbata*, *Ephemera simulans* **(Figure 9.2); Order Trichoptera, again only in a small number of species**

Exposure and Severity Ratings

- **Exposure Level: 2–3**
  - Locally uncommon (2) in aquatic zones
  - During seasonal emergence swarms, may be moderate (3) and highly concentrated

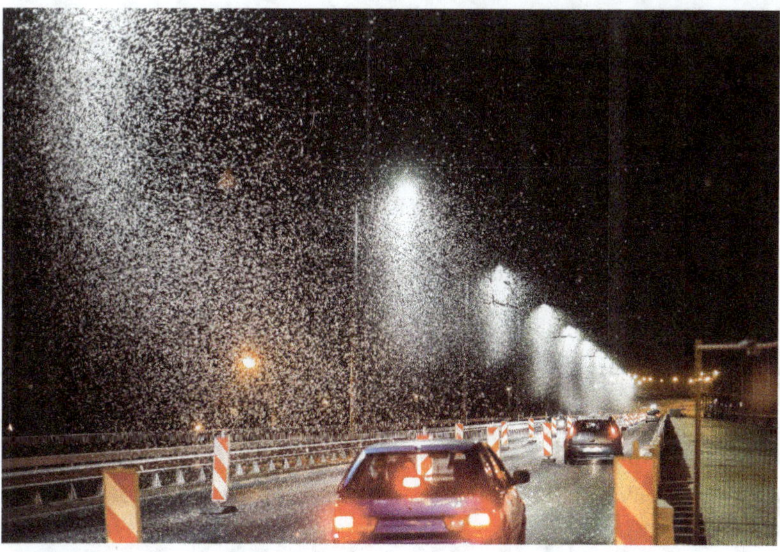

FIGURE 9.2   Mayflies and caddisflies. Mayfly swarm in construction zone on a road.

- **Severity Level: 1–4**
  - Typically presenting minimal (1) harm
  - During seasonal emergence swarms, may range from moderate (3) to severe (4) harm, especially in regard to allergies, slip/trip/fall hazards, driving and visibility hazards, and equipment fouling

References: Edmunds et al. (1976), Dublon and Sumpter (2014), Cavallero (2026)

Mayflies and caddisflies are aquatic insects best known for their brief adult lifespan and spectacular synchronized emergences near freshwater sources such as rivers, lakes, and reservoirs. As nymphs, they serve as indicators of good water quality and play vital roles in aquatic food webs.

However, during peak emergence events – especially near large rivers like the Mississippi and Ohio – mayflies can become entomological hazards by:

- Creating slick roadways due to crushing by vehicles
- Causing vehicle accidents, including motorcycle crashes and pileups
- Overwhelming lighting systems, triggering mass accumulations on bridges and buildings
- Inducing respiratory allergies or eye irritation due to airborne fragments of dead insects

Mayflies do not bite or sting, nor do they transmit disease, but their sheer biomass can create operational and, potentially, health complications for environmental workers, utility crews, and transportation authorities.

Symptoms

While individual exposure is almost exclusively harmless, mass emergences may cause:

- Slick roadways due to crushing by vehicles, which may cause administrative closure of roads
- Vehicle accidents, including motorcycle crashes and pileups
- Sneezing, coughing, itchy eyes, and allergic reactions from airborne particulates
- Eye irritation from body fragments or scale dust
- Loss of traction when walking or driving through piles of insects
- Anxiety or distraction among workers encountering insect swarms

Populations may reach millions per square kilometer during synchronized emergence nights.

Occupational Exposure

Ecologists and environmental professionals may encounter high-density aquatic insect swarms when:

- Working near large, clean rivers or lakes during spring or summer evenings
- Performing bridge or road inspections, especially under artificial lights

- Maintaining lighting systems or power infrastructure near water
- Conducting wetland or riparian habitat surveys during emergence windows
- Assisting with traffic management or cleanup after emergence events

Both mayflies and caddisflies are strongly phototactic and can clog vents, lights, or instrumentation.

Prevention

While difficult to avoid during emergence season, mitigation strategies include:

- Adjusting work schedules to avoid dusk-to-midnight peaks during emergence periods
- Using yellow or shielded lights to reduce attraction
- Wearing safety goggles and masks if airborne debris is present
- Applying non stick coatings or physical barriers to protect vulnerable equipment
- Alerting transportation crews and field teams about emergence forecasts

In floodplain regions, awareness of seasonal timing is key to preparation.

What To Do If Affected

- For eye or respiratory irritation, use saline eyewash and antihistamines as needed
- Avoid driving on roads which are impacted by tarantula migrations
- Keep abreast of road closures
- If driving is necessary, reduce speed, increase following distance, and make all maneuvers (steering, braking, accelerating) in a slow and gradual manner

Most effects are temporary and environmental, rather than directly biological.

Mormon Crickets

Entomological Agents: Order Orthoptera, Family Tettigoniidae: *Anabrus simplex* **(Mormon cricket) (Figure 9.3)**

Exposure and Severity Ratings

- **Exposure Level: 3**
  - Moderately (3) common in western rangeland and mountains from WA and MT south to CA and NM
  - Large swarms occur periodically (approximately 8- to 15-year cycles)
  - Mormon crickets do not occur outside of the western rangelands
- **Severity Level: 1–4**
  - Bite: mild (1) pain but harmless
  - Swarming impact results in moderate (3) to severe (4) harm on driving (slippery roads), contaminated gear, and morale

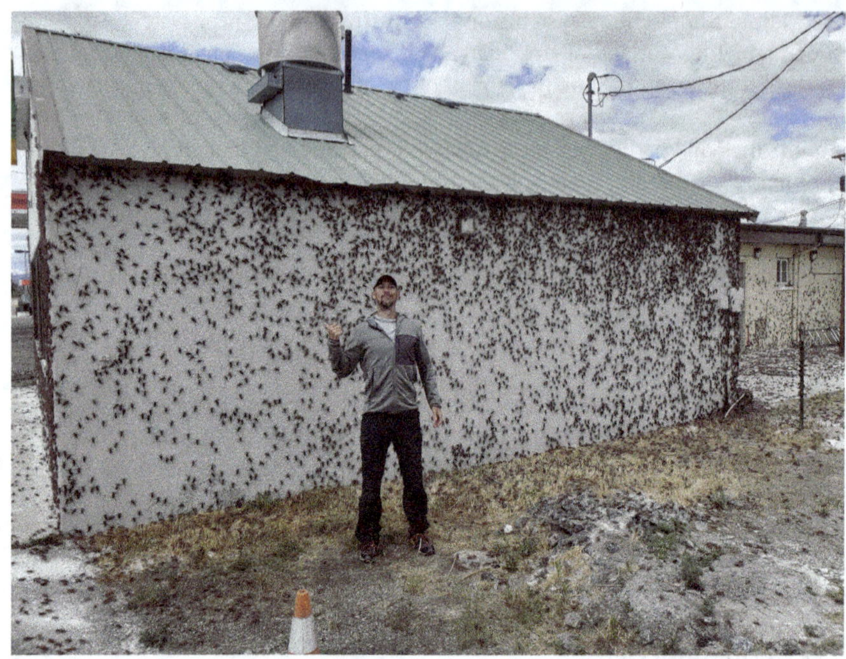

FIGURE 9.3   Mormon crickets. Swarm of Mormon crickets on building.

References: Wakeland (1959), Edel et al. (2024)

Despite its name, the Mormon cricket is not a true cricket but a large, flightless katydid found across the western United States, especially in sagebrush steppe, grasslands, and rangeland ecosystems. These insects are known for their mass migratory outbreaks, during which they form large bands of tens of millions of individuals that march across landscapes, often crossing roads, fields, and pastures.

In outbreak years, they pose significant nuisance and safety issues as they can be found in densities up to 100 individuals/m². Hazards include slick roads from crushed bodies, fouling of structures and field gear, and large-scale agricultural damage.

While road hazards are the most frequent hazard associated with Mormon crickets, they can reach lengths of 5–8 cm and are equipped with strong, chewing mandibles capable of painful bites if handled carelessly. While they are not venomous and do not seek out humans, they will bite in self-defense, especially when restrained or accidentally contacted.

Symptoms

- Creating slick roadways due to crushing by vehicles, which may cause administrative closure of roads
- Causing vehicle accidents, including motorcycle crashes and pileups
- Painful bite, comparable to a large grasshopper or katydid, see p. 121–122

Bites typically occur only when insects are handled bare-handed or become trapped in clothing or equipment.

Occupational Exposure

Exposure to ecologists and environmental professionals occurs most commonly in:

- Range management, ecological fieldwork, or entomological surveys in the western United States
- Roadside surveys, driving, or hiking in outbreak areas
- Vegetation sampling or herbivory monitoring
- Campgrounds or structures where swarms mass
- State or federal pest management work involving Mormon cricket control

Swarming often peaks in late spring and summer, with tens of thousands of individuals per hectare.

Prevention

- Wear gloves when collecting or handling Mormon crickets
- Avoid walking or driving through dense aggregations, especially on hot asphalt
- Use sticky barriers or exclusion fencing around tents and field stations if needed
- Keep boots, cuffs, and clothing sealed, as crickets may crawl inside
- Clean field gear and shoes regularly – insects may defecate or regurgitate when handled
- Inform staff of risks associated with swarm behavior, especially road slickness and psychological aversion

Field workers often report distress or disgust, especially during dense outbreaks

What To Do If Affected

- Treat bites as described on p. 121–122

- Avoid driving on roads which are impacted by Mormon cricket migrations
- Keep abreast of road closures
- If driving is necessary, reduce speed, increase following distance, and make all maneuvers (steering, braking, accelerating) in a slow and gradual manner

No venom or disease transmission is involved.

CICADAS (PERIODICAL AND ANNUAL)

Entomological Agents: Order Hemiptera, Family Cicadidae: *Magicicada* spp., *Neotibicen* spp., and others
  Exposure and Severity Ratings (Figure 9.4)

- **Exposure Level: 2–4**
    - Minimal (2) in most years and regions (due to low density or only annual species)

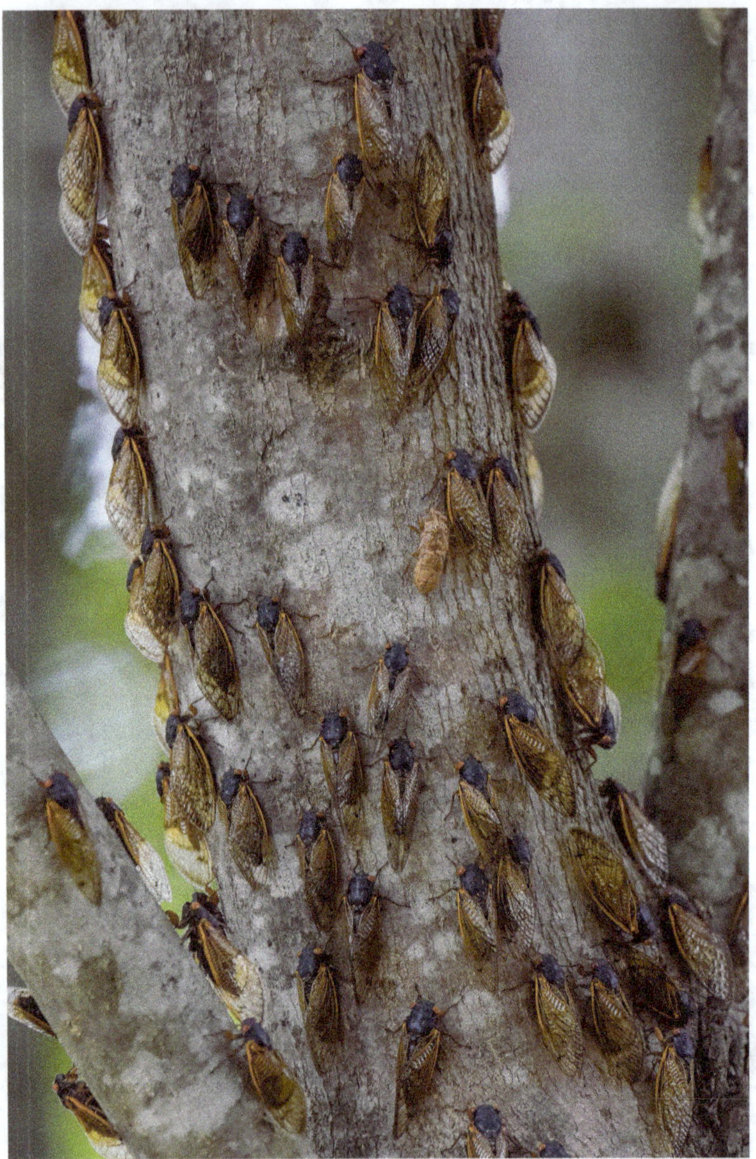

FIGURE 9.4 Cicadas. Swarm of periodical cicadas on tree.

- High (4) during periodical emergence years (13- or 17-year broods), especially in the eastern United States; locations vary by year but have become somewhat predictable
- **Severity Level: 1–2**
  - Minimal (1) for direct harm: no bites or stings
  - Mild (2) when emergence results in noise hazards, falling debris, or operational interference

Reference: Kritsky (2004)

Cicadas are large, non-biting, plant-feeding insects best known for their noisy mating calls and, in some species, synchronized mass emergences. Periodical cicadas (*Magicicada* spp.) emerge by the millions every 13 or 17 years, depending on brood, and can significantly affect outdoor operations through their sheer numbers and the environmental impacts of oviposition and carcass buildup.

Larvae feed underground on the roots of trees. When it is time to emerge as adults, they crawl up just about any stationary vertical surface and leave their shed skin (called exuvium) behind. When mass emergences occur, there can be hundreds of exuviae littering trees, fence posts, walls, etc.

Although harmless medically – no biting or stinging, and little in terms of allergens – their auditory output can exceed 100 dB at close range, posing a potential noise hazard to workers. Flying cicadas can strike people or equipment, and dead cicada accumulations, including their exuviae, can attract scavengers, increase odor, or affect sanitation in sensitive areas.

Symptoms

Cicadas do not bite, sting, or transmit disease, but they may:

- Cause temporary hearing discomfort or disruption due to loud choruses
- Create startle responses when flying into people
- Induce panic or discomfort in noise-sensitive individuals
- Lead to slip/fall risks or clogging when dead individuals accumulate on walkways, machinery, or filters
- Rarely, trigger allergies from shed skins or dust from carcasses

Occupational Exposure

Ecologists, construction crews, arborists, and other field professionals may encounter large cicada populations when:

- Working during emergence years of periodical cicadas (brood years vary by location)
- Conducting vegetation surveys or utility work in deciduous forests
- Setting up long-term monitoring equipment in rural or wooded areas
- Participating in education/outreach during high-visibility emergence events
- Maintaining infrastructure near dense tree cover (especially oaks, maples, hickories)

Prevention

While cicadas are not dangerous, certain precautions can minimize disruption:

- Monitor brood maps and emergence years via United States Forest Service, United States Department of Agriculture, or university extension data
- Wear hearing protection when working in dense forests during peak mating calls
- Secure food and waste containers in emergence areas to avoid secondary nuisance species

- Shield equipment and sensitive surfaces from insect debris
- Use mesh netting on exposed or sensitive outdoor gear
- Avoid unnecessary nighttime lighting, which may attract cicadas

What To Do If Affected

- Use earplugs or earmuffs in areas with intense calling
- Gently remove cicadas that land on personnel or equipment; there is no need to swat
- Sweep or hose down surfaces where dead cicadas accumulate
- Document large emergences in project notes to explain potential delays or disruptions
- Reassure field crews that cicadas are harmless and temporary

TERMITES

Entomological Agents: Order Blattidae, Infraorder Isoptera, Families Rhinotermitidae, Heterotermitidae, and Kalotermitidae (Figure 9.5)
   Exposure and Severity Ratings

- **Exposure Level: 2–3**
    - Uncommon (2) in most environments
    - Moderately common (3) in humid climates, especially around wood structures or debris piles
    - May occasionally swarm; such swarms have been reported on weather radar in New Orleans
    - Formosan termites rarely found north of 35°N in North America

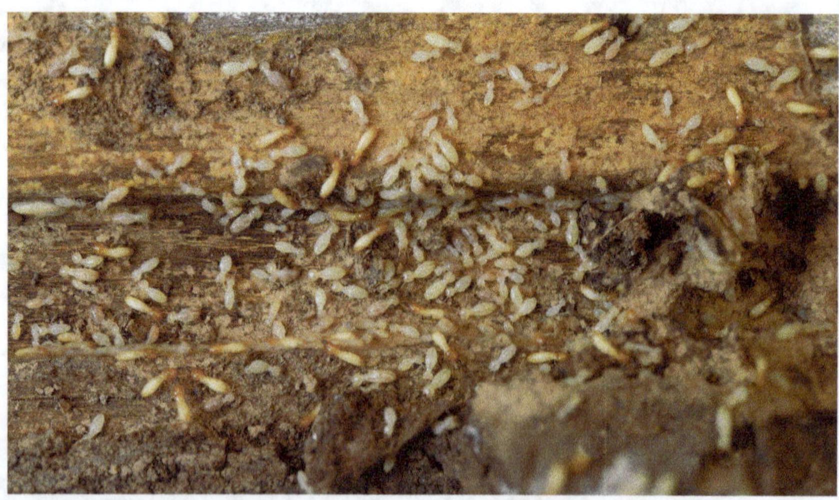

FIGURE 9.5   Termites. Termite infestation in wood.

- **Severity Level: 1–4**
  - Typically, a minimal (1) nuisance when present in low numbers, escalating to Moderate (3) or Severe (4) risk when structural or operational integrity is compromised
  - Increased risk of slips and falls when adults are swarming
  - North American species may attempt to bite but cannot break the skin
  - Nests may harbor molds and other allergens

Reference: Forsythe (2004)

Termites are best known for their ability to digest cellulose, making them highly destructive to wood and plant-based materials. Although they do not bite or sting humans, their colonies, which can number in the tens or hundreds of thousands, can undermine buildings, boardwalks, outdoor infrastructure, equipment sheds, and even field laboratory setups. Their presence is most concentrated in warm, humid regions but may occur wherever untreated wood accumulates.

Species vary in behavior: subterranean termites (e.g., *Reticulitermes* spp.) build extensive mud tubes and attack wooden structures from below; the mud tubes often indicate the presence of termites when on drywall installations. Drywood termites (*Incisitermes* spp.) and the Formosan termite (*Coptotermes formosanus*) infest furniture, fence posts, trees, or walls without needing soil contact. A mature Formosan termite colony may eat up to 400 g of wood per day, but damage may go unnoticed until major collapse or equipment failure occurs.

Termite nests may harbor molds, fungi, or other allergens that could trigger allergic reactions in some individuals.

Additionally, many termite species swarm during mating season. When this happens, millions of individuals called "alates" (winged males and females) emerge at the same time, often in spring or after rains. Being phototactic, these alates are attracted to lights and may congregate in well-lighted locations, causing slippery conditions as they are stepped on and crushed and their wings cover ground surfaces.

Symptoms

North American termites do not pose direct medical risks to humans, but their presence can result in:

- Structural weakening or failure of buildings, bridges, or boardwalks
- Compromised field stations, storage units, or trail signage
- Electrical shorts or malfunctions due to mud tube encasement of wiring
- Operational delays due to required structural repairs
- Unexpected collapses or trip hazards in rotted wooden platforms
- Slip and fall hazards from crushed bodies and shed wings during swarming events

Occupational Exposure

Environmental professionals may encounter termites when:

- Conducting long-term research in forested or tropical settings
- Working in boardwalks, viewing platforms, or educational kiosks

- Operating or storing gear in wooden sheds, boxes, or untreated equipment containers
- Surveying damaged wood for wildlife, fungi, or other ecological assessments
- Installing infrastructure in wetland, savanna, or mangrove ecosystems
- Working near lights during swarming events

Exposure risk increases with moisture, age of wood, and duration of field site occupation.

Prevention

To reduce termite-related hazards:

- Avoid storing wooden gear directly on soil or leaf litter
- Treat wooden infrastructure with borate or other preservatives
- Elevate wooden platforms and use termite barriers where possible
- Inspect for mud tubes or frass near structures or stored gear
- Rotate site use and inspect frequently for hidden infestations
- Use non-cellulose-based materials (metal, plastic) where feasible for long-term field equipment or structures

What To Do If Affected

- Cease use of any structure showing visible weakening or termite damage
- Remove and replace infested wood; do not reuse or relocate it
- Report structural issues to site managers or park authorities
- Engage pest management professionals for colony elimination when appropriate
- For critical sites (labs, bridges, buildings), consider long-term monitoring stations or soil treatment
- Seek medical attention for serious falls due to slips

Although medically harmless, termites can cause expensive and dangerous operational disruptions. Proper design, maintenance, and vigilance are essential to ensure safety and continuity in fieldwork environments.

Non-Biting Gnats

Entomological Agents: Order Diptera, Family Chironomidae (Figure 9.6) Exposure and Severity Ratings

- **Exposure Level: 2–3**
  - Moderate (3) exposure increasing to frequent (4) near water bodies
  - Periodic explosive emergence events
- **Severity Level: 1–2**
  - Exposure to one or a few individuals is minimal (1) nuisance and irritation
  - Exposure to mass emergence is a mild (2) risk to allergies, slip/trip/fall hazards, or operational delays

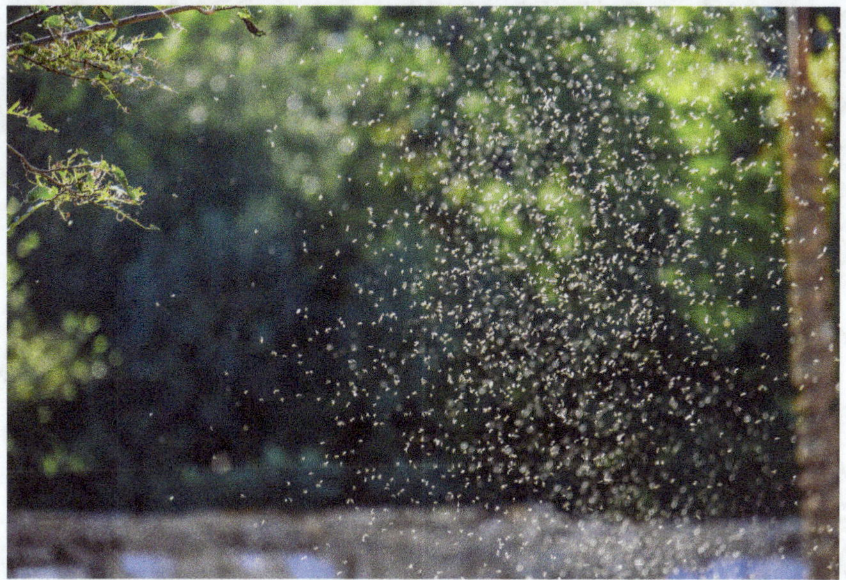

FIGURE 9.6   Non-biting midges. Swarm of non-biting midges.

References: Henson (1966), Dublon and Sumpter (2014)

Non-biting gnats are small, mosquito-like flies that breed in aquatic environments and often emerge in enormous, synchronized swarms. Though harmless in terms of biting or disease transmission, their sheer numbers can cause significant disruption, especially near lakes, reservoirs, treatment facilities, or wetlands.

These insects are highly phototactic, swarming around lights and often coating surfaces, vehicles, and buildings. Dead midges can form thick mats that clog air filters, damage electronics, and create slip hazards on roadways or docks. Their shed skins and body fragments can trigger asthma and allergy symptoms, especially in sensitive individuals.

Certain genera (e.g., *Chironomus*, *Tanytarsus*) are especially notorious for large emergences near urban waterfronts and hydroelectric structures.

Symptoms

While not dangerous individually, midges can cause:

- Eye and respiratory irritation due to airborne insect scales or decomposing carcasses
- Allergic reactions, including coughing, sneezing, wheezing, and eye redness
- Nuisance swarming, which can obstruct vision and distract workers
- Slick surfaces from crushed insect bodies
- Overloaded HVAC systems, causing decreased air quality in buildings or vehicles

Mass emergences can significantly affect worksite safety and efficiency.

Occupational Exposure

Ecologists and environmental professionals may encounter midges when:

- Working near lakes, marshes, reservoirs, or slow-moving rivers
- Conducting nighttime or early morning operations near aquatic habitats
- Performing utility maintenance, water quality sampling, or dam inspections
- Operating around treatment lagoons, aeration basins, or similar infrastructure
- Engaging in urban mosquito monitoring, often misidentifying midges as target species

Exposure may be seasonal or year-round, depending on local climate and water temperature.

Prevention

While midge swarms cannot be completely avoided, mitigation strategies include:

- Avoiding nighttime work near aquatic sources during peak emergence
- Using non-attractive lighting (e.g., amber LED or sodium vapor)
- Installing screens or air curtains on sensitive equipment and ventilation systems
- Wearing goggles and masks in dense swarms
- Designing workspaces to reduce standing light and reflective surfaces near water
- Employing maintenance protocols to clean insect buildup regularly

Long-term control may require environmental engineering to reduce larval habitat near critical infrastructure.

What To Do If Affected

- Rinse eyes, face, and nasal passages with clean water if irritation occurs
- Use antihistamines or corticosteroid sprays for allergic symptoms
- Clean work surfaces and clear ventilation systems after heavy emergence
- For severe allergic or respiratory effects, seek medical evaluation
- Report mass emergence events to site managers or public health authorities

Although midges are not medically dangerous, their impact on comfort, safety, and operations can be substantial.

MOTH FLIES AND DRAIN FLIES

Entomological Agents: Order Diptera, Family Psychodidae: *Clogmia*, *Psychoda*, and related genera (Figure 9.7)
  Exposure and Severity Ratings

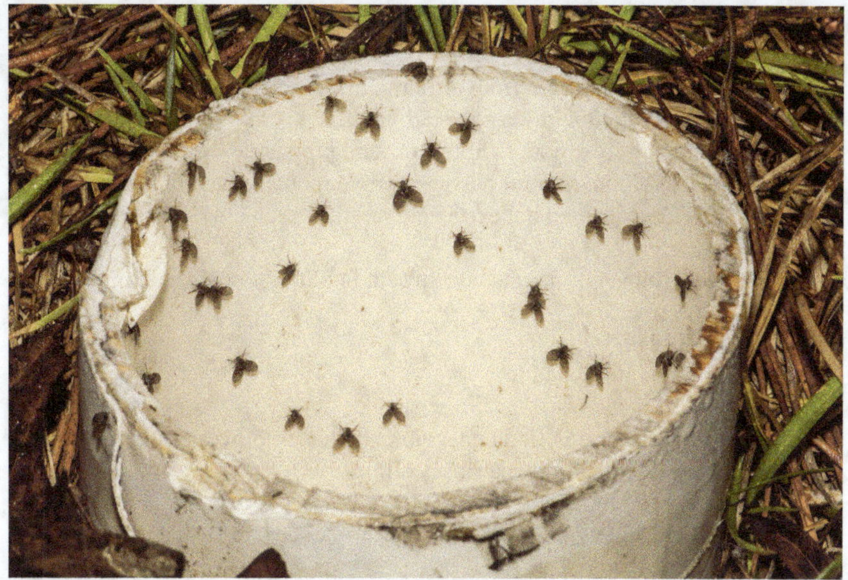

FIGURE 9.7 Moth flies and drain flies. Moth flies in a plastic drain.

- **Exposure Level: 2**
  - Rare (1) in most natural settings
  - Can be uncommonly (2) encountered in poorly maintained drainage areas
  - Populations can spike quickly, especially indoors
- **Severity Level: 1–2**
  - Nuisance or minor allergic irritation: minimal (1) to mild (2)
  - Minimal (1) contamination of sensitive work areas

Reference: Theuret and Gerry (2014)

Moth flies, commonly called drain flies or filter flies, are small, fuzzy-winged flies often found in moist, organic-rich environments such as drains, sewage systems, compost bins, and leaky pipes. They are harmless in terms of biting or disease transmission, but they can pose occupational nuisances when water drainage issues are not properly addressed, especially in clinical labs, research settings, food preparation areas, and animal facilities.

These flies reproduce in organic biofilm, such as that found inside plumbing, and populations can surge rapidly in the presence of neglected drainage areas. Their moth-like appearance makes them appear easy to control, but they are surprisingly quick and hard to exclude from restrooms, sewage systems, and other drains.

While usually considered cosmetic pests, moth flies have been implicated in allergic responses, and their presence may indicate violation of sanitation standards in certain workspaces.

Symptoms

- No biting or envenomation
- Allergic rhinitis or asthma from airborne insect scales or frass
- Eye or throat irritation in sensitive individuals
- Contamination of restroom facilities or food prep areas
- Rarely, colonization of nasal passages or wounds in severely incapacitated individuals (documented but extremely rare)

The psychological impact of insects in restroom facilities can also be significant.

Occupational Exposure

Drain flies are commonly found in:

- Bathrooms, floor drains, and under sinks in labs or offices
- Animal care facilities and veterinary clinics
- Greenhouses and moist field stations
- Health care settings, where their presence may concern patients or violate inspection standards
- Food service areas, where organic matter and moisture combine
- Research labs with leaky sinks or poor sanitation in shared spaces

They are active at night but may be observed resting on walls near sinks and drains during the day.

Prevention

To eliminate and prevent infestations:

- Clean drains regularly with enzymatic or microbial treatments to remove biofilm
- Use wire brushes or plumbing snakes to physically remove buildup
- Eliminate standing water and repair leaks in pipes and under sinks
- Use tight-fitting drain screens
- Install dehumidifiers in chronically damp rooms
- Keep windows and vents screened in tropical or greenhouse areas

Prevention relies on environmental sanitation, not insecticides.

What To Do If Affected

- Identify and clean breeding sources, typically in plumbing or organic waste
- Vacuum or wipe down surfaces to remove adult flies and particulates
- If allergic symptoms occur, use air purifiers and antihistamines as needed
- For contamination-sensitive areas (e.g., culture labs or clinical rooms), consult facilities or infection control staff
- Report persistent infestations to building maintenance

Outbreaks can usually be resolved with plumbing and janitorial intervention, not pest control.

Lovebugs

Entomological Agents: Order Diptera, Family Bibionidae: *Plecia americana* **and** *P. nearctica* **(Figure 9.8)**
Exposure and Severity Ratings

- **Exposure Level: 4**
  - Frequently (4) encountered throughout the southeastern United States from Texas to Georgia, less so in states from Missouri to North Carolina
- **Severity Level: 1–2**
  - No biological effects as they do not bite or sting
  - Operational nuisance/disruption may be mild (1) to moderate (2) due to visual, mechanical, and logistical issues

References: Leppla (2009), Dublon and Sumpter (2014)

Lovebugs, especially *Plecia nearctica*, are small, black flies with an orange thorax, notorious for flying in copulating pairs. They are native to Central America and now common in the southeastern United States, particularly Florida, Louisiana, Mississippi, and Texas. There are typically two major adult emergences per year, in late spring (April–May) and late summer (August–September).

Lovebugs do not bite or sting, but they can swarm in enormous numbers, creating problems for outdoor workers, motorists, and field researchers. When crushed, their bodies release acidic fluids that can damage vehicle paint, clog radiators, or foul lab and sampling equipment.

Despite being ecologically benign and even beneficial as decomposers in their larval stage, lovebugs are a major nuisance species during flight season.

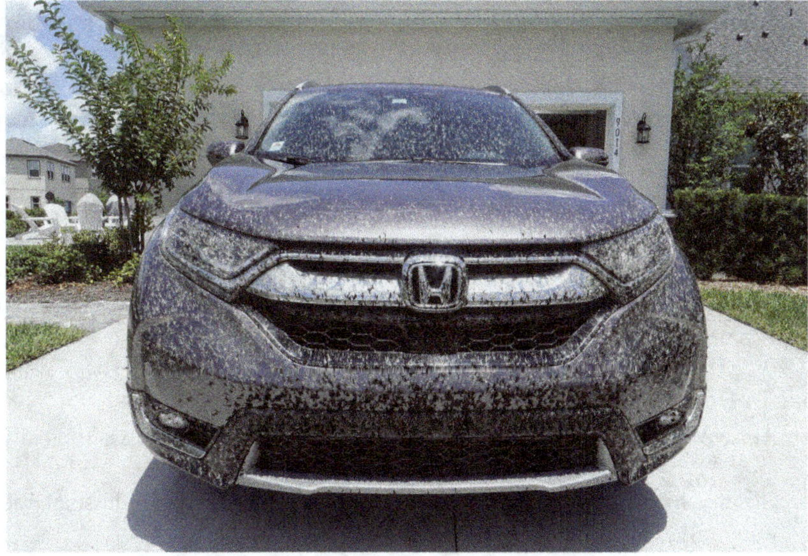

FIGURE 9.8 Lovebugs. Car covered in lovebugs.

Symptoms
- Visual obstruction when swarms cluster around faces, eyes, or equipment
- Irritation from inhaling or ingesting airborne insects during fieldwork
- Fouling of traps, notebooks, nets, and sampling equipment
- Vehicle hazards:
  - Reduced visibility on windshields
  - Clogged air intakes and radiators
  - Etching or staining of paint if remains are not cleaned quickly
- Psychological distraction due to swarm density and fly persistence

Though not harmful biologically, they may cause secondary hazards due to distraction or surface damage.

Occupational Exposure
Most problematic for:

- Field biologists and ecologists working in lowland or wetland habitats during emergence
- Transportation, such as researchers driving long distances during swarms
- Outreach or interpretation staff in parks or preserves during public events
- Entomological samplers whose traps become saturated with non-target *Plecia* adults
- Aircraft and drone operators, whose optics may be obscured by body residue

Emergences are synchronized and highly regional, often linked to soil moisture and temperature.

Prevention
- Schedule field activities around known emergence periods, where possible
- Wear head nets, sunglasses, or face shields to reduce inhalation or eye contact
- Install bug screens on radiators or field station air intakes
- Use coarse filters on collection traps if operating during swarms to reduce contamination
- Advise participants about the nuisance nature and lack of health threat to reduce concern

Long-term control is not feasible, but mitigation and personal protection are highly effective.

What To Do If Exposed
- Rinse equipment or skin if fluids are irritating, though effects are typically mild
- Clean vehicles promptly after driving through swarms; use mild soap and water (allowing crushed bodies to remain can harm paint)

- Clean optics and electronics as soon as feasible
- No medical attention is needed unless allergic reaction to airborne fragments occurs (rare)

Symptoms, if any, are inconsequential and resolve quickly.

NON-STINGING ANTS

Entomological Agents: Order Hymenoptera, Family Formicidae: *Lasius, Camponotus, Formica, Prenolepis, Tapinoma, Tetramorium, Monomorium, Linepithema humile,* **and many others (Figure 9.9)**

Exposure and Severity Ratings

- **Exposure Level: 4–5**
  - Frequent (4) to ubiquitous (5)
- **Severity Level: 1**
  - No direct medical effect, but can cause minimal (1) to mild (2) logistical and psychological disruption

Reference: Fisher and Cover (2007)

The majority of ant species encountered during field operations do not sting or bite but can interfere with equipment, food supplies, and personnel comfort. Some, like the odorous house ant (*Tapinoma sessile*) or the Argentine ant (*Linepithema*

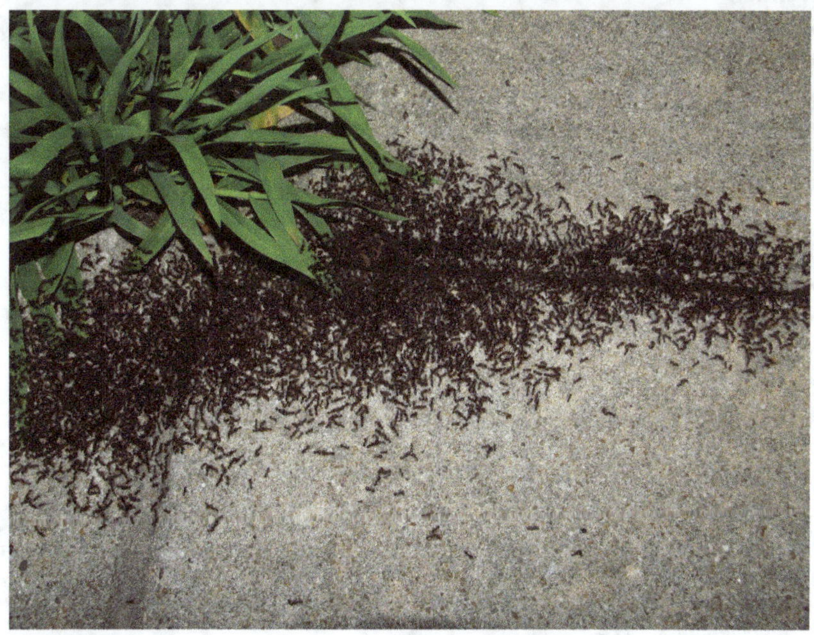

FIGURE 9.9   Non-stinging ants. Swarm of pavement ants, *Tetramorium caespitum.*

humile), invade in large numbers, disrupting field camps, data loggers, and sensitive electronic equipment. Others may crawl on personnel, causing distraction, or nest in coolers, sample containers, or vehicles.

These ants pose no venomous or disease risk, but their high abundance and resource-seeking behavior can cause significant downtime and frustration during fieldwork, especially in humid, coastal, or forested areas. Occasionally, *Camponotus* (carpenter ants) may cause structural damage by chewing on gear but are not hazardous to personnel.

Symptoms
- Ants in food, tents, clothing, or bedding
- Electrical failures from ant nesting or chewing in equipment
- Psychological stress or distraction during high-infestation events
- Loss of sample integrity from ant contamination

Occupational Exposure
Non-stinging ants may be a problem for ecologists and environmental professionals at:

- Campsites or gear stored near leaf litter, rotting logs, or moist soil
- Open food storage or trash near trails, traps, or field stations
- Work near buildings or vehicles previously infested
- Long-term monitoring equipment left in field

Prevention
- Store food in sealed containers
- Avoid placing gear near logs, stumps, or ground nests
- Regularly inspect electronics, cases, and tents
- Apply perimeter barriers (e.g., diatomaceous earth – although D.E. is useless in damp or wet situations – or ant baits) if returning to same site
- Keep personal gear off ground and shake out before use

What To Do If Infested
- Remove ants physically and relocate gear
- Clean equipment with mild detergents or alcohol
- Apply safe ant bait or repellents for extended work at the site
- Check electronics and pack gear in sealed tubs if returning to camp
- Document severe infestations in health and safety logs for future planning

REFERENCES

Cavallero MC. 2026. Nuisance status of a net-spinning caddisfly (Trichoptera: Hydropsychidae): Survey responses of residents on the Colorado River in Bullhead City, Arizona. *J. Med. Entomol.* 63: tjaf172.

Cranshaw W. 2011. A review of nuisance invader household pests in the United States. *Am. Entomol.* 57: 165–169.

Dublon IAN, Sumpter DJT. 2014. Flying insect swarms. *Curr. Biol.* 24: R828–R830.

Edel C, Rühr PT, Frenzel M, van de Kamp T, Faragó T, Hammel JU, Wilde F, Blanke A. 2024. Bite force transmission and mandible shape in grasshoppers, crickets, and allies is not driven by dietary niches. *Evolution* 78: 1958–1968.

Edmunds Jr GF, Jensen SL, Berner L. 1976. *The Mayflies of North and Central America.* University of Minnesota Press, St. Paul, MN.

Fisher BL, Cover SP. 2007. *Ants of North America: A Guide to the Genera.* University of California Press, Los Angeles, CA.

Forsythe P. 2004. *A Review of Termite Risk Management in Housing Construction.* Forest & Wood Products Research and Development Corporation, Surrey Hills, NSW, Australia.

Henson EB. 1966. Aquatic insects as inhalant allergens: A review of American Literature. *Ohio J. Sci.* 66: 529–532.

Kritsky G. 2004. *Periodical Cicadas: The Plague and the Puzzle.* Indiana Academy of Science, Indianapolis, IN.

Leppla NC. 2009. Living with Lovebugs. Fact Sheet ENY840, University of Florida, Institute of Food and Agricultural Sciences, Gainesville, FL.

Lim CSH, Lim SL, Chew FT, Ong TC, Deharveng L. 2009. Collembola are unlikely to cause human dermatitis. *J. Insect Sci.* 9: 3.

Theuret D, Gerry A. 2014. Moth or Drain Flies. Pest Notes Publication 74167, University of California Statewide Integrated Pest Management Program.

Wakeland C. 1959. Mormon Crickets in North America. Technical Bulletin 1202, US Department of Agriculture, Agricultural Research Service.

Appendix A
Example Standard
Operating Procedure

This appendix is intended to provide an example of language that may be used in a Standard Operating Procedure (SOP) document addressing entomological health and safety. Individual health and safety teams can and should modify it as appropriate for their corporate circumstances.

ENTOMOLOGICAL HEALTH AND SAFETY STANDARD OPERATING PROCEDURES

OBJECTIVE

This SOP document outlines general safety practices and risk mitigation strategies for managing exposure to medically and operationally significant arthropods during field operations. It is intended to support safe work practices for personnel conducting fieldwork, environmental assessments, ecological surveys, construction inspections, or any occupational activity that may place them in contact with entomological hazards.

GENERAL

Field personnel may be exposed to arthropod-related hazards ranging from minor nuisance bites to medically significant envenomation and vector-borne diseases. Entomological exposure may also result in allergic reactions, psychological distress, mechanical interference with equipment, or logistical disruptions. This SOP provides general guidance to minimize such risks and should be supplemented by a site-specific Health and Safety Plan (HASP) that includes a biological hazard assessment and mitigation strategy.

OCCUPATIONAL EXPOSURE AND HAZARDS

The level of entomological risk depends on task type, site conditions, and seasonality. The following activities are associated with elevated risk:

- Vegetation surveys, soil sampling, and wetland delineation
- Stream, pond, or marsh sampling (especially during peak mosquito activity)
- Forest, shrubland, and grassland work involving dense vegetation
- Ground disturbance (e.g., augering, excavation, or geotechnical drilling)

- Inspections of crawlspaces, attics, hollow trees, or abandoned structures
- Overnight field deployments or work during dawn/dusk hours

Potential hazards include:

- Bites or stings from mosquitoes, ticks, ants, wasps, spiders, bees, and flies
- Contact with urticating hairs or allergenic body parts (e.g., caterpillars, cockroaches)
- Mechanical disruption from swarming insects or arthropod-infested gear
- Psychological discomfort from repeated nuisance exposure
- Transmission of pathogens or parasites by biological vectors
- Exposure to contaminated water or animal waste attracting arthropods

PERSONAL PROTECTIVE EQUIPMENT (PPE)

PPE should be selected based on the specific entomological risk profile of the site and task. Common PPE used for protection against entomological health and safety hazards includes:

- Long-sleeved shirts and full-length pants
- Treated or fine-weave field clothing to deter insect entry
- Permethrin-treated outerwear or gaiters (if approved by company policy)
- Insect repellent (e.g., DEET or picaridin-based) for exposed skin
- Head nets and gloves when insects are abundant
- Tucked-in pant legs and shirt hems to reduce access points
- Light-colored clothing to help detect crawling arthropods (many insects are also attracted to darker colors)
- Antihistamines or epinephrine auto-injectors (as medically indicated)

TRAINING

All personnel working in environments with potential entomological hazards shall receive training in:

- Recognition of medically significant arthropods common to the region
- Proper use and limitations of insect repellents and PPE
- Identification of symptoms from bites, stings, allergic reactions, or vector-borne illnesses
- Immediate response procedures for exposure or injury
- Site-specific controls outlined in the HASP

FIRST AID AND MEDICAL RESPONSE

This SOP does not provide medical advice. All injuries or exposures must be reported, and proper medical evaluation sought as soon as possible. General guidelines include:

- **For Insect Stings or Bites**: Wash area with soap and water, apply a cold compress, and monitor for signs of allergic reaction

- **For Ticks**: Remove with fine-tipped tweezers, grasping as close to the skin as possible, then clean the site with soap and water and record the location/date for follow-up
- **For Allergic Responses**: Follow individual emergency allergy protocols, including the use of prescribed epinephrine auto-injectors, if applicable
- Seek emergency medical attention for systemic symptoms, difficulty breathing, or suspected anaphylaxis

EMERGENCY COMMUNICATIONS

All field teams must maintain access to a means of communication (e.g., mobile phone, satellite device, or radio) to report emergencies. Incident protocols should be outlined in the HASP and include:

- Location of nearest medical facility
- Emergency medical services contact numbers
- Protocols for reporting stings, bites, or suspected vector exposure
- Chain of communication from field personnel to project and safety managers

ADDITIONAL HAZARDS AND ENVIRONMENTAL FACTORS

Entomological risks may coincide with:

- Extreme heat or sun exposure, which may exacerbate insect activity and health symptoms
- Dense vegetation or debris that obscures nests or harborage
- Flood-prone areas where mosquitoes or biting flies are abundant
- Structural features (confined spaces, crawlspaces, equipment, sheds) that may harbor infestations

Fieldwork should be delayed or modified during conditions that elevate the risk of serious exposure, such as swarming insect periods or known disease outbreaks.

LIMITATIONS

This SOP provides general guidance and is not exhaustive. It must be implemented alongside site-specific safety planning and does not override regulatory or medical requirements. This document is not a medical manual, and references to treatments are informational only. All health concerns must be addressed by licensed medical professionals.

REFERENCES AND RELATED DOCUMENTS

- Site-Specific Health and Safety Plan
- Biological Hazard Assessment or Risk Matrix
- Insect Repellent Safety Data Sheets (SDS)
- Vector Control Agency or Public Health Department bulletins

Appendix B
Example Job Hazard Analysis

This appendix is intended to provide an example of the language that may be used in addressing the entomological hazards portion of a job hazard analysis (JHA). It does not address any other aspects of the JHA. Individual health and safety teams can and should modify it as appropriate for their corporate circumstances.

The particular job used for an example here involves aquatic ecology/biomonitoring in streams using benthic invertebrate samplers and electrofishing gear.

ENTOMOLOGICAL HAZARDS – AQUATIC ECOLOGY FIELD SAMPLING

Field personnel engaged in benthic macroinvertebrate sampling and electrofishing in aquatic habitats may encounter a variety of arthropods that pose occupational health and safety risks. While most arthropod interactions are harmless, certain species can bite, sting, or transmit disease-causing agents. During activities in riparian habitats surrounding streams, the following potential entomological hazards should be considered:

Ticks may be present in grassy or shrubby streamside areas. Though tick activity tends to decline by late summer, tick bites remain possible in the fall and even through the winter in the southern United States, and field teams should follow standard tick prevention practices, including the use of Environmental Protection Agency (EPA)-approved repellents, wearing long sleeves and permethrin-treated clothing, and performing tick checks after fieldwork.

Mosquitoes may be present near stagnant or slow-moving water, especially in backwater areas. While the risk of West Nile virus transmission has dropped, localized outbreaks continue to occur, especially in late summer and early fall. Insect repellent containing DEET or picaridin is recommended. Workers should also minimize exposed skin and reapply repellent as needed.

Biting flies, including black flies (Simuliidae) and deer flies (Tabanidae), may be encountered near flowing water. While bites are generally painful but non-medical, they can cause significant distraction or discomfort during sampling operations. Protective clothing, insect repellent, and awareness of swarm behavior can help reduce exposure.

Stinging insects such as yellowjackets (*Vespula* spp.) and paper wasps (*Polistes* spp.) are seasonally active and may be especially aggressive in the fall as colonies reach maturity and forage for sugars and proteins. Be alert around vegetation, equipment, or trash where wasps may congregate. Workers with known sting allergies should carry epinephrine auto-injectors and inform team members of their condition.

Aquatic insects, such as toe-biters (Belostomatidae), may be present in sampling equipment or handled inadvertently. Though not dangerous from a disease standpoint, these insects can deliver painful defensive bites if mishandled. Caution should be taken when removing samples from samplers or examining organisms by hand.

To mitigate risks:

- Apply insect repellent before entering the field and reapply per label instructions
- Wear light-colored, long-sleeved clothing and tuck pants into socks or boots to deter crawling arthropods
- Avoid disturbing known insect nesting areas and check field gear before loading or handling
- Conduct tick checks at the end of each sampling day and follow established tick removal protocols

While the likelihood of severe arthropod-related illness or injury is low, maintaining situational awareness and adhering to preventive measures will help ensure a safe and productive field campaign.

Appendix C
Example Health and Safety Plan

This appendix is intended to provide an example of the language that may be used in addressing the entomological hazards portion of a health and safety plan (HASP). It does not address any other aspects of the HASP. Individual health and safety teams can and should modify it as appropriate for their corporate circumstances.

The particular project used for an example involves aquatic ecology/biomonitoring in streams using benthic samplers and electrofishing gear; the site involves a river, a mid-sized stream, and an irrigation ditch in Pueblo County, Colorado, with sampling intended for the month of September.

ENTOMOLOGICAL HAZARDS – AQUATIC ECOLOGY FIELD SAMPLING

Fieldwork in riparian and aquatic environments presents potential exposure to biting, stinging, or disease-vector arthropods. During this project, team members will conduct benthic invertebrate sampling (using a kick net sampler) and electrofishing surveys at three freshwater sites near Pueblo, Colorado. Sites include a large river, a mid-sized creek, and an irrigation ditch. Each site will be accessed for approximately 4–6 hours during daylight in September. Although the overall risk of serious entomological injury or illness is low, preventive measures are necessary to minimize discomfort, allergic responses, or rare vector-borne infections.

Potential arthropod exposures include ticks, mosquitoes, biting flies, stinging wasps/bees, and aquatic insects capable of defensive biting. While tick activity generally declines in early autumn, *Dermacentor* and *Ixodes* species may still be encountered in brushy or grassy margins. Workers should wear long sleeves and permethrin-treated clothing, apply Environmental Protection Agency (EPA)-registered repellents (e.g., DEET or picaridin), and perform tick checks at the end of each day. If a tick is found attached, it should be removed using the approved method outlined in the Tick Removal Standard Operating Procedure (SOP) and reported to the site supervisor.

Mosquitoes may be active near slow-moving water and shaded stream margins, especially around the irrigation ditch. While the risk of West Nile virus in Pueblo County is considered low, workers should avoid bites by using repellents and minimizing exposed skin. Similarly, biting flies such as black flies and deer flies may be present at riverine sites; although not medically significant, their bites can be painful and distracting. Aquatic hemipterans, including giant water bugs, may be present in samples and can deliver painful defensive bites. Handling of live organisms should be done with care and appropriate tools.

Stinging insects, especially yellowjackets and paper wasps, may pose a higher risk in September, when colonies are large and foraging activity peaks. Workers should remain alert near shrubs, refuse, and equipment where these insects may nest or scavenge. Field crew personnel with known insect sting allergies are encouraged to notify the field lead, carry an epinephrine auto-injector, and ensure that team members are aware of emergency procedures.

The Site Health and Safety Officer (SHSO) may review entomological risks during daily briefings, and project leads are encouraged to consult with local ecologists and field staff for current, site-specific arthropod awareness, as they may be aware of species or seasonal activity not captured in this plan. If unusual arthropod activity is observed (e.g., large nests, dense swarms, or biting outbreaks), the SHSO may modify work plans or recommend alternate protective measures.

By following these precautions, teams can effectively reduce entomological risks while conducting aquatic ecological monitoring. For task-specific guidance, refer to the Job Hazard Analysis (JHA) and detailed SOPs on arthropod exposure management.

E

F

G

H

For Product Safety Concerns and Information please contact our EU
representative GPSR@taylorandfrancis.com
Taylor & Francis Verlag GmbH, Kaufingerstraße 24, 80331 München, Germany